RABBIT NUTRITION

AND

NUTRITIONAL HEALING

THIRD EDITION

Lucile Moore

Illustrated by Evonne Vey

Front cover photo by Amanda Gilmore
Back cover art by Evonne Vey

The information contained in this volume is intended to help you provide care for your rabbit; however, this information is not intended for diagnostic purposes. A veterinary professional should be consulted for any diagnostic questions regarding a particular rabbit's health. The author, illustrator, contributors, and publisher are not responsible for the use or misuse of any information in this book and are not liable or responsible to any person or group with any loss, illness or injury caused or alleged to be caused by the information in this book.

This book is dedicated to
Evonne Vey
who wouldn't stop pestering me
until I wrote the first edition,
and whose illustrations greatly
add to the volume.

and to the memory of
White Rabbit
beloved companion lost far too
soon.

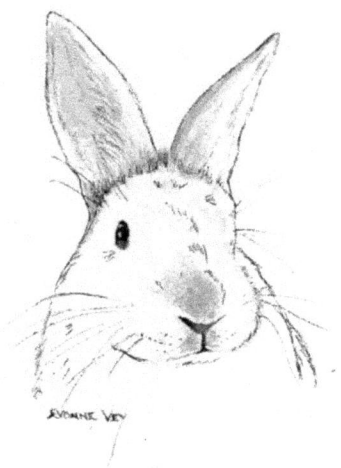

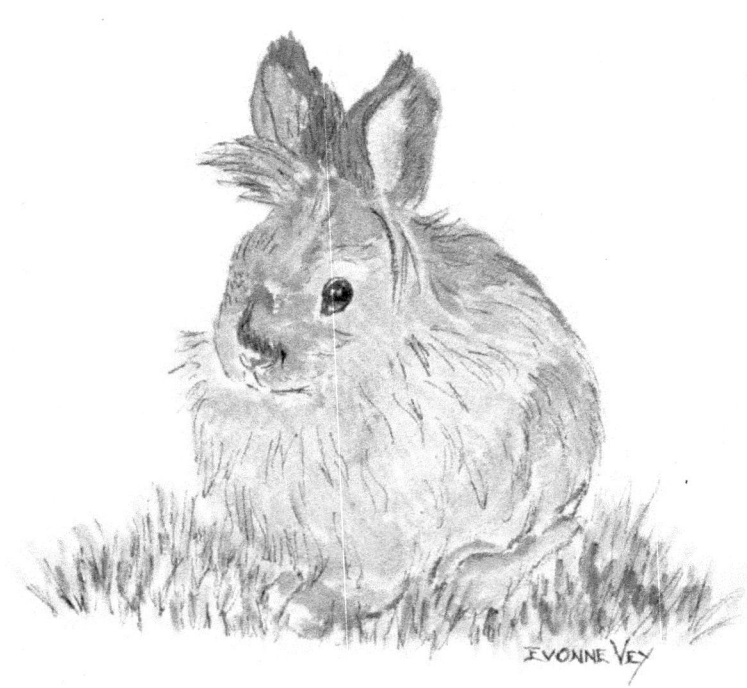

TABLE OF CONTENTS

Preface   1

Contributors   3

Introduction   5

1. What Does a Wild Rabbit Really Eat?   9

2. The Rabbit Digestive System   16
    The digestive process   17
    Digestive system of young rabbits   25

3. Carbohydrates   30
    Monosaccharides and disaccharides   32
    Oligosaccharides   36
    Polysaccharides (glycans)   39
    Understanding carbohydrates and rabbit digestion   52

4. Fat and Protein   60
    Fat   60
    Protein   66

5. Vitamins and Minerals   77
    Vitamins   79
    Minerals   91
    Drug and nutrient interactions 104

6. Pellets, Hay, Grass, and Mycotoxins   118
    Pellets   119
    Homemade treats   129
    Hay   131
    Balanced diet   137
    Fresh grass   138

Other fresh foods   141
  Foraging   145
  Water   147
  Mycotoxins   152

7. Phytochemicals and Plants   166
  Phytonutrients (phytochemicals)   167
  Cultivated plants   182
  Gardening for rabbits   197

8. Wild Plants and Toxic Plants   212
  Fifteen generally rabbit-safe wild plants   213
  Toxic Plants   225

9. Prebiotics, Probiotics, and Other Feeding Issues   232
  Prebiotics and probiotics   232
  Cleanliness   239
  Weather   240
  Thought, energy and intuition   246

10. Factors Affecting Rabbit Diet and Disease   259
  Life stages and diet   260
  Rabbit breeds and diet   272
  Community rabbits   274
  Diet and disease   278

Appendix I: Possible Signs of Nutritional Deficiencies and Excesses   308

Appendix II: Bunny-safe Treats   310

Acronyms and Abbreviations   312

Index of Tables   314

General Index   315

Preface

After I wrote the first edition of this book, a person who looked at the manuscript warned me that I was giving my potential readers "too much credit" and that they were not going to understand what I wrote or my purpose in writing it. I am happy to report that the response from readers showed me that for the most part my readers did appear to understand the gist of the book and my reasons for writing it. In fact, when this rabbit nutrition book went out of print, the many requests I received to have it available in print again were what led to this print edition.

Of course not everyone agreed with everything I wrote; that goes with the territory for nonfiction writers and is not necessarily a negative. I believe that disagreement can be positive when it generates thoughtful discussion. Because one of my goals is to present information that may not be found on the websites and literature of all rabbit organizations, I even expected some people to attack my views quite strongly, and a few did take umbrage because not all the information I present reflects common feeding recommendations.

Still, I was rather shocked when—after the second edition had already been out for some time – I was flat-out libeled on the website of a large house rabbit organization, and by a member who admitted she had never seen or read the book and was not even sure it was out yet. I think I speak for most nonfiction writers when I say that I don't mind people taking issue with something I write, but I would prefer to be quoted correctly and in context and by a person who has actually read the work in question!

Yet what bothered me most about the virulent attack was not the libelous statements, which I could easily prove were not true, but an accurate accusation that was made: I had, the person complained, changed my ideas from my first books and had a "new stance" on rabbit nutrition. Yes, I had changed my stance on some topics since my first books. I spent over 2,000 hours searching the scientific literature on rabbit diet and nutrition before I wrote the first edition of this book and many more hours before the second. I would hope that anyone who put that amount of time into studying rabbit diet or any other topic would change at least a few of their ideas. If a person did *not* change any of their thinking after devoting that much time to a topic I would be concerned because to me it would indicate that either the person had a very closed mind or was so arrogant as to think he or she had all the answers before the study began.

Because of the amount of reading I have done in the field I have been exposed to information that the majority of people involved with companion rabbits have not, including most vets. (Rabbit nutrition is an area in which the vast majority of studies and publications are done by biologists, not veterinarians.) It is part of my purpose in writing this book to share that information with readers so that they and their rabbits can benefit.

I believe that the more information a person has, the better decisions regarding their rabbit's care can be made. The core of my philosophy regarding rabbits is that they are individuals. I understand why some rabbit organizations publish guidelines regarding diet, and they can be a good place to start. I provide guidelines myself. But at some point, whether because of environment, genetics, disease, or age, the guidelines will need to be modified. I hope the information I make available to readers in this volume will help them make those diet modifications for their rabbit when they are needed.

Let me end this preface as I did that of my second edition: I neither expect nor desire every reader to agree with all the information I present in this book. But I hope that it may cause thoughtful readers to consider that there is no single 'right answer' when it comes to rabbit nutrition and health; that each rabbit is an individual and what works for one may not be best for another.

Lucile Moore, PhD
January 2019

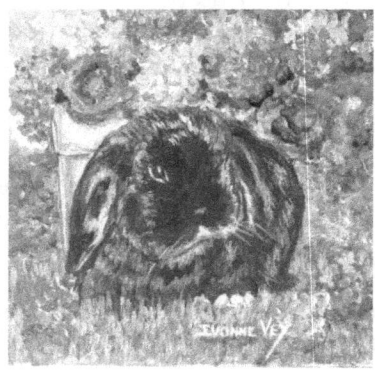

Contributors

Christine Carter is the author of *The Wonderful World of Pet Rabbits*. Christine's work received acclaim in her native Australia because of its wealth of practical knowledge about rabbit care and feeding. She is especially knowledgeable about weeds, grasses, cultivated plants, and other rabbit foods. Christine has been working in the field of rabbits since 1987.

Lisa Hodgson is the publisher and editor of the British quarterly *Bunny Mad!*, the only retail magazine outside the US devoted to rabbits and rabbit welfare. *Bunny Mad!* is available worldwide singly or through subscription, and is also sold at Dobbie's Garden centres and Pets at Home shops in the UK.

Lisa has been active in rabbit welfare and advocacy for over a decade, particularly in the area of promoting awareness of rabbits' unique qualities and needs. Lisa is also dedicated helping rescue rabbits throughout the world by fundraising for rescues through the magazine.

Elizabeth Sharp became interested in nutrition and natural healing while recovering from a life-threatening basal skull fracture. When she brought her first companion rabbit, Sarah, into her life, Liz extended her interest in natural foods and natural healing to rabbit care. Liz has worked in various technical areas of the medical field for over twenty-five years.

Kathy Smith has been a recognized and respected voice in the field of companion rabbits since 2001 when the first edition of *Rabbit Health in the 21st Century* came out (originally titled *Rabbit Health 101*) and received a positive review in *Exotic DVM* veterinary magazine. The second edition in 2003 brought further acclaim. Kathy also authored *King Murray's Royal Tail* and *Mithril's Magic* and coauthored *When Your Rabbit Needs Special Care* and *Touched by a Rabbit*. Her articles have appeared in the annual *Rabbits USA*, the British quarterly *Bunny Mad!*, and numerous rabbit newsletters, both in print and online.

Kathy worked for 25 years in the pharmaceutical industry as an analyst reviewing study data, with an emphasis on adverse events. This has given her unique insight into many aspects of drug therapy as it applies to our companion rabbits. The many rabbits she has shared her home with over the years have provided motivation for ongoing study and inspiration for her writing. They have also served as her greatest teachers in life.

Debby Widolf has been an educator for the House Rabbit Society (HRS) since 1998, was manager of the Rabbit Department at Best Friends Animal Society for nine years, was a speaker at the 2010 No More Homeless Pets Conference, and a speaker at the HRS national conference in 2014.

Debby now devotes her time to the cause of community rabbits, and in 2016 started the website and Facebook page dontdumprabbits.org. Her passion and mission is to work with individuals and groups to stop the abandonment of domestic rabbits and to find solutions for community rabbits that need sanctuary. She can be reached via her website, www.dontdumprabbits.org

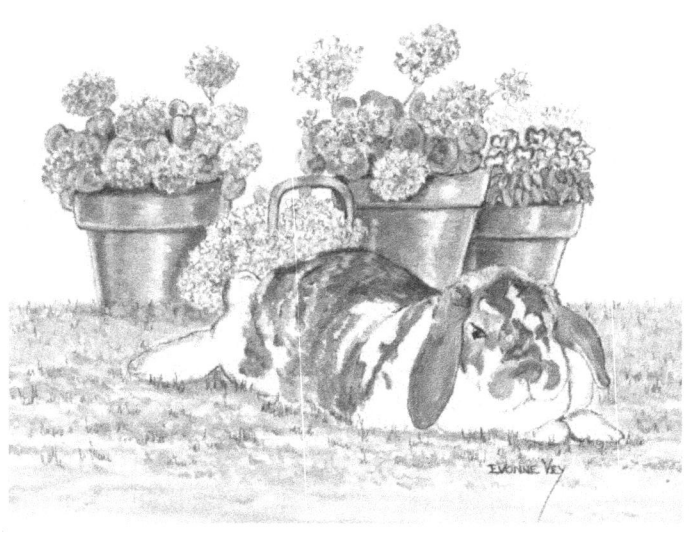

Introduction

The primary changes in this third edition of *Rabbit Nutrition and Nutritional Healing* are in the chapters specifically about diet (chapters 6 and 10), although there are minor changes and additions throughout. I added topics to Chapter Six, and rewrote Chapter Ten to be less technical, but I did not rewrite the entire book. Kathy Smith and Debby Widolf both contributed several excellent new pieces for this edition (found in chapters five, six and ten), and Lisa Hodgson generously allowed me to reprint another article from *Bunny Mad!* magazine.

When I wrote the first edition I made the decision not to interrupt the flow of the text with constant references and footnotes, and instead listed references at the end of each chapter. Most readers have been satisfied with this compromise between technicality and readability, but a few have commented that they wish I had been more precise with my references. I wish to illustrate why I was not. Take this sentence:

> "Both soluble and insoluble fiber affect the microflora of the gut, the rate of passage of digesta, and play a role in maintaining the integrity of the mucosa and the mucosal immune response."

If I were to put references into the sentence it would look something like this:

> "Both soluble and insoluble fiber affect the microflora of the gut [11, 16, 39, 42, 59], the rate of passage of the digesta [3, 6, 9, 29, 36, 42, 67, 95, 98], and play a role in maintaining the integrity of the mucosa [14, 15, 69, 72] and the mucosal immune response. [15, 46, 72]

While a very small minority of readers might actually prefer the second option above, I felt the vast majority would prefer the first. Not to mention that the second option would add greatly to the length and expense of the book! I believe that those who wish to find a reference to a particular topic will be able to make a good guess by reading the titles of the journal articles cited at the end of each chapter.

In the second edition I explained why I respectfully disagreed with a reader with some science background who felt I should not include as many anecdotes. The reader felt that despite the explanation I give about anecdotal versus scientific evidence too many readers would assume cause/effect relationships where they might not exist. After careful consideration I chose to leave the anecdotes for the following two reasons:

   1) Despite great strides in knowledge of rabbit physiology and medicine over recent years, rabbit health and medicine is still in its infancy. In my opinion, anecdotal evidence serves a particularly important role when a discipline is young, bringing *possible* cause/effect relationships to the attention of research scientists.

   2) Some of my most interesting information comes from veterinarians who give it under condition of anonymity because they have not done any studies on a particular subject but have observed certain patterns over many years of practice. I feel it is useful to share some of these observations with my readers.

There is still a misconception among many that anecdotal evidence is "bad" and formal scientific evidence "good." Nothing could be further from the truth. Anecdotal evidence comes from personal observations, often of a possible cause/effect relationship. Such anecdotal evidence can lead to questions that are then put to the test of studies based on the scientific method, hopefully (but not always) leading to scientific evidence that will support the person's theory. Each type of evidence has its place, and both are valuable. It should also be noted that scientific evidence is not always valid or good—it depends upon how well the study was designed and carried out, how well the data derived from the study was analyzed, and how that analysis was applied in reaching the conclusions presented. However, I do agree that readers should be careful not to assume cause/effect relationships from anecdotal evidence.

Another caution I must repeat from the first edition is that regarding the tables on nutrient content in this volume: listed values are not firm, but are simply averages. Data on any nutrient can (and does) vary considerably, depending upon what soil the plant grew in, what part of the plant was analyzed, how old the plant was, and what method of analysis was used, among other factors. Repeatedly I found published values for the same nutrient in the same plant species that varied several hundredfold. Due to its very nature, nutrition is far from an exact science—the values given must be taken as relatives, not absolutes.

As always, I owe thanks to those who helped make this volume what it is. Firstly I thank my contributors – Kathy Smith, Debby Widolf, Lisa Hodgson, Christine Carter, and Elizabeth Sharp—for so generously donating their time and talents. (Their bios are at the beginning of this third edition.) Secondly I owe thanks to the person without whom the first edition of this book would never have come to be, and whose illustrations add so much to what would otherwise be a rather dry volume: Evonne Vey, my illustrator. Finally, I thank all the rabbits who have shared my life and from whom I have learned so much.

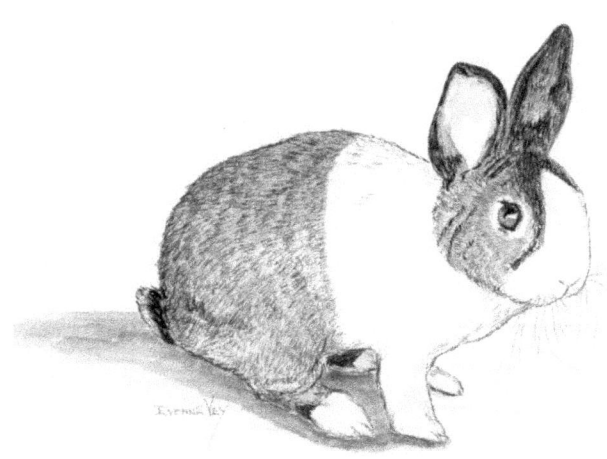

8

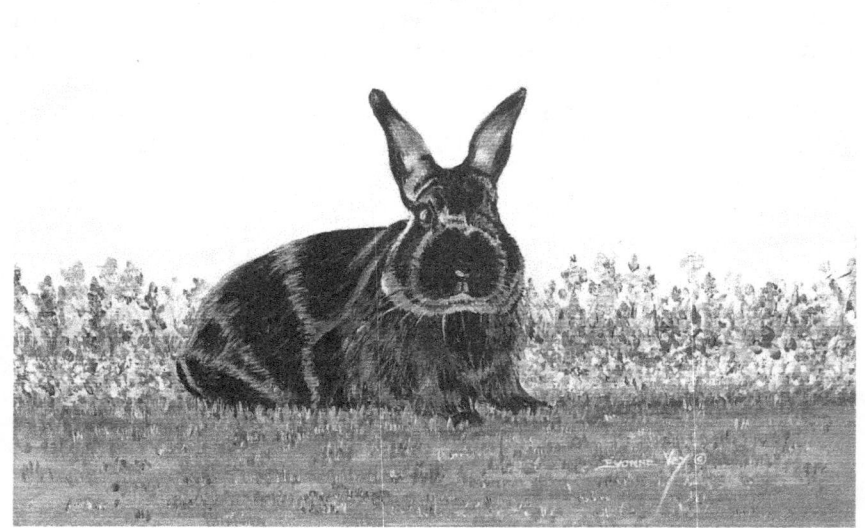

Chapter 1

WHAT DOES A WILD RABBIT REALLY EAT?

How often do we hear a spokesperson for a rabbit organization, an individual expert, or a veterinarian expound on the merits of a particular diet, claiming it is closest to that of a wild rabbit? Yet the same claim may be made for very different rabbit diets. How can we know who is telling the truth? Is it really possible to mimic a wild rabbit's diet when we feed our domestic rabbits? Should we even try?

Those with knowledge of wild animal feeding habits or those who live in the country realize the issue of a wild rabbit's diet is not as simple as some of the experts would make it out to be. I live where there are cottontail rabbits and jackrabbits (hares). While these two lagomorphs belong to different species than the rabbit from which our domestic rabbits (*Oryctolagus cuniculus*) are descended, the major factors that affect diet are the same. At the time of this writing, it has been a year of very low rainfall where I live, and the rabbits have had fewer annual herbaceous plants to choose from than during the previous year of high rainfall, when there was an abundance of annuals. I have sometimes observed jackrabbits munching on young prickly-pear cactus pads with soft spines in early spring of drought years! And even in years of normal precipitation there are few herbaceous plants available in the winter and both the cottontails and jackrabbits have much less choice of food.

Obviously there are many variables that will affect a wild animal's diet, including weather, temperature, time of year, and the particular habitat in which the animal lives. A wildlife biologist may refer to *availability* and *palatability* when talking about the food resource of a species. These are categories used to describe factors that affect what foods wild animals—including rabbits—will eat.

Availability refers to what is there for the rabbit (or other animal) to eat. Availability may be affected by many factors, including rainfall, temperature, season of the year, the plants that are able to grow in a rabbit's particular habitat, and whether the rabbit can access the plant. Researchers studying wild rabbits of *Oryctolagus cuniculus* (the species from which our domestic rabbits are descended) diet in one habitat found that the winter diet of wild rabbits included large amounts of woody shrubs while in the summer it was comprised mainly of grasses. They also found that the rabbits' diet was diverse, including cereals (grasses that produce grains; e.g., wheat), grass stems and leaves, forbs (herbaceous plants with broad leaves), acorns, and browse (tender parts of shrubs and trees), the proportions of which varied with rainfall and season. For example, the amount of cereals in the rabbits' diet was lower in the winter than in other seasons. Altogether, the overall nutrient quality of the rabbits' winter food was lower than required for maintenance, and the researchers postulated that the lower nutrient content might be a factor in rabbit survival.

The results of the above study were reflected in another where wild *Oryctolagus* diet was found to be flexible, with the rabbits switching foods in different seasons. In late spring and through the summer the rabbits of this study relied strongly on seeds. The quality of a rabbit's available diet has also been found to affect the size of digestive organs.

In yet another study, researchers discovered that wild rabbits in a pine forest consumed a diet that did not change significantly from winter to summer, while the diet of wild rabbits in a scrubland habitat did change significantly between the seasons. They also found that the plants available to the rabbits in a nearby pine forest differed from those available to rabbits in the scrubland throughout the year. In other words, wild *O. cuniculus* were eating very different diets in two habitats that were not a long geographical distance apart.

Palatability refers to how well an animal likes to eat a food that is available. For example, if a stalk of grass and a young low-fiber broad-leafed herbaceous plant are both available to a wild rabbit, which will it eat? Most often (although not always) it will be the young low-fiber herbaceous plant! Researchers have found that when given a choice, wild rabbits usually choose succulent low-fiber plants. Rabbits usually choose tender leaves over stems. This holds true for grass as well as forbs, and when eating grass, rabbits will seek young green blades rather than older grass or dried grass. They will choose cultivated grasses (barley, rye, wheat, corn) over wild grasses if they are available. Rabbits will also sometimes select flowers, seeds, and fruits, and have been observed to cut down long stems in order to reach them. When plant availability allows, rabbits have been found to adjust their diets to consume needed fiber, water, and nutrients.

Although many may assume grass always comprises the bulk of a wild rabbit's diet, in fact the percentage of a rabbit's diet that is grass can vary widely and in various studies has been found to be as low as 30% to more than 75 percent. One researcher suggested that overgrazing by large herbivores such as horses, deer, and sheep was a primary factor in the high percentage of grass (about 66% in this particular study) in wild rabbit diets. Researchers have also found that when rabbits do eat grass they select grasses with the lowest silica content, and hypothesize that some grasses have evolved high silica levels as a defense against predation by herbivores such as rabbits. Mature grasses have less nutritional value than young grasses, and dried grasses (hay) even less.

When the more palatable grass and forbs are not available, rabbits often turn to woody shrubs, eating the more tender parts at the tips. However, a decline in the availability of more nutrient-rich plants usually leads to a corresponding decline in health that ultimately results in an increase in mortality. Rabbits, with their high metabolism, need higher-quality forage than larger herbivores, and their health declines and mortality increases when forced to subsist on low-quality forage.

In taste tests, rabbits have been found to respond positively to the sugars in starches, and they frequently choose high-starch plants to eat. In one study it was found that acorns (a relatively high-starch food) were an important part of the diet of a wild rabbit population year-round.

Another researcher commented on the number of studies that have shown many populations of wild rabbits consume high-carbohydrate foods and postulates that the development of a taste preference for the sugars in starches may be an evolutionary adaptation that helps ensure wild rabbits consume enough carbohydrates to meet their energy needs. This preferential selection of *nutrient-dense* foods (nutrient-rich low-fiber plants) when they are available may help rabbits fulfill nutritional requirements that high-fiber but less palatable foods do not meet. Animals that choose their foods for high nutrient content in this manner are called *concentrate selectors.*

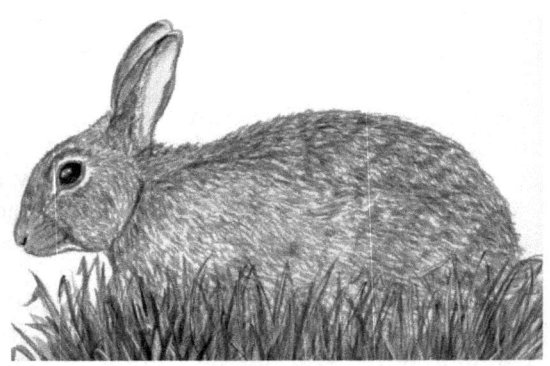

Clearly it is not that easy to determine exactly what comprises a wild rabbit's diet, as there are too many factors that affect it. It would be very difficult indeed to mimic a wild rabbit's diet when we feed our rabbits. Perhaps we should instead ask ourselves "Does it matter what a wild rabbit eats and how closely the diet we feed our domestic rabbits mirrors that of a wild rabbit?" To a great extent I don't think it does, because our domestic rabbits are not wild rabbits. They lead very different lives, in general lead longer lives, and have different energy needs.

Still, there a few points about wild rabbit diet that we should perhaps note:

- A wild rabbit's diet is often variable, and therefore our domestic rabbits may be able to adapt to eating different foods and differing amounts of those foods without suffering unduly negative effects. Moreover, they may need to consume a variety of foods to maintain optimal physical health.

- Wild rabbits usually eat diets high in fiber if for no other reason than that in many habitats the succulent low-fiber foods they may prefer are not always available, and the rabbit digestive tract has evolved to require a certain amount of fiber.

- Wild rabbits *may* consume—depending upon

habitat and other variables—a relatively large amount of high-carbohydrate foods (e.g., acorns) year round. This fact points to the possibility that domestic rabbits may also be able to consume some high-carbohydrate foods without undue negative effects.

- Wild rabbits require certain nutrients for body maintenance, just as other species do, and there is evidence that a diet low in these nutrients may affect survival. It may be extrapolated that a lack of adequate nutrition in a domestic rabbit's diet could also affect that domestic rabbit's survival.

In the following chapters we will explore the mysteries of rabbit diet—how the rabbit digestive system functions, what nutrients rabbits require, how much of those nutrients they need, and what foods contain them. We will also look at what problems may arise if rabbits have deficiencies of those nutrients and how they can be corrected. It is my hope that after perusing this book readers will be able to make more informed decisions regarding the feeding of their rabbits.

References

Alves, J., J. Vingada, and P. Rodrigues. 2006. The wild rabbit (*Oryctolagus cuniculus* L.) diet in a sand dune area in central Portugal: a contribution toward management. *Wildl. Biol. Pract.* 2(2): 63–70.

Bonino, Never and Laura Borrelli. 2006. Seasonal variation in the diet of the European wild rabbit (*Oryctolagus cuniculus*) in the Andean region of Neuques, Argentina. *Ecol. Austral.* 16 (1): 7–13.

Broussis, P. and J. L. Chapais. 1998. Deferred seasonal increase in testes weight under poor nutritional conditions in a sub-Antarctic population of rabbits (*Oryctolagus cunuiculus*). *J.Z.* 245(3): 285–291.

Cotterill, J.V., R. W. Watkins, C. B. Brennan, and D.P. Cowan. 2006. Boosting silica levels in wheat leaves reduces grazing by rabbits. *Pest Manage. Sci.* 63(3): 247–253.

Duffy, S.G., J .S. Fairley, and G. O'Donnell. 1996. Food of rabbits *Oryctolagus cuniculus* on upland grassland in Connemara. *Bio. and*

Env.: Proc. Royal Irish Acad. 96B(2): 69-75.

Ferreira, C. and P. C. Alves. 2009. Influence of habitat management on the abundance and diets of wild rabbit (*Oryctolagus cuniculus algirus*) populations in Meditaerranean ecosystems.

Gasmi-Boubaker, A., R. M. Losada, H. Abdouli, and A. Riguiero. 2012. Importance of Mediterranean forest products as food resource of domestic herbivores: the case of oak acorn. *Eur. Fed. Anim. Sci.* 129: 123-126.

Hunt, J. W., A. P. Dean, R. E. Webster, G. N. Johnson, and A. R. Ennos. 2008. A Novel Mechanism by which Silica Defends Grasses against Herbivory. *Ann. Bot.* 102(4): 653–656.

Laska, M. 2002. Gustatory responsiveness to food-associated saccharides in European rabbits, *Oryctolagus cuniculus*. *Physiol. & Behav.* 76: 335–341.

Marques, C. and M. L. Mathias. 2001. The diet of the European wild rabbit, *Oryctolagus cuniculus*, in coastal habitats of Central Portugal. *Mamm.* 65(4): 437–450.

Martin, M. C., P. Marrero, and M. Nogales. 2003. Seasonal variation in the diet of wild rabbits *Oryctolagus cuniculus* in a semiarid Atlantic island (Alegranza, Canarian Archipelago). *Acta Theriologica* 48: 399–410.

Martin, R. C., L. E. Twigg, and L. Zampichelli. 2006. Seasonal changes in the diet of the European rabbit (*Oryctolgaus suniculus*) from three different Mediterranean habitats in south-western Australia. *Wldlf. Res.* 34(1): 25-42.

Martins, H., J. A. Milne, and F. Rego. 2002. Seasonal and spatial variation in the diet of the wild rabbit (*Oryctolagus cuniculus* L.) in Portugal. *J. Zool.* 258: 395–404.

Rogers, P. M. 1981. Ecology of the European wild rabbit *Oryctolagus cuniculus* (L.) in Mediterranean habitats. *J. Ap. Eco.* 18: 355–371.

Rogers, P. M., C. P. Arthur, and R. C. Soriguer. 1994. The rabbit in continental Europe. In: *The European Rabbit: The history and biology of a successful colonizer.* (eds. H. V. Thompson and C. M. King.) Oxford: Oxford University Press.

Sibley, R. M., K. A. Monk, I. K. Johnson, and R. C. Trout. 1990. Seasonal variation in gut morphology in wild rabbits (*Oryctolagus cuniculus*). *J. Zool.* 221(4): 605-619.

Somers, N., T. Milotic, and M. Hauffmann. 2012. The impact of sward height, forage quality and competitive conditions on forgaging behaviour of free-ranging rabbits *(Oryctolagus cuniculus* L.) *Belg. J. Zool.* 142(1): 74-85.

Soriguer, R. C. 1988. Alimentacion del conejo (*Oryctolagus cuniculus* L. 1758) en Donana, SO Espana. *Acta Vert.* 15(1): 141-150.

Wallace-Drees, J. M. and B. Deinum. 1985. Quality of the Diet Selected by Wild Rabbits (*Oryctolagus cuniculus* (L.)) in Autumn and Winter. *Neth. J. Zool.* 36(4): 438–448.

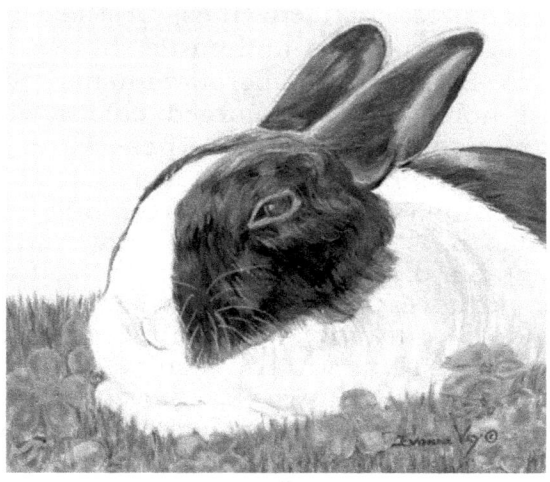

Chapter 2

THE RABBIT DIGESTIVE SYSTEM

Rabbits are herbivores, which are animals adapted to obtain nutrients directly from plant materials. Because no mammals produce all the enzymes necessary to break down the structural material of plants (e.g., cellulose), herbivores have large populations of microorganisms (which do produce such enzymes) in their guts. Some herbivores, such as sheep and cattle, have a specialized *rumen* which houses the microorganisms. Others, like rabbits and horses, have enlarged colons and cecums where the microorganisms live. These latter herbivores are called *hindgut fermenters*.

Although rabbits, like horses, are hindgut fermenters and their digestive systems are often compared to equines, there are notable differences between them. Rabbits have larger colons and cecums in relation to body size than do horses. In horses microbial fermentation occurs in the colon; in rabbits it occurs in the cecum. In rabbit digestive systems large-particle fiber is removed from the body rapidly and is not fermented; in horses large-particle fiber passes through the system more slowly than it does in rabbits, and is fermented. This means that the structural components of plants are more completely digested by horses: for example, the digestion of the structural components of alfalfa hay is about 14% in rabbits and is 41% in horses. Yet rabbits require more energy for their body size than do horses. Therefore the rabbit has had to develop other ways to meet their high-energy requirements: high voluntary feed intake (VFI), feeding frequently (up to 30 times a day), digesting and utilizing non-fibrous carbohydrates quickly, eliminating indigestible lignified materials rapidly, and moving those fibrous materials that are digestible by microflora to the cecum where the nutrients are made available through fermentation.

As stated in the first chapter, rabbits are *selective feeders* and given a choice will often choose to consume low-fiber, succulent, nutrient-dense, high-sugar foods. Selecting these foods enables rabbits to meet the energy requirements of their high metabolic rate. However, since these preferred foods are not always available, rabbits have evolved to extract some nutrition from more difficult-to-digest complex carbohydrates (e.g., pectin, hemicellulose, cellulose) by means of the populations of microorganisms in their cecum. The microorganisms are able to break down structural plant material that the enzymes in the rabbit gut are unable to digest well. This adaptation enables rabbits to take advantage of and utilize energy from a wide range of plants including grasses, twigs, bark, shrub leaves, herbaceous plants, fruits, and seeds.

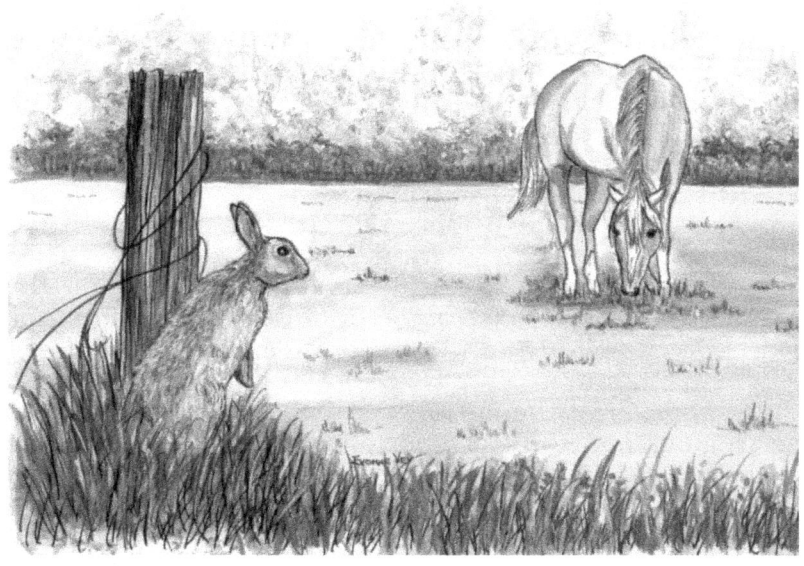

THE DIGESTIVE PROCESS

Digestion in the rabbit[1] begins after food is taken into the mouth with the aid of a large tongue and mobile lips,

---

[1] This explanation of digestion in the rabbit refers to that of adult rabbits. The specialized digestion of young rabbits will be discussed at the end of this chapter.

razor-sharp incisors cutting the material into manageable pieces for the cheek teeth to grind. Rabbit teeth are different from human teeth in that they grow continuously and do not have a true anatomical root. Rabbit incisors may grow 2–3 mm/week, and must be worn down and kept sharp through use. Rabbit molars and premolars grow at a slower rate but must also be worn down through use.

During the mastication process, the food is moistened with saliva from four pairs of salivary glands that secrete the enzyme amylase that begins the digestion of starch. Because plant structural material is so difficult for mammals to digest, most herbivores crush it thoroughly in their mouths to begin breaking the plant material down, and rabbits are no exception. A normal healthy adult rabbit will chew from 120–200 times per minute in a side-to-side motion, concentrating first on one side and then the other as the food is ground with molars and premolars. However, a hungry rabbit may chew food less thoroughly or even swallow it whole. At worst, these scenarios can potentially lead to a blockage in the stomach at the pylorus and at best could lead to less wear of the molars and limit the nutrition the rabbit's digestive system will be able to extract from the under-chewed food.

Swallowed food enters the rabbit's large, thin-walled stomach. This organ accounts for about 15% of the volume of the rabbit's gastrointestinal (GI) tract, and is the largest for its body size of any monogastric (one-stomached) mammal. The stomach has a well-developed *cardiac sphincter* at the entrance which prevents food from being regurgitated. In a special area of the stomach termed the *fundus,* there are specialized parietal cells which secrete acid, producing the conditions under which pepsin works best, and chief cells, which secrete the pepsinogen that breaks down protein. Once in the stomach, ingested food is mixed with the hydrochloric acid, pepsinogen, and water, resulting in what is termed *chyme.* This fluid mixture (which normally also contains ingested hair) remains in the stomach about 3–6 hours; the acid and pepsinogen continuing the process of breaking down the plant material that was begun in the rabbit's mouth. Rabbits' stomachs do not completely empty, and are still half-full after not eating for 24 hours.

The pH of an adult rabbit's stomach is extremely acid, between 1-2 (a human's has a pH of 2–3). The mucus lining of the stomach, which is viscous and has a neutral pH, protects the stomach from the strong acid. It used to be thought that the rabbit's upper intestine was sterile because of this. However, recent studies have shown that some bacteria do inhabit the upper intestine, possibly from digesting cecotrophs (soft, partially-digested fecal pellets). The total length of the small intestine is about 3 meters, and it is in the small intestine that readily-digestible materials such as sugars, starch, fats, and soluble proteins are extracted and absorbed, volatile fatty acids (VFAs) being the main substance created from the breakdown of those compounds. Absorption occurs at the tips of microvilli (finger-like structures that increase the absorptive surface), which protrude through the mucous lining of the intestine. This mucous lining is extremely important, creating an environment in which the nutrients can be absorbed while acting as a barrier to pathogenic organisms and destructive enzymes.

The chyme then exits through the small, muscular pylorus to the upper small intestine, the duodenum, where it forms an acute angle near the liver. (This angle is where intestinal obstruction often occurs.) Bicarbonate is secreted into the duodenum, neutralizing the extremely acid chyme that exits the stomach and creating the more alkaline environment preferred by other enzymes. Although horses do not have gall bladders, rabbits do, and the gall duct opens into the duodenum. The rabbit gall bladder mostly secretes biliverdin instead of bilirubin (secreted by most mammals), which breaks up large globules of fat into smaller ones. The pancreatic duct also opens into the duodenum, releasing amylase for digesting starch, lipase for processing fats, protease for converting proteins, and chymotrypsin.

The middle section of the small intestine, termed the jejunum, is the largest section. Here excess bicarbonate is absorbed and the readily digestible plant materials (sugars, soluble protein, and starch) continue to be extracted and absorbed. Aggregates of lymphoid tissue called Peyer's patches are found along the walls of the jejunum and the second half of the ileum, and induce immune response in the mucosal tissues of the gut. Peyer's patches and related

Figure 2:1. The rabbit digestive system

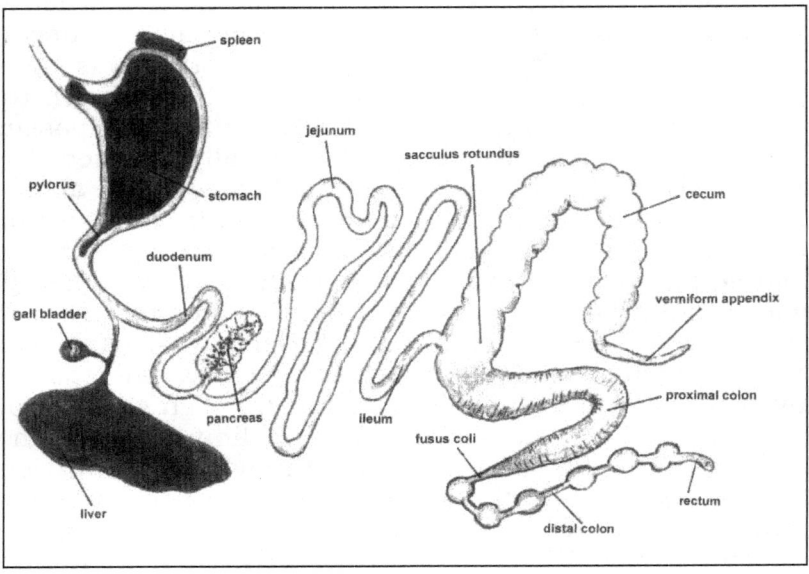

intestinal lymphoid tissues are termed "gut-associated lymphoid tissue," or GALT. GALT tissues recognize foreign antigens in the digesta and initiate the immune response. When areas of lymphoid tissue are damaged, undamaged Peyer's patches "reseed" the damaged areas, thus restoring the immune system.

Both the duodenum and jejunum have specialized cells that secrete a polypeptide hormone called motilin, which stimulates gastrointestinal smooth muscle. (Motilin is released in response to fat; carbohydrates inhibit its release. It is not present in the cecum, but reappears in the colon and rectum.)

The chyme takes about 10–20 minutes to pass through the jejunum, and then enters the last section of the small intestine, the *ileum*, which it passes through in about 30–60 minutes. The ileum ends in a thick-walled, enlarged area that is found only in rabbits: the *sacculus rotundus*, which is essentially a junction for the ileum, colon, and cecum. The sacculus rotundus has large amounts of lymphoid tissue and microvilli that are shorter and thicker than those of the ileum. A muscular valve in the sacculus rotundus controls movement of digesta from the ileum and prevents it from moving backwards into the small intestine. (This is the second most common place for foreign body impaction to occur.) A weaker valve allows chyme into the cecum. It has been suggested the sacculus rotundus is a transitional region where ingesta is prepared for the cecum. Like Peyer's patches, the sacculus rotundus may also play a role in the immune response of the digestive system.

The colon and cecum together constitute the hindgut. Contractions of the upper (proximal) colon, which is about 35 cm long, separate large-particle fiber (that over 0.5 mm, including most lignified fiber) from small-particle fiber and non-fibrous materials. Water content of the ingesta increases slightly in the upper colon, and a loose, discontinuous layer of mucus encourages the growth of "good" bacteria, which produce short-chain fatty acids that are absorbed and used for energy.

The *fusus coli*, a particularly muscular area containing few microvilli, is located between the proximal (upper) and distal (lower) colon and regulates the contractions of the colon and controls the production of hard and soft feces. The large particle fiber separated in the upper colon is moved quickly through the center of the colon to its distal (lower) end by peristaltic contractions as water is removed and absorbed, and into the rectum where the material is formed into hard fecal pellets that are expelled from the anus about four hours after the food is eaten. Mucus in the distal colon forms a thin layer that helps provide lubrication for feces. Soluble fiber and other more digestible materials are moved back along the colonic walls and haustra by antiperistaltic contractions of the colon.

Leng suggests that since the largest fibrous components are the most likely to be lignified, more may be removed, decreasing the lignin in the cecum relative to that of the whole diet and that excreted in hard feces. Since phenolic compounds from lignin have been shown to suppress bacterial growth and reduce digestibility of cellulose and starch, Leng suggests that the removal of the lignified fiber as hard feces may help improve the efficiency of bacterial growth in the cecum.

The cecum is essentially a large fermentation vat where microorganisms break down digestible fiber. The rabbit's cecum is the largest, per body size, of any mammal, accounts for up to 40% of the volume of the rabbit's GI tract, and has about ten times the capacity of the rabbit's stomach. The thin-walled organ ends in a narrow *vermiform appendix*, unique to rabbits. The vermiform appendix contains lymphoid tissue and may play a role in the immune response of the digestive system. It also secretes bicarbonate and water that buffer the semi-fluid cecal contents to a neutral pH. (Although in actuality the pH of the cecal contents changes from more alkaline in the morning to more acid in the afternoon as the populations of various microorganisms fluctuate.) The digesta routed to the cecum remains in that organ for about four hours. It is here—the more neutral pH being favorable for growth of bacteria—that microorganisms produce enzymes to break down structural plant material, releasing *volatile fatty acids* (VFAs) in the process. These fatty acids produced from the microbial breakdown of the plant carbohydrates are a major source of energy to the rabbit. The primary bacterial inhabitants of the cecum are those belonging to the genus *Bacteroides*, although small amounts of other bacteria such as *Escherichia coli* or clostridia may be present, along with a few ciliated protozoa and yeasts. Antibiotics, which kill the beneficial microbes along with targeted microbes, can alter the balance of the cecal microflora and allow pathenogenic species to proliferate.

Acetic acid (60–80%), butyric acid (8–20%), and proprionic acid (3–10%) are the primary VFAs produced by cecal fermentation, and account for about 40% of the energy that is required for body maintenance by the rabbit. After the cecal mixture has fermented about four hours, during which time some of the VFAs are absorbed by the cecum, small amounts of the cecal contents are periodically forced into the colon where more VFAs and some water are absorbed by the colonic walls. In the fusus coli the cecal material is formed into soft pellets. As the soft pellets move through the rectum toward the anus, lysozymes (enzymes that digest bacterial cell walls) and a mucous membrane are secreted by the colonic wall.

Approximately eight hours after food was initially consumed, soft, mucus-covered feces called cecotrophs (or cecotropes) are expelled from the anus and consumed by the rabbit. This process of consuming fecal material is termed coprophagy, or more specifically for material from the cecum, cecotrophy. (Both terms are correct.) Cecotrophs contain food residues, microorganisms and the products of microbial fermentation (including amylase), high levels of the B-vitamins and potassium, and twice the protein and half the fiber of hard feces. It is through their consumption that more of the nutrients from difficult-to-digest plant materials are made available to the rabbit.

Swallowing cecotrophs whole leaves their protective mucous covering intact as they enter the acidic stomach. Once in the stomach, the cecotrophs remain in the area called the fundus, which has a higher pH than the rest of the stomach The cecotrophs stay in the fundus for several hours, and remain intact for about six hours. Toward the end of this time in the stomach the cecotrophs disintegrate and begin to be digested, glucose being converted to carbon dioxide and lactic acid. These products, along with amino acids and vitamins, are mostly absorbed in the small intestine. Lysozymes, which were incorporated into the cecotrophs in the colon, begin the breakdown of the bacterial protein in the cecotrophs while they are still in the stomach, and the constituent amino acids are subsequently absorbed in the small intestine.

Production of the two kinds of feces is primarily governed by the different times the two different fiber mixtures enter the colon. The composition of the hard feces reflects the rabbit's diet—as dietary fiber increases so does the fiber in the hard feces. The difference in the nutrient absorption/excretion of the two feces phases may be summarized as follows:

- Hard feces phase: Water, sodium, and potassium absorbed in the proximal colon; water, VFA's and electrolytes absorbed in distal colon.

- Soft feces phase: Sodium, chloride, and VFAs are absorbed while potassium is excreted.

According to one researcher, concentrate-fed rabbits do not need to consume cecotrophs as do forage-fed rabbits, since complete nutrition is supplied in the concentrate. Rabbits given concentrate foods may consume fewer cecotrophs for this reason.

Urine

Although the topic of urine would normally be addressed in a discussion of the urogenital system and not the digestive system, I am mentioning it here because the appearance of rabbit urine may sometimes cause concern, especially to new rabbit owners. Rabbit urine normally contains some particulates, and the color may vary from clear to a dark reddish color, depending upon various factors.

Because of the rabbits' unique calcium metabolism, they excrete a large proportion of their dietary calcium in their urine, some of which precipitates out as calcium carbonate. Along with ammonium magnesium phosphate crystals, this is what gives rabbit urine its cloudy or gritty quality. Some precipitate is normal and a sign that the rabbit is receiving adequate dietary calcium. Rabbits needing more calcium (e.g., growing rabbits, pregnant rabbits, lactating rabbits) may have clear urine, as may anorexic rabbits.

Under certain conditions (e.g. lack of exercise, dehydration), calcium carbonate crystals or other precipitates may accumulate as bladder "sludge" or aggregate to form uroliths. Jenkins suggests there is a difference between calciuria (calcium crytals in urine) and sludge, which Jenkins calls micro urinary calculi, or MUC, which contain calcium-based calculi, not just crystals. Jenkins states that these calculi form in response to cystitis or other conditions, and that rabbits on low-calcium diets may actually have greater amounts of MUC. For a more in-depth discussion of calcium in rabbit diets see the calcium entry in Chapter Five.

Pigmented urine in rabbits is usually caused by *porphyrins*. Porphyrins are a large class of organic compounds which are able to bind metals. When rabbits eat certain foods high in some plant porphyrins, or are on some antibiotics, the levels of porphyrins excreted in their urine temporarily increase, causing the urine to turn orange-red to reddish-brown. Some foods that may cause this change in urine color include acorns, alfalfa, beets, broccoli, cabbage, carrots, and dandelion greens. Several rabbits being fed the same foods may have differing colors of urine due to factors such as stress and hydration. For example, urine color may be more pronounced if the rabbit is not drinking adequate liquids.

Colored rabbit urine may sometimes be caused by other compounds. A dark brown urine color may be caused by the presence of myoglobin (a protein pigment similar to hemoglobin). Blood from the reproductive tract or urinary tract may cause voided urine to appear reddish. Hematuria (blood in the urine) can be caused by a variety of conditions. A veterinarian may do a dipstick test or use a Wood's lamp (plant porphyrins will fluoresce, hemoglobin will not) to determine whether a red coloration is from blood.

Ketones are another aspect of urine composition affected by nutrition. Ketone bodies (acetone, actoacetic acid, and beta-hydroxybutyric acid) appear in rabbit urine when the metabolism is severely impaired, usually from malnutrition or starvation; that is, rabbits that do not eat enough or do not eat food that is high enough in nutrition over a period of time. Rabbits with severe dental disease and rabbits on hay-only diets that have impacted cecums will commonly have ketones in their urine. If the nutrition problem is not corrected, eventually more ketone bodies may be produced than can be handled by the rabbit's metabolism, eventually leading to hepatic lipidosis and death.

DIGESTIVE SYSTEM OF YOUNG RABBITS

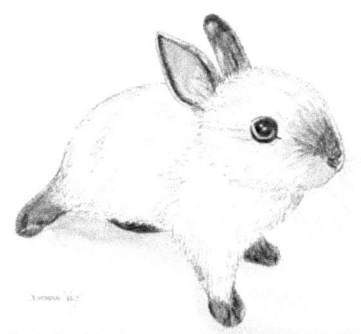

The digestive system of very young rabbits is critically different from that of adult rabbits. Nursing rabbits depend upon the protein and fat in their mother's milk and normally have distended stomachs filled with milk curd. This curd has a high pH of 5.0–6.5, which would encourage bacterial growth were it not for the presence of "milk oil," ocanoic and decanoic fatty acids that are produced from an enzymatic reaction with the doe's milk. These fatty acids have an antimicrobial action that protects the young rabbits until weaning.

As the milk consumption of the young rabbit (kitten)

decreases, its gastrointestinal microflora increases. Up to 14 days of age, the predominant bacterial genus present is usually *Streptococcus*, although some *Bacterioides*, *Escherichia coli*, *Clostridium*, *Endosporus*, and *Acuformis* are often also present. At about 2–3 weeks of age the young rabbits (kittens) begin to consume their mother's cecotrophs (this helps them begin to develop gut microflora), and gradually the bacteria involved in fermenting fibrous carbohydrates (primarily *Bacterioides*) become dominant in the cecum as solid foods are added to the diet (solid food intake begins at approximately 17 days and increases until weaning at approximately one month of age). The distal colon develops particularly rapidly, and along with the cecum provides early immune defense. From 3–9 weeks of age the kittens gradually develop the mature gastrointestinal tract: the cecum increases in size until it is the largest organ of the GI tract at about 5–6 weeks of age, and the stomach slowly develops a more acid pH until it reaches the acidic pH of the adult stomach. The pancreas is not fully developed before eight weeks, and since pancreatic enzymes normally digest starch in the small intestine, dietary starch in young rabbits goes into the cecum where it can cause imbalances of the microflora.

The digestive health of rabbits at any age depends upon a delicate balance between the microflora and the protective mucosal tissues lining the gut. However, rabbit kittens are particularly vulnerable to digestive problems during the time just prior to weaning through weaning and shortly afterwards as their immune systems, particularly that of the gut, develop rapidly. In one study it was found that bacterial fibrolytic enzymes increased by 30% ten days after weaning.

The digestive system, especially the cecum, continues to develop and come to maturity from 3-5 weeks of age. If the kitten should receive any *sudden* changes to its diet—particularly if it suddenly receives a high-starch diet—pathogenic bacteria such as *Clostridium* can gain dominance in the gut, leading to sickness and death. High protein diets may also increase mortality in young rabbits, for the protein is incompletely digested in the intestine, allowing protein to enter the lower GI tract where it may cause a negative alteration in the microflora (dysbiosis). For this reason, it is suggested by many rabbit experts that rabbits prior to and through weaning should be given a diet that is consistent and composed of low-protein, low-starch, high-fiber foods containing high levels of pectins and xylans (hemicellulose).

Conversely, the doe's diet needs to have higher protein and higher energy content because of milk production. Therefore, it is recommended that rabbit kittens be prevented from eating the mother's diet at weaning. Alternatively, the doe's diet can be changed to one low in protein and high in fiber about ten days prior to weaning her kits.

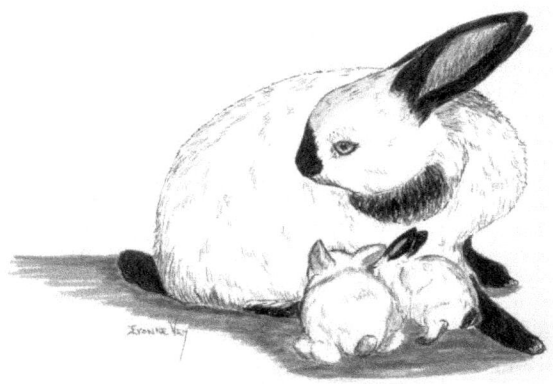

References

Besoluk, K., E. eken, and E. Sur. 2006. A morphological and morphometrical study on the sacculus rotundus and ileum of the Angora rabbit. *Veter. Medicina* 51(2): 60-65.

Brewer, N.R. 2006. Biology of the Rabbit. *J. Am. Asso. Lab. An. Sci.* 45(1): 8–24.

BSAVA Manual of Rabbit Medicine and Surgery. Second edition. 2006. Edited by Anna Meredith and Paul Flecknell. Glouster: British Small Animal Veterinary Association.

Brooks, Dale L. 2004. Nutrition and Gastrointestinal Physiology. In: *Ferrets, Rabbits, and Rodents Clinical Medicine and Surgery,* 2nd Ed. Katherine E. Quesenberry and James W. Carpenter, eds. St. Louis:Saunders.

Cheeke, Peter R. 2010. Nutritional Management of Rabbits and Principles of Rabbit Nutrition. Convention notes, 2010 ARBA National Convention.

Debray, L., I. LeHuerou-Luon, T. Gidenne, and L. Fortun-Lamothe. 2003. Digestive tract development in rabbit according to the dietary energeytic source: correlation between whole tract digestion, pancreatic and intestinal enzymatic activities. *Comp. Biochem Physio.* 135(3): 443–455.

Dorier, A., Y. Piery, and Cl. Bacques. 1989. Etude en Microscopie Optique et Electronique a Balatage de l'Evolution Structurale des Parois du Caecum et du colon, Durant la Periode Perinatale, Chez le Lapin (*Oryctolagus cuniculus* L.) *Anat. Histol. Embryol.* 18(2): 183-192.

Fortun-Lamothe, L. and S. Boullier. 2004. Interactions between gut microflora and digestive mucosal immunity, and strategies to improve digestive health in young rabbits. *Proceedings:* 8th World Rabbit Congress, Puebla.

Gidenne, T., L. Debray, L. Fortune-Lamothe, and I. Le Huerou-Luron. 2007. Maturation of the intestinal digestion and of microbial activity in the young rabbit: impact of the dietary fibre:starch ratio. *Comp. Biochem. Phys.* 148(4): 834-844.

Harcourt Brown, Frances. 2002. *Textbook of Rabbit Medicine.* Oxford: Butterworth Heinemann.

Harkness, J. E., P. V. Turner, S. VandeWoude, and C. L. Wheeler. 2010. *Biology and Medicine of Rabbits and Rodents.* Fifth edition. Singapore: Blackwell Publishing.

Hotchkiss, Charlotte Evans. 1994. Mucus secretagogue activity in cecal contents of rabbits with experimentally-induced mucoid enteropathy. Dissertation, University of Florida. 232 pp.

Irlbeck, N.A. 2001. How to feed the rabbit (*Oryctolagus cuniculus*) gastrointestinal tract. *J. Anim. Sci.* 79(E.Suppl.): 343–346.

Jeklova, E., L. Lenka, H. Kudlackova, and M. Fladyna. 2007. Functional development of immune response in rabbits. *Vet. Immunol. and Immunopath.* 118(3-4): 221-228.

Jenkins, J. R. 2010. Evaluation of the Rabbit Urinary Tract. *J. Exo. Pet Med.* 19(4): 271-279.

Johnson-Delaney, C. A. 2006. Anatomy and Physiology of the Rabbit and Rodent Gastrointestinal System. *Proceedings:* Association of Avian Veterinarians.

Lavrenic, A. 2006. The effect of rabbit age on *in vitro* caecal fermentation of starch, pectin, xylan, cellulose, compound feed and its fibre. *Animal* 1: 241–248.

Leng, R. A. 2008. Digestion in the rabbit—a new look at the effects of their feeding and digestive strategies. *Proceedings*: MEKEARN Rabbit Conference: Organic rabbit production from forages (Eds: Reg. Preston and Nguyen Van Thu), Catho University, Vietnam.

McWilliams, D. A. 2001. Nutritional Pathology in Rabbits: Current and Future Perspectives. Paper: Ontario Commercial Rabbit Growers Asso. Congress.

Makala, L. H. C., N. Suzuki, and H. Nagasawa. 2002. Peyer's Patches: Organized Lymphoid Structures for the Induction of Mucosal Immune Responses in the Intestine. *Pathobiol.* 70(2): 55–68.

The Merck Veterinary Manual. Ninth edition. 2005. Edited by Cynthia M. Kahn. Whitehouse Station: Merck and Co., Inc.

Mestecky, J. and C. O. Elson. 2008. Peyer's Patches as the Inductive Site for IgA Responses. *J. Immun.* 180: 1293–1294.

Murray, M. J. 2005. Rabbit Gastro-Intestinal Disease. *Proceedings:* North American Veterinary Conference, Orlando, Florida.

Oglesbee, Barbara L. 2006. *The 5-Minute Veterinary Consult: Ferret and Rabbit.* Ames: Blackwell Publishing Professional.

Partridge, G. G. 1989. Nutrition of farmed rabbits. *Proc. Nutr. Soc.* 48: 93-101.

Saunders, Richard A. and Ron Rees Davies. 2005. *Notes on Rabbit Internal Medicine.* Oxford: Blackwell Publishing.

Snipes, R. L., W. Clauss, A. Weber, and H. Hornicke.1982. Structural and functional differences in various divisions of the rabbit colon. *Cell Tiss. Res.* 225(2): 331-346.

V arga, Molly. 2014. *Textbook of Rabbit Medicine.* Second edition. Oxford: Butterworth Heinemann Elsevier.

Chapter 3

CARBOHYDRATES

Carbohydrates (saccharides) can be one of the most difficult areas of rabbit nutrition to understand. Confusion may arise because common usage of terms varies and in some cases does not conform to the actual meaning of the word. For example, variations of the following statement appear on many rabbit websites and in many articles and books on rabbits: "Rabbits should be fed a low-carbohydrate high-fiber diet." Yet technically this statement is contradictory, for fiber *is* carbohydrate (Figure 3:1).

Reduced to basic terms, carbohydrates are neutral chemical compounds primarily composed of carbon, hydrogen, and oxygen, the H and O usually in the ratio of 2:1. They occur as single molecules, short chains, or complex chains, and are primarily produced by green plants where they are found in the cell wall and cell contents. Cell walls contain the polysaccharides hemicellulose and cellulose, as well as lignocellulose, and are about 40-70% digestible by microflora inhabiting mammal digestive systems. Cell contents include sugar and starch saccharides as well as protein and other compounds. These contents are about 90% digestible and provide rapidly available energy.

In one way or another all mammalian life is dependent upon carbohydrates because they are one of the two main energy-giving compounds (fats being the other) that mammals break down and use to fuel cell function. Mammals may consume carbohydrates directly by eating foodstuffs such as vegetables, fruits, and grains or may consume them indirectly by eating the flesh of mammals whose diet consists primarily of green plants. In general, herbivores must consume more food to meet their energy needs than do omnivores and carnivores. Because of their small body size and high metabolic rate, rabbits have relatively high energy needs even when compared to many other herbivores, especially the larger ones.

We know the simpler carbohydrates as "sugars." Some of the more complex ones are *starches*, *gums*, and *cellulose*. Sugars include the *monosaccharides*, which contain one carbohydrate molecule (e.g., glucose, fructose, galactose), and the *disaccharides* (e.g., sucrose, lactose, maltose), which contain two sugar molecules. The *oligosaccharides* (e.g., raffinose, stachyose) have chains of 3–10 molecules, and the *polysaccharides* (e.g., starch, pectin, cellulose) have chains of more than 10 molecules. The bodies of mammals must break down the more complex carbohydrates before the energy can be used. The ability of a particular mammal to break down a certain kind of carbohydrate will affect the place of foods containing that carbohydrate in the mammal's diet. Carbohydrates not broken down by enzymes produced by the rabbit are broken down by enzymes produced by the microflora in the rabbits gut. The main end-products from the breakdown of carbohydrates are *short-chain fatty acids* (SCFAs), also called *volatile fatty acids* (VFAs).

There is an unfortunate perception among some rabbit owners that "complex" carbohydrates (especially fiber) are better for and are more necessary in a rabbit's diet than the "simple" carbohydrates. The reality is that both are necessary for optimal health in a rabbit. But how much, and of what kind? For some of the answers to those questions we may look at scientific studies that have been done on the subject of rabbit nutrition. Much valuable information on rabbit diet has come from these studies and found its way into the literature on feeding show and pet rabbits. But there is a problem with applying the results of these studies too literally, because most of this research on rabbit nutrition was done by scientists interested in advancing knowledge for rabbit production, especially meat production. The vast majority of these studies were done on rabbits 80 days old or less, because production rabbits are normally slaughtered by about that age.

Those who bred rabbits for show were among the first to realize that the available information on rabbit diet needed to be adapted to apply to their particular rabbits depending upon breed, age, and varying environmental and physical conditions. Show rabbits may be kept for several years, and in order to win awards the rabbits must be in top condition. Rabbits that are obese, too thin, have poor coats, mites, bad teeth, or other defects are either disqualified or receive no awards. Proper nutrition is essential if the rabbits are to be in prime physical form.

Years later, as rabbits became more popular as pets, those with companion rabbits also became interested in discovering just what diet was healthiest for their rabbits and would maximize the years they would enjoy with their pets.

Despite the interest of these two groups, research on the subject of rabbit nutrition tailored to longer-lived rabbits remains rare. It is not that the results of studies on short-lived rabbits cannot ever be applied to longer-living show or companion rabbits, but it should be done so with an understanding of the changes occurring in a rabbit's digestive system with age, differing energy requirements for rabbits kept under different environmental conditions, and the special nutritional requirements of particular breeds.

MONOSACCHARIDES AND DISACCHARIDES

Sugars of one kind or another are found in almost every food we and/or our rabbits eat. Glucose is present in most plant and animal tissues. Lactose and galactose are found in milk; fructose in honey and many plant materials, including grass and fruits. Sucrose, which we eat in the refined form of "table sugar," is naturally present in fruits and vegetables.

In a rabbit's digestive system most of the monosaccharides and disaccharides are digested in the stomach and small intestine. The disaccharides are first broken down into simple sugars by hydrolysis, or a breaking of the bonds holding the monosaccharide units together. Normally little or no undigested sugars reach the cecum and they are therefore unlikely to cause imbalances in the microflora of that organ. (However, it is possible that when unusually large amounts are consumed some sugars may reach the cecum undigested and could potentially cause the microflora of the cecum to alter, resulting in digestive problems.) How much sugar is safe for a rabbit to ingest? As with most dietary issues, the answer depends partly upon the age, health, activity, normal diet, and breed of the rabbit. Very young rabbits in particular can develop fatal digestive problems if given too much of a sugar they do not yet have the ability to process. Very young rabbits still on their mother's milk have a high ability to digest the milk sugars, lactose and galactose, but little ability to digest fructose. After they are weaned, the ability of rabbit kittens to digest the milk sugars decreases and their ability to digest fructose—which would normally be entering their diet about this time—increases. The instability of the cecal microflora at this critical juncture makes young rabbits very susceptible to digestive problems—loss of appetite, diarrhea, enterotoxemia, death—as they transition from their mother's milk to solid foods. High glucose and/or fructose may allow pathogens such as *Clostridium spiroforme* and *Escherichia coli* to proliferate and colonize the cecum. Toxins from these organisms, such as iota toxin, are often lethal to kits. Mortality rates of 14–20% are not uncommon after weaning.

In a very early study done on the assimilation limits of various sugars in *adult* rabbits, the researchers found the sugar tolerances of the rabbits they studied to be, from least tolerance to greatest: sucrose, levulose (fructose), glucose, maltose. Although this study is very old and it has to be taken into consideration that little was understood about rabbit digestion at the time and that the methods were not what they would be today, the data collected is still worth looking at. I found the study particularly interesting because it is one of very few in which adult rabbits were studied over a period of several months (nine), thus providing information on older rabbits than are usually used as subjects in nutrition studies. In a recent study, the effect of replacing varying percentages of feed ingredients with dates (high in sugar) was investigated, and the researchers found that the dates had no deleterious effects on the rabbits.

In my opinion, *adult* rabbits may be able to tolerate more sugar in their diet than some sources on rabbit diet recommend, although a consistent high-sugar diet would undoubtedly be unhealthful. Certainly there is adequate science to show that concentrate feeds (often sweetened with sugar beet molasses, which is about 50% sugar, mostly sucrose) do not harm the flora and function of the rabbit digestive system. It further appears that many adult rabbits are able to tolerate *occasional* high doses of sugar without undue harm.

I have reasons for believing adult rabbits may be able to tolerate high-sugar foods occasionally. When I visited my parents' house 3 of my rabbits stayed in my mother's

34

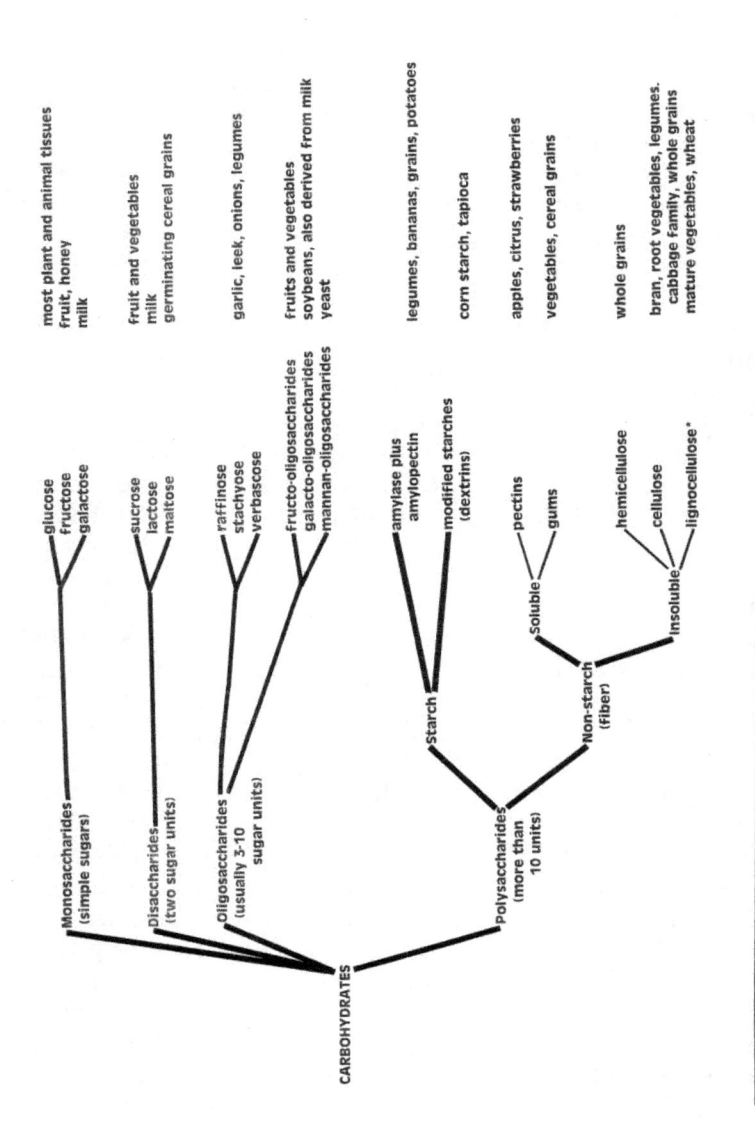

Category	Subcategory	Examples	Sources
Monosaccharides (simple sugars)		glucose, fructose, galactose	most plant and animal tissues, fruit, honey, milk
Disaccharides (two sugar units)		sucrose, lactose, maltose	fruit and vegetables, milk, germinating cereal grains
Oligosaccharides (usually 3-10 sugar units)		raffinose, stachyose, verbascose	garlic, leek, onions, legumes
		Fructo-oligosaccharides, galacto-oligosaccharides, mannan-oligosaccharides	fruits and vegetables, soybeans, also derived from milk, yeast
Polysaccharides (more than 10 units)	Starch	amylase plus amylopectin	legumes, bananas, grains, potatoes
		modified starches (dextrins)	corn starch, tapioca
	Non-starch (fiber) — Soluble	pectins	apples, citrus, strawberries
		gums	vegetables, cereal grains
	Non-starch (fiber) — Insoluble	hemicellulose	whole grains
		cellulose	bran, root vegetables, legumes, cabbage family, whole grains
		lignocellulose*	mature vegetables, wheat

Fig. 3:1 Simplified carbohydrate tree

* lignin is not a carbohydrate, but because of the importance of the cellulose/lignin complex in rabbits' diet, lignocellulose is included in this carbohydrate tree.

bedroom. I usually took care to see that my mother's closet door was closed while they were there, as I knew my mother stored food on the floor of the closet. But one time several years ago I must have left it open just enough that they could push the door aside, for hours later I found the three rabbits—a Holland Lop, American Fuzzy Lop, and Dutch—happily devouring a ripped-open 5-pound sack of sugar, or sucrose. As near as I could tell, the rabbits had eaten from two tablespoons to ¼ cup of refined sucrose apiece. It was a weekend and no vet was available. From the information I had read on rabbits at that time I was sure there was no hope—my three rabbits were all going to die. I made sure they had plenty of hay and water and waited for the terrible end...and waited...and waited. Nothing happened. None of the three rabbits developed loose stools, passed excessive cecotrophs, had a gastrointestinal slowdown, or appeared to be in any pain or discomfort.

In the scientific world, the above is what is termed "anecdotal evidence." It is only my personal experience and observation; not the results of a controlled scientific study. But here again I found the old study on sugar tolerance in rabbits interesting. The researchers kept track of the cases of diarrhea among the rabbits given the various oral doses of sugars, and in my opinion it was surprisingly low, and appeared non-fatal, for the same rabbits were sometimes mentioned later in the study. One rabbit received over 40 doses of sugar over the nine month period and never had diarrhea. Moreover, the researchers stated that the rabbits remained in "good nutritive condition."

Why were my pet rabbits and the rabbits of the studies able to tolerate these high intakes of sugar without serious ill effects? It is possible that it was because the normal diet of both the experimental rabbits and the diet of my rabbits contained a certain amount of sugar. The first experimental rabbits were given barley and corn – both fairly high-sugar – and the rabbits of the more recent study as well as my rabbits received commercial feeds (which contain sweeteners such as molasses) and limited fruit. As was explained in Chapter 2, the digestive systems of rabbits handle foods better if the rabbits are accustomed to consuming those foods and have populations of microflora that have adapted to them. Age may have also been a factor given that there is evidence young rabbits are much more susceptible to digestive ills from high-sugar content foods, and my and the study rabbits were older.

This is NOT to say that I believe rabbits should be fed high-sugar diets. I do not. Great care should be taken to prevent rabbit kits, in particular, from consuming high-sugar foods. But I do believe many *adult* rabbits, although not all, can consume most commercial pellets with no harm from the sugar content and can *occasionally* be given fairly high-sugar foods such as a small piece of carrot, apple, or a few dried cranberries without ill effects. I normally give all my adult rabbits one such treat each evening, and have had no digestive problems result in my rabbits from this practice. Christine Carter, author of *The Wonderful World of Pet Rabbits,* feels that while owners should be wary of giving rabbits dried fruits because of additives, sugar content should not be a reason to avoid fresh fruits. Christine states: "Personally, I can vouch that sweet tasting fruit and vegetables do not cause a problem when fed to bunnies in sensible amounts."

OLIGOSACCHARIDES

Oligosaccharides are sugars composed of several monosaccharide units, usually considered to be 3–10 units (although some sources give 3–6 or 3–9), and include the fructo-oligosaccharides, galacto-oligosaccharides, and mannanoligosaccharides. Oligosaccharides are not completely digested by the enzymes secreted by mammals, and the undigested portions become food for the microorganisms of the digestive system, which produce the enzymes to break the sugars down to simpler units. Fructo-oligosaccharides (FOS) occur naturally in many vegetables, galacto-oligosaccharides (GOS) occur in soybeans and can be derived from milk, and mannanoligosaccharides (MOS) are derived from yeast.

In humans it has been found that FOS and GOS can increase the populations of and "friendly" bacteria while reducing "unfriendly" bacteria, and they are sometimes sold as food supplements for this reason. MOS is often added to feeds for livestock to promote intestinal health. Studies have been done on the effects of these oligosaccharides on rabbits, but it is difficult to make a final judgment as to their possible benefit as a feed supplement because results from different studies vary. Some researchers have found no significant effect on cecal function when MOS was added to the diet of young rabbits. But other researchers obtained results that might be interpreted to show MOS may have a positive effect on the rabbit digestive system by increasing the production of volatile fatty acids (VFAs), especially butyrate, and reducing the pH of the cecum, thus making the cecum a less favorable environment for pathogenic bacteria. Other effects found in various studies include increased absorption of magnesium, improved elimination of toxic compounds, and lower mortality rates in recently-weaned rabbits.

Fructans (fructo-oligosaccharides and inulin) are non-starch plant storage carbohydrates that are found in various plants, including grasses, Jerusalem artichokes, globe artichokes, asparagus, chicory root, green beans, jicama, and plants of the onion family. The two compounds are chemically similar, but fructo-oligosaccharides are composed of shorter chains than inulin, which is a more complex carbohydrate and is actually a polysaccharide rather than an oligosaccharide. In some studies, adding FOS to the diets of rabbits resulted in increased VFAs in cecal contents and a reduction of cecal ammonia, both considered positive effects. Rats, another hindgut fermenter, showed improvement in muscle tone, body weight, and cognitive processes in some studies where chicory-derived fructans were added to the diets.

In a study done on young rabbits, rabbits fed chicory before weaning had improved cecum function while those fed chicory after weaning had a higher food intake and weight gain than rabbits not fed chicory. In another study where chicory was added to the diet of rabbits, researchers concluded that adding 10% chicory root to the diet of the rabbits beneficially affected fermentative activity in the cecum.

Other researchers compared a control diet containing low inulin to a diet with added fruto-oligosaccharide and a diet with added inulin. The diets were given to rabbits from 8–9 weeks old. Digestibility of both the fructo-oligosaccharide and inulin was 100 percent. Both the

Table 3.1 Sugar and starch content of selected foods. *Values compiled from multiple sources.*

Food	% Sugar	% Starch	Food	% Sugar	% Starch
acorns	0	33.9	molasses*	60.0	0
almonds	4.8	2.7	oats, rolled	2.0	64.9
apples	10.39	1.1	oranges	14.0	0
banana	11.6	4.65	papaya	18.0	0
barley	0.8	55.38	peach	12.2	0
bread, white	0.75	50.5	peanuts	6.2	6.4
brewer's yeast*	0	21.0	pineapple	9.6	1.97
chicory	0.7	0.2	plum	8.9	0
cracker, saltine	0	14.0	pumpkin	1.96	4.64
cranberries, dried	65.0	0	raisins	70.0	0
cucumber	1.67	0.1	raspberries	4.42	1.02
dates, dried	65.3	0	soybeans*	5.6	4.8
endive/escarole	0.25	0	spinach	0.43	0.1
grapes	15.0	0	sunflower seeds	2.62	5.64
hay, alfalfa	7.0	2.0	tomato	2.7	0.5
hay, grass	8.0	2.5	walnuts	1.1	0.7
kale	1.34	0.1	watermelon	6.2	0.95
lettuce, romaine	1.19	0.6	wheat bran	22.1	27.0
mango	19.9	0.45	zuchinni	0	0.1

*Used as ingredients in some commercial rabbit foods

fructo-oligosaccharide and inulin lowered the cecal pH, the inulin to a greater degree than the fructo-oligosaccharide. (Lowering of cecal pH is thought to make the cecal environment less friendly to bacteria such as clostridia.) The researchers did not find significant increases in VFA concentration among the diets, but the proportions of VFAs did change, especially in the rabbits fed inulin.

However, another researcher did *not* find that added inulin improved the environment of the cecum, and in this particular study the highest incidence of diarrhea occurred in the group of rabbits with inulin added to their diet. The rabbits in the first study were younger, and the age difference may account for some of the difference in the findings. In still another study on the effects of FOS on young rabbits, the researchers found no statistical difference in mortality or diarrhea incidence in those rabbits given FOS.

Raffinose, stachyose, and verbascose are oligosaccharides found in legumes (e.g., peas, beans, alfalfa) and plants of the onion and cabbage families. These are the compounds that cause "gas" or flatulence in mammals. Because the enzyme needed to break these compounds down (alpha galactosidase) is not secreted by the mammalian digestive tract, mammals are dependent upon the microflora of their digestive tracts to break this group of oligosaccharides down for them. In specialized herbivores this will usually occur in the rumen or cecum, in humans it occurs in the large intestine.

While many references on rabbit diet from the United States warn rabbit owners not to provide excessive amounts of foods containing these oligosaccharides to their rabbits because of the gas formed from their breakdown, cabbages and other member of that plant family (e.g., cauliflower, broccoli, Brussels sprouts) are commonly fed to rabbits in some European countries. I believe the ability of a rabbit to process these foods without excessive gas depends upon the amount and frequency it is given to the rabbit, as many rabbits appear to be able to tolerate small amounts in their diets and appear to relish them. If small amounts of the vegetables were given fairly often, the rabbit's microflora would most likely adjust. But again, the decision to give or not to give vegetables from the cabbage family should be made based on the health, age, and sensitivities of each individual rabbit.

POLYSACCHARIDES (glycans)

Polysaccharides are the most complex of the carbohydrates and comprise the largest group of saccharides. They can be divided into *starch* and non-starch, or *fiber* (Figure 3:1). Unlike some of the simpler carbohydrates, polysaccharides (other than starch) are not absorbed in the stomach and upper intestine, which do not secrete the enzymes necessary for their breakdown.

Instead, they are digested in the rabbit's cecum, where microorganisms produce the needed enzymes. Most of the research that has been done on rabbit nutrition in the area of carbohydrates has been on the polysaccharides.

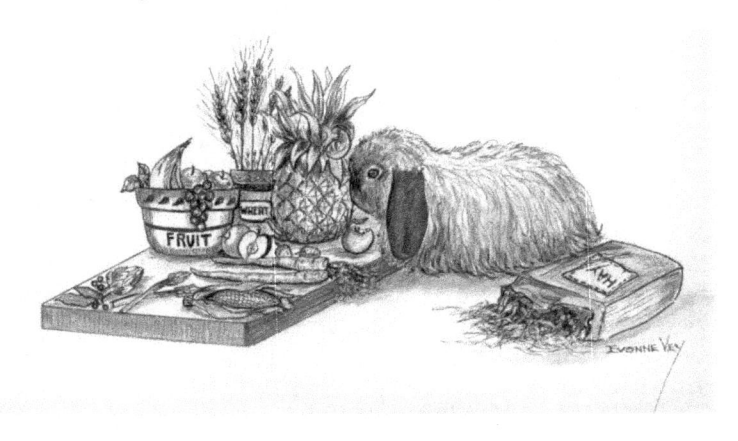

Starch

Starch (amylum) is the primary storage carbohydrate in green plants, and is found in stems, seeds, and underground plant organs such as tubers, corms, and rhizomes. It is composed of amylose, a straight glucose polymer (molecule formed by the bonding of two or more smaller molecules), and amylopectin, a more complex, highly branched polymer. Amylose usually comprises from 20–30% of starch, and is soluble in warm water. Amylopectin, which usually comprises about 70–80% of starch, is insoluble in water.

There is a misconception by some people that wild *Oryctolagus* do not have diets that are high in starch. As we saw in the first chapter, the diets of wild rabbits depend upon the habitat, weather, and other factors. Acorns, which were found to be a food of year-round importance for some populations of wild *Oryctolagus*, are a high-starch food, about 57-60% of acorn dry matter. Another researcher found that rabbits have a taste preference for maltose and polycose and suggests this may add to the taste sensation for starch plants in rabbits. He postulates that rabbits may have specialized taste receptors for starch that are an evolutionary adaptation to the diet of wild rabbits, which several researchers have found to be high in starch.

What is called the "whole-tract digestibility" of starch has been found to be almost complete in the rabbit digestive system, unlike more complex polysaccharides, which are only partially digested while passing through the rabbit's digestive tract. Amylase in the saliva starts breaking starch down, but most starch is digested in the stomach and small intestine and any remaining starch is usually digested in the cecum where it is broken down to lactate and VFAs. The amount of starch broken down before it reaches the cecum appears to depend upon the type; researchers investigating the starch concentration in the ileum for three kinds of starch: barley, pea, and maize, found the lowest ileal concentration for barley and higher for pea and maize. Retention time in the whole tract was higher when the ileal starch concentration was higher, as was the quantity of digested fiber.

There have been many studies on *young* rabbits that found a high incidence of digestive disorders (enterotoxemia) and mortality with high-starch diets during the time around weaning when young rabbits' foods change from milk to plant carbohydrates. (In one study amylase activity increased by 59% at weaning while the activity of the sugar enzymes maltase, sucrase, and lactase decreased activity by 30, 48, and 72% respectively.) Since the pancreas is not fully developed until around eight weeks, and pancreatic enzymes normally digest starch in the small intestine, high amounts of rapidly digestible sugars and starch in the diet of young rabbits may cause an overload in the cecum, resulting in overgrowth of cecal bacteria, some of which may produce toxins. (Interestingly, however, in one study where young rabbits were fed diets with similar fiber composition but differing sugar and starch amounts, the diets with *low* starch and higher sugar resulted in higher mortality of young rabbits than those with *high* starch and low sugar.)

For many years it was assumed this sensitivity to starch levels also applied to adult rabbits. However, some more recent studies show *adult* rabbits appear to digest starch well and without ill effects, most of the starch being digested before it ever reaches the cecum (although microbes in the cecum have been found to be able to digest starch). In one study on the digestibility of starch as it passed though the ileum, the ileal digestibility was more than 93% for starch at all the levels of dietary fiber tested (meaning most starch is broken down and absorbed by the time it leaves the small intestine). Researchers conducting another study concluded that starch does not significantly affect fermentation in the cecum, and yet another group of researchers conducting *in vitro* studies using cecal inoculums from different-aged rabbits concluded that starch is not an important substrate for the microorganisms of the cecum at any age. Researchers have hypothesized that hydrolysis of starches in the rabbit digestive tract may even be modified according to the type of starch, thus controlling the rate of its passage and cecal fermentation.

Starch is a valuable food that provides easily-digested nutrition and quick energy. It also often occurs in conjunction with other valuable nutrients, such as cellulose, hemicellulose, and pectin. While it may be possible for adult rabbits to receive a starch overload, adult rabbits in good health can most likely consume some high-starch foods without ill effects. I give my rabbits *occasional* small high-starch treats such as pieces of dried bread. Christine Carter, author of *The Wonderful World of Pet Rabbits,* also feels that giving rabbits occasional treats of dried bread is not harmful:

> A bit of bread—rabbits are particularly fond of bread and known to behave as though they are addicted to it. Should your bunny exhibit the following behaviour when presented with some bread, it is a pretty clear indication that he is an addict:
> *Alone in his hutch, he quickly snatches up the piece of bread and runs around in a panic as if another bunny or someone is going to seize it from him. He will settle in a far corner or hidey-hole and munch away while staying on high alert—keeping an eye out for the threat of an imaginary, phantom 'bread thief'. Mother rabbits are also loath to share a bit of bread with their babies.*
> Ensure bread for your bunny is dry and crusty by drying it on a windowsill or toasting it. My family prefers to eat bread that does not contain preservatives or emulsifiers and so the bunnies are fed left over Italian or Lebanese bread. Wholemeal breads containing bran or seeds are obviously more nutritious than refined white bread. Check that bunny

bread has no mould spots. Do not overfeed bread, as it is not a natural rabbit food and should hence be fed only as a small treat.

Dextrins

Dextrins, the other starch carbohydrates, are modified starches that are produced by the hydrolysis, or breakdown, of starch molecules. They are formed naturally during digestion or may be formed intentionally in a manufacturing process. Cornstarch is a dextrin, as is powdery tapioca starch.

Non-starch polysaccharides (fiber)

Although some rabbit owners consider "fiber" to be synonymous with grass hay, fiber comes in many different forms, one or another of which may be dominant in a particular plant or plant tissue. Fiber cannot be digested in the mammalian stomach and upper intestine because mammals do not produce the enzymes to break these compounds down. They must rely upon microorganisms that have the enzymes to break them down. In the rabbit this occurs in the cecum, where fiber is a main energy source for cecal microorganisms. Volatile fatty acids (VFAs) are an important product of carbohydrate hydrolysis, and they are one of the substances that give cecotrophs their distinctive odor. The type and amount of fiber affects the amount of microbial protein in cecotrophs.

Fiber can be divided into two major categories: soluble and insoluble. Soluble fiber includes pectins and gums; insoluble fiber includes cellulose, hemicellulose, and lignocellulose. Lignin itself is actually a phenolic compound, not a carbohydrate, but since it often forms a complex with cellulose in cell walls it is usually included in discussions of plant fiber/carbohydrates. Both soluble and insoluble fiber affect the microflora of the gut, the rate of passage of digesta, and play a role in maintaining the integrity of the mucosa and the mucosal immune response. Too little fiber in the diet can lead to GI hypomotility, decreased cecotroph production, and increased retention time in the cecum. Too much can negatively affect the intestines and mucus and lead to prolonged retention in the stomach and sometimes the cecum.

SOLUBLE FIBER

Soluble fiber can be dissolved in water. It is sometimes considered less important than insoluble fiber in the rabbit diet, but there is no scientific evidence that supports this assumption. Soluble and insoluble fiber have different effects upon the digestive system of the rabbit and are both necessary for optimal health. In general, soluble fiber absorbs water and slows the movement of food through the digestive system, allowing time for nutrients to be absorbed and possibly helping regulate glucose and cholesterol levels in the blood. Increasing soluble fiber increases dietary nutritive values. However, too high a proportion of pectins and gums in the diet may contribute to cecal impaction.

Pectins are carbohydrates that are mostly found in material (the middle lamellae) between plant cells where they help hold adjacent cells together. Pectin occurs in plant tissues other than fruit, but we most often associate it with that plant organ. Fruit provides a good example of the importance of pectin, for it is the degradation of pectin as fruit becomes older (or is treated by chemicals) that causes the fruit to become soft. Several commercial rabbit feeds contain fairly high amounts of pectin, often from the inclusion of sugar beet pulp, which is about 25% pectin, or dehydrated alfalfa, which is also high in pectin. Legumes contain 5–10% and grasses 3–4% pectin.

Pectin is about 75% digestible by the rabbit digestive system. Studies on cecal micro-organisms have found high populations of bacteria able to break down pectin, the most important of which are bacteria of several species in the genus *Bacterioides*. The fermentation of pectin in the cecum appears to occur more rapidly in young rabbits than adults. It has been shown there is even some pectinolytic activity in the upper gastrointestinal tract of rabbits, possibly from their consumption of microorganism-containing cecotrophs. There have been many studies on the effects of pectin on the rabbit digestive system. Overall, it has been shown that pectin does not have a negative effect on the health of the rabbit digestive system, and may have several positive effects, especially at weaning.

One group of researchers suggested that giving rabbits

foods with pectin at weaning may help adult digestive tract microflora to develop at this critical time. Researchers found that adding hemicellulose and pectin led to higher weight gain, increased digestibility, and increased content of VFAs. The latter is considered a benefit because VFAs help the absorption of water and sodium, thereby possibly preventing diarrhea at times sugars are not fully digested in the stomach and ileum before they reach the cecum. It has been found in some studies that higher VFA concentrations lower the pH of the cecum, making the cecal environment less favorable to pathogenic bacteria (although the results of still other studies have not always shown an increase in cecal pH with increased VFA). One researcher reported that only pectin content of the diet is related to cecal pH, although other researchers suggested that hemicellulose may also increase the pH of the cecum. Researchers doing an *in vitro* study found that giving rabbits a diet of commercial feed also promoted high SCFA (SCFAs and VFAs are the same thing) concentrations.

Gums are soluble polysaccharides of multiple sugar subunits linked together. Like pectin, gums help hold adjacent cells together. Also like pectin, they absorb water and add bulk to the cecum. True gums are found in high concentrations in vegetables. Alginates, carrageenans, and agars are polysaccharides closely related to gums and are sometimes included in this category of soluble fiber.

There have not been many studies done specifically on the effects of gums on rabbit digestion, although gums—being a natural vegetable constituent—are found in many of the feeds given to rabbits, and would be included in studies on the soluble fiber fractions of feed. In general, one may assume the effects of gums on rabbit digestion are similar to those of pectins.

INSOLUBLE FIBER
The category of insoluble fiber includes complex carbohydrates that are not easily broken down and are important constituents of the structural part of plants, especially the cell wall. Hemicellulose, cellulose, and lignocellulose are insoluble fibers. They account for most of the total biomass on earth.

Table 3:2 Percent soluble and insoluble fiber content of selected foods. *Values compiled from multiple sources.*

Food	soluble fiber %	insoluble fiber %	Food	soluble fiber, %	insoluble fiber, %
almonds	1.10	10.10	kiwi	0.8	2.6
apples	0.69	1.74	lettuce	0.4	1.6
apricots	0.9	0.85	mango	0.70	1.07
banana	0.5	1.26	nectarine	0.98	1.06
bell pepper	0.63	1.0	oats, rolled	3.36	3.12
blueberries	0.6	2.2	oranges	1.57	1.0
bread, white	1.30	1.36	pear	1.02	1.85
bread, whl/wheat	1.51	5.21	pineapple	0.08	1.27
broccoli	0.44	3.06	plum	1.12	1.76
cabbage	0.46	1.79	pomegranate	0.11	0.49
cantaloupe	0.3	0.8	raisins	0.9	2.17
carrot root	0.99	3.29	raspberries	1.8	4.8
cauliflower	0.6	2.95	spinach	0.77	3.03
cherries	0.6	0.7	strawberry	0.85	1.7
cucumber	0.2	0.94	sunflower seeds	4.2	6.3
dates, dried	1.28	3.56	tomato	0.12	1.13
grapes	0.24	0.36	walnuts	2.26	4.53
hay, alfalfa	8.2	28.0	watermelon	0.13	0.30
hay, grass	7.1	37.0	wheat bran	2.33	26.3

Hemicellulose is a modified form of cellulose that is more complex than cellulose because the structure is branched and contains a mixture of several kinds of sugars. Hemicellulose (HC) binds with pectin and cellulose to form networks of cross-linked fibers that bind the substances together. Hemicellulose is found in the highest concentrations in plant endosperm. (What are called "ivory nuts," the seeds of some palm trees with a high HC content, are sometimes carved into jewelry.) Hemicellulose composes about 20–30% of grasses, 8–12% of alfalfa, and is found in fairly high concentrations in apples, banana, beets, cabbage, corn, green leafy vegetables, pears, and peppers.

Structurally hemicellulose is weak and is easily broken apart by dilute acids or bases. Mammals do not produce the enzymes necessary to digest this fiber, and it is broken down by microflora. Hemicellulose is not completely fermented in the rabbit cecum, but is the most digestible of the insoluble fibers. Like pectin, hemicellulose is fermented more rapidly in the cecum of rabbits at weaning than in older rabbits.

Many of the effects of hemicellulose in rabbit diets appear to be similar to those of pectin. Researchers have found that a higher hemicellulose/pectin to starch ratio lowered mortality in young rabbits and led to increased cecal fermentation activity. Like pectin the

inclusion of HC in foods at weaning may help promote the development of adult cecal microflora, and the kits may be less susceptible to digestive upsets.

Cellulose fiber consists of glucose molecules linked to form straight chains of sugar. Unprocessed cotton is nearly pure cellulose. Cellulose has as much nutritive content as starch, but is only digestible by cecal microorganisms that produce the enzyme cellulase. Therefore, while starch is usually completely digested in the rabbit digestive system (and all the nutrients utilized), cellulose is only about 30–40 % digestible after going through a rabbit's digestive system twice through cecotrophy (it is only about 14% digestible on the first pass), meaning that most of the nutrients of cellulose are not utilized by the rabbits. The cellulose content of both grasses and legumes is about 15–30 percent.

Enzymes that degrade cellulose are not present in a rabbit's cecum before weaning. In one study the enzyme amounts were discovered to increase from weaning to 36 days of age, but cellulose-degrading activity in the cecum remained low, suggesting to the researchers that cellulose is not an important nutrient for the microflora of the cecum at any period of rabbits' lives.

In some studies it has been found that when large amounts of cellulose are included in the diets of rabbits during or after weaning, fermentation activity in the cecum is poorly developed, and the resultant unabsorbed and unfermented carbohydrates may increase fecal output, thereby increasing the loss of nitrogen, energy, water, and electrolytes. Some positive effects of high cellulose in the diet of rabbits at weaning included increased elimination of toxic substances.

Cellulose often occurs with lignin in plant cell walls, forming a complex called *lignocellulose*. Lignin itself is a phenolic compound, not a carbohydrate, but because of its presence in the cell walls between molecules of cellulose, hemicellulose, and pectin, it is usually included in discussions of fiber. It is present in most plants, giving strength and rigidity to the vessels used for conducting water in the plant. Spruce bark contains about 15–20% lignin, legumes 6–10%, grasses about 3–7%, and a banana about 0.2% lignin. Lignocellulose is present in larger quantities in mature plants than in young ones. Growing grasses and forbs contain about 3-8% lignin, but the mature plants will have up to 12% lignin.

Lignin is nearly indigestible, even by the microflora of the rabbit cecum, and therefore is not an important source of nutrition, although the presence of lignin in a rabbit's diet can affect the digestion of nutrients present in other plant materials. Lignin decreases the digestibility of crude protein and decreases the amount of VFAs.

Studies on high lignin content diets in rabbits have found that high lignin diets may have a negative effect on milk production in lactating does, but in young rabbits high dietary lignin content reduces diarrhea and has a positive effect on digestive disorders. In one study where rabbits were fed diets with acorns (acorns have a relatively high lignin content) replacing fractions of the regular diet, the digestibility of the overall diet decreased in adult rabbits. For growing rabbits, those fed the acorn diet had no diarrhea. Several researchers have found that lignin and cellulose reduce diarrhea and have favorable effects on digestive disorders in young rabbits. One researcher recommended that young rabbits have 6 grams of lignin per day in their diets to help minimize digestive problems.

Adding some lignin increases the speed at which digesta moves through the cecum, and may result in lower cecal pH and lower cecum weight along with faster passage time of cecal contents, (thereby limiting fiber digestion), but also resulting in *higher* stomach weight and retention time. Since fiber is not digested in the stomach and ileum, this last could possibly lead to a functional blockage in these organs if excessive amounts were to be consumed. However, it has also been found that very high amounts of small-particle lignin reverse this, increasing retention time in the cecum and decreasing digestibility, potentially leading to cecal impaction.

Fiber Terms

The different terms used in discussing fiber can be confusing to the uninitiated. *Crude fiber* usually refers to the total indigestible fiber, and is a term often seen on feed ingredient tags. Many of the studies done on the role of fiber in rabbit diets refer to acid detergent fiber (ADF) and neutral detergent fiber (NDF) rather than specific fibers such as cellulose or pectin. These terms actually refer to processes by which fiber fractions are separated out of foods. ADF measures the content of indigestible fiber, silica, and insoluble nitrogen. A diet high in ADF is lower in digestible energy than a diet high in NDF. NDF (sometimes also called "cell walls") measures the combined content of cellulose, hemicellulose, lignin, tannins, and cutins. NDF is mostly excreted in hard feces. NDSF, or neutral detergent soluble fiber, refers to compounds found in the inner cell wall of plants that are not covalently bound to lignin and are therefore easily fermented: pectins, beta-glucans, and gums. Digestible fiber (DF) may be found by subtracting one value from another. The acronym "DF" is also sometimes used for the term "dietary fiber," which can refer to all fiber. Low-digestible fiber (lignin and cellulose) may be represented by the acronym "LDF" as may the term "low dietary fiber." As you can see from the last two examples, a particular author's definition of an acronym should always be checked.

The interactions between the different kinds of fiber and fermentative activity in the rabbit digestive system are very complex and still not completely understood, despite the many studies that have been done on the different fibers and their role in rabbit digestion, especially in young rabbits. The details of such studies will have little interest to most readers of this volume, but a summary of the conclusions and results may be helpful in understanding the role of fiber in rabbit diet.

Decreasing dietary crude fiber levels leads to a decrease in intestinal transit time, along with an increase of cecal volume and a decrease in the carbohydrate supply for energy. At the other extreme, if fiber content is increased to a point where insufficient dietary energy is consumed, this also results in an increase in the proportion of energy that is derived from protein and promotes proteolytic bacteria and ammonia production.

In general, decreasing the amount of indigestible fiber in the diet of young rabbits has been found to lead to a decrease of cecal VFAs in rabbits up to two weeks old (although at ten weeks there is little change), higher cecal pH, increased digestibility of fiber, increase in the proportion of protein in cecotrophs, lower cecal fermentation, decreased cecotroph production, and higher mortality from diarrhea during the cecotrophy period. (In the hard feces phase there is increased cecal fermentation with a reduction of indigestible fiber in the diet.) However, too much indigestible fiber can also cause digestive problems if the dietary protein level is higher than the digestible energy, leading to the growth of excessive amounts of proteolytic microflora and creating imbalances of the digestive microflora as well as excessive ammonia. For young rabbits not more than 16% indigestible fiber is recommended.

Increasing digestible fiber in the diet of young rabbits stimulates the fermentative process, increasing microbial activity in the cecum, increases the proportion of protein in cecotrophs, and increases the digestibility of less digestible fiber. Increasing digestible fiber did not lead to an increase in cecotroph production, although it does lead to an increase in the protein content of the cecotrophs. Digestible fiber is important to the development of the gut immune system, as increasing digestible fiber in young rabbits has been found to improve mucosal integrity and functionality. Increasing soluble fiber in the diet of growing rabbits has also been found to be associated with lower mortality from digestive illnesses.

Soluble fiber, which is highly fermentable, promotes the development of more favorable conditions for fermentative activity, and leads to the production of more gas. The less digestible, slowly fermentable fibers produce less gas and decrease retention time in the cecum, but also lead to a lower rate of microbial protein synthesis. It should be remembered that the microflora in the cecum do not exist specifically to digest fiber, rather, the microbial populations use the easiest available substrate (soluble or small-sized particles) for their energetic needs.

Lignin in rabbit diets has been found to significantly decrease the digestibility of crude protein, ADF and NDF, gross energy, and dry matter content. More simply stated, diets with high lignocellulose content are less digestible than those with lower lignocellulose content, and the amount of nutrients and energy rabbits obtain from their diet is decreased. It also increases retention time in the stomach, potentially allowing the development of functional blockages. Although small amounts of dietary lignin decrease retention time in the cecum, excessive amounts of ground or short particle lignin *increase* cecal retention time, potentially leading to cecal impaction.

Fiber particle size, as well as amount, has been found to have an effect on the digestive system of adult rabbits, smaller particles (less than 0.3mm) go into the cecum. Too much small-particle fiber leads to slower passage time but does not improve the digestibility of the cell walls. Excessive amounts can lead to cecal dysbiosis and impaction. Long fiber, or that over 0.3-0.5mm, is shunted away from the cecum and passes rapidly through the rabbit digestive tract with few nutrients being extracted. However, this longer fiber plays an important role in digestion, and rabbits need long-particle fiber as well as short-particle fiber. Adult rabbits that receive too little long fiber may chew their fur. The balance of short fiber and long fiber is critical; both are necessary for good digestive health.

It is not only fiber type, amount, and particle size that affect rabbit digestion. The botanical origin of the fiber also influences digestion and cecal fermentative activity. Providing fiber from a single botanical origin has been found to be detrimental to both cecal fermentation activity and general health. Rabbits receiving commercial feeds, which are comprised of multiple plant species, will have enough variety in their diet, but rabbits on hay-only diets may not, particularly if they are fed only limited varieties of grass hay.

Dietary Fiber Recommendations

Growing rabbits (4-12 weeks): 16-20% crude fiber (11-12% NDSF, 28-30% NDF), 6g lignin.

Lactating does: 12-14% crude fiber.

Adult rabbits, crude fiber levels from 14-16% are

recommended, higher for wool rabbits (18-20%) and overweight rabbits (18-20%).

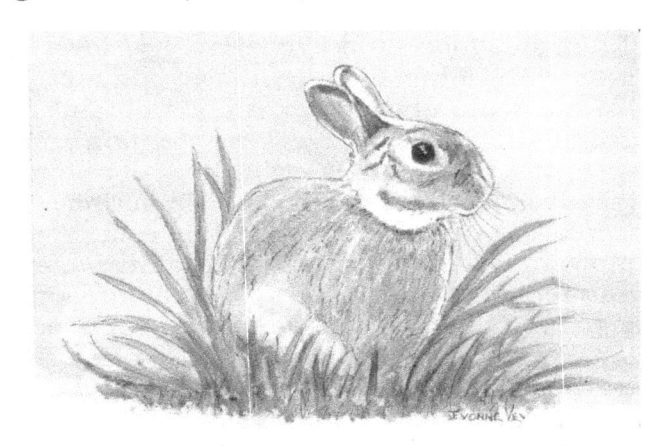

UNDERSTANDING CARBOHYDRATES AND RABBIT DIGESTION

Trying to sort out all the results of the different studies done on the effects of carbohydrates in the diets of rabbits can appear overwhelming, particularly where results of different studies may appear contradictory. But there are a few conclusions that can be drawn with some certainty:

- Carbohydrates affect the digestive system of young rabbits very differently than they affect the digestive system of adult rabbits.

- Young rabbits appear to be detrimentally affected by high sugar and/or starch levels, and more positively affected by both high soluble fiber levels (which encourage development of adult microflora in the cecum) and high non-soluble fiber (lignin and cellulose) that speed digesta through the digestive tract and reduce diarrhea.

- If the levels of non-soluble fiber are increased to the detriment of soluble fiber such as pectin during and after weaning, the microflora of the cecum may be poorly developed and lead to unabsorbed nutrients and poor weight gain. In other words, giving young rabbits one kind of fiber only is not good; they require both soluble and insoluble fiber. However, excessive amounts of either digestible or indigestible fibers increases mortality.

- Adult rabbits, with their fully developed population of cecal microflora, appear able to handle most sugars and starches much better than young rabbits. Adults may require significant amounts of these compounds in order to receive energy and nutrition in their diet, although excessive amounts may be harmful.

- Adult rabbits are not efficient at utilizing nutrients in crude fiber; they utilize only about half as much as does a guinea pig or horse.

- As indicated by cecal bacteria population, soluble fiber is important and may help absorption of nutrients. Rabbits absorb more nutrients from soluble fiber than insoluble fiber. Insoluble fibers are not completely digested by the rabbit, and also increase the speed of digesta passage through the digestive tract, possibly decreasing the amount of nutrients that are absorbed. It is the balance of insoluble and soluble fiber that is important for optimal digestive health; there is interplay between the two types of fiber.

- Lignin may have a beneficial effect on young rabbits when included at 6g of lignin per day, but lignin reduces the nutrients and energy rabbits obtain from their diet. Increasing lignin in a rabbit's diet at first decreases cecal retention time, but at very high levels of short particle lignin cecal retention time increases. High levels of inclusion may lead to both functional blockages in the stomach and cecal impaction.

- Although adult rabbits do require indigestible fiber in their diets (pressure and irritation from indigestible fiber help stimulate gut movement), if the rabbit does not also receive enough energy-rich digestible sugars, starches, and digestible fiber, it could become malnourished. In other words, an adult rabbit fed unlimited hay but little low-fiber high-nutrient food could develop serious nutrient deficiencies and even die. Rabbits given unlimited hay and not enough nutrient-dense foods may eat voraciously but develop pot bellies and other signs of nutrient deficiencies.

Perhaps the most important fact to remember about fiber in the rabbit diet is this: *both diets that have too little crude fiber and diets that provide too much crude fiber can have harmful effects on rabbits.* It has been found that if rabbits receive diets containing less than 6-10% crude fiber they are susceptible to digestive problems such as gastrointestinal hypomotility and enteritis. Yet if rabbits are given diets with more than 20-22% crude fiber it can lead to mucoid enteropathy and cecal impaction, possibly because of imbalances in the cecal microflora that develop when a high percentage of the cecal contents are less-digestible fiber. Too much fiber can also lead to energy deficits that in turn can lead to excessive ammonia and toxicity, expecially in small breeds. Rabbits require diets providing necessary nutrients *in balance*.

References

Al-dobaib, S. N., M. H. Khalil, M. Hashad, and A. N. Al-Saef. 2007. Growth, carcass, and caecal traits in v-line and crossbred rabbits fed diets containing discarded dates. *World Rabbit Sci.* 15: 81–90.

Alvarez, J. L., I. Marguenda, P. Garcia-Rebollar, C. de Blas, A. Corujo and A. I. Garcia-Ruiz. 2007. *World Rabbit Sci* 15(1): 9–18.

Bellier, R. and T. Gidenne. 1996. Consequences of reduced fibre intake on digestion, rate of passage and caecal microbial activity in the young rabbit. *British J. Nutr.* 75: 353–363.

Bennegadi, N., T. Gidenne, and D. Licois. 2001. Impact of fibre deficiency and sanitary status on non-specific enteropathy of the growing rabbit. *Anim. Res.* 50(5): 401–413.

Bonai, A., Zs. Szendro, L. Maertens, Zs. Maties, H. Febel, L. Kametler, G. Tornyos, P. Horn, F. Kovacs, and M. Kovacs. 2008. Effect of inulin supplementation on caecal microflora and fermentation in rabbits. *Proceedings*: 12th World Rabbit Congress, Verona.

Bovera, F., A. Lestingi, S. Marono, F. Iannaccone, S. Nizza, K. Mallardo, L. de Martino, and A. Tateo. 2012. Effect of dietary mannan-oligosaccharides on *in vivo* performance, nutrient digestibility and caecal content characteristics of growing rabbits. *J. anim. Phys. Anim.*

Nutr. 96(1): 130-136.

Carabano, R., I. Badiola, S. Chamoro, J. Garcia, A. I. Garcia-Ruiz, P. Garcia-Rebollar, M. S. Gomez-Conde, I. Gutierrez, N. Nicodemus, M. J. Villamide, and J. C. de Blas. 2008. Review: New trends in rabbit feeding: influence of nutrition on intestinal health. *Span. J. Agri. Res.* 6 (special issue): 15-25.

Castellini, C., R. Cardinali, P.G. Rebollar, A. Dal Bosco, V. Jimeno, and M. E. Cossu. 2006. Feeding fresh chicory (*Chicoria intybus*) to young rabbits: Performance, development of gastro-intestinal tract and immune functions of appendix and Peyer's patch. *Anim. Feed Sci Technol.* 134(1–2): 56–65.

Chiou, P. W., B. Yu, and C. Lin. 1998. The effect of different fibre components on growth rate, nutrient digestibility, rate of digesta passage and hindgut fermentation in domestic rabbits. *Lab. Anim.* 32: 276-283.

Debray, L., I. LeHuerou-Luon, T. Gidenne, and L. Fortun-Lamothe. 2003. Digestive tract development in rabbit according to the dietary energeytic source: correlation between whole tract digestion, pancreatic and intestinal enzymatic activities. *Comp. Biochem Physio.* 135(3): 443–455.

Falcao-e-Cunha, L., H. Peres, J. P. B. Friere, and L. Castro-Solla. 2004. Effects of alfalfa, wheat bran, or beet pulp, with or without sunflower oil, on caecal fermentation and on digestibility in the rabbit. *An. Feed Sci. Tech.* 117 (1–2): 131–149.

Fortun-Lamothe, L. and S. Boullier. 2004. Interactions between gut microflora and digestive mucosal immunity, and strategies to improve digestive health in young rabbits. *Proceedings:* 8th World Rabbit Congress, Puebla.

Garcia, J., C. deBlas, R. Carrabano, and P. Garcia. 1994. Effect of chemical composition of alfalfa hay on several digestive measurements in growing rabbits. *Proceedings*: World Rabbit Congress, Dijon.

Garcia, J., T. Gidenne, L. Falcao-e-Cunha, and C. de Blas. 2002. Identification of the main factors that influence caecal fermentiation traits in growing rabbits. *Anim. Res.* 51(2): 165–173.

Gasmi-Boubaker, A., H. Abdouli, M. R. Mosquera-Losada, L. Tayachi, M. Mansouri, and I. Zaidib. 2007. Cork oak (*Quercus suber* L.) Acorn as a Substitute for Barley in the Diet of Rabbits: Effect on *In vivo* Digestibility, Growth, and Carcass Characteristics. *J An. Vet Ad.* 6(10):1219–1222.

Gidenne, T. 1992. Effect of fibre level, particle size and adaptation period on digestibility and rate of passage as measured at the ileum and in the faeces in the adult rabbit. *Br. J. Nutr.* 67(1): 133–46.

Gidenne, T. 2003. Fibres in rabbit feed for digestive trouble prevention: respective role of low-digestible and digestible fibre. *Liv. Prod. Sci.* 81(2–3): 105–117.

Gidenne, T., P. Arveux, and O. Madec. 2001. The effect of the quality of dietary lignocillulose on digestion, zootechnical performance and health of the growing rabbit. *Anim. Sci.* 73(1): 97–104.

Gidenne, T. and R. Bellier. 2000. Use of digestible fibre in replacement to available carbohydrates: Effect on digestion, rate of passage and caecal fermentation pattern during the growth of the rabbit. *Liv. Prod. Sci.* 63(2): 141–152.

Gidenne, T., B. Carre, M. Segura, A. Lapanouse, and J. Gomez. 1991. Fibre digestion and rate of passage in the rabbit: effect of particle size and level of lucerne meal. *An. Food Sci. Tech.* 32(1-3): 215-221.

Gidenne, T., L. Debray, L. Fortune-Lamothe, and I. Le Huerou-Luron. 2007. Maturation of the intestinal digestion and of microbial activity in the young rabbit: impact of the dietary fibre:starch ratio. *Comp. Biochem. Phys.* 148(4): 834-844

Gidenne, T. and F. Lebas. 2002. Role of dietary fibre in rabbit nutrition and in digestive troubles prevention. *Proceedings:* 2nd Rabbit Congress of the Americas. Habana City, Cuba.

Gidenne, T., V. Pinheiro, and L. Falcao-e-Cunha. 2000. A comprehensive approach of the rabbit digestion: consequences of a reduction in dietary supply. *Liv. Prod. Sci.* 64(2–3): 225–237.

Gidenne, T. and J. N. Perez. 1993. Effect of dietary starch origin on digestion in the rabbit: 2. Starch hydrolysis in the small intestine, cell wall degradation and rate of passage measurements. *Anim. Feed Sci. Technol.* 42(3–4): 249–57.

Gomez-Conde, M. S., S. Chamorro, P. Eiras, P. G. Rebollar, A. Perez de Rozas, C. de Blas, and R. Carabano. 2007. Neutral detergent-soluble fiber improves gut barrier function in twenty-five-day-old weaned rabbits. *J. Anim. Sci.* 85(12): 3313-3321.

Goodrich, B. S., E. R. Hesterman, K. S. Shaw, and R. Mykytowycz. 1981. Identification of some volatile compounds in the odor of fecal pellets of the rabbit, *Oryctolagus cuniculus*. *J. Chem. Eco.* 7(5): 817-827.

Gutierrez, I., A. Espinosa, J. Garica, R. Carabano, and J. C. De Blas. 2002. Effect of levels of starch, fiber, and lactose on digestion and growth performance of early-weaned rabbits. *J. Anim. Sci.* 80(4): 1029–

1037.

Johnson-Delaney, C. A. 2006. Anatomy and Physiology of the Rabbit and Rodent Gastrointestinal System. *Proceedings:* Association of Avian Veterinarians.

Laska, M. 2002. Gustatory responsiveness to food-associated saccharides in European rabbits, *Oryctolagusa cuniculus*. *Physiol.Behav.* 76: 335–341.

Lavrenic, A. 2006. The effect of rabbit age on *in vitro* caecal fermentation of starch, pectin, xylan, cellulose, compound feed and its fibre. *Animal* 1: 241–248.

Leng, R. A. 2008. Digestion in the rabbit—a new look at the effects of their feeding and digestive strategies. Proceedings MEKEARN Rabbit Conference: Organic rabbit production from forages (Eds: Reg. Preston and Nguyen Van Thu), Catho University, Vietnam.

Li, B. W., K. W. Andrews, and P. R. Pehrsson. 2002. Individual Sugars, Soluble, and Insoluble Dietary Fiber Contents of 70 High Consumption Foods. *J. Food Comp. Anal.* 15: 715–723.

Lowe, J. A. Pet Rabbit Feeding and Nutrition. 2010. *In: Nutrition of the Rabbit.* Carlos de Blas and Julian Wiseman, eds. Wallingford: CABI Publishing.

McWilliams, D. A. 2001. Nutritional Pathology in Rabbits: Current and Future Perspectives. Paper: Ontario Commercial Rabbit Growers Asso. Congress.

Maertens, L., J. M. Aerts, and J. DeBoever. 2004. Degradation of dietary oligofructose and inulin in the gastro-intestinal tract of the rabbit and the effects of caecal pH and volatile fatty acids. *World Rabbit Sci.* 12: 235–246.

Mendel, L. B. and M. R. Jones. 1920. Studies on carbohydrate metabolism in rabbits. *J Biol. Chem.* 42(3):491–506.

The Merck Veterinary Manual. Ninth edition. 2005. Edited by Cynthia M. Kahn. Whitehouse Station: Merck and Co., Inc.

Morisse, J. P., G. le Gall, R. Maurice, J. P. Cotte, E. Boilletot. 1992. Effect of a fructo-oligosaccharides mixture on some intestinal and plasmatic parameters in young rabbits. *Rivista Zootecnia e Veterinaria* 20(1): 57-61.

Mourao, J. L., A. Alves, and V. Pinheiro. 2004. Effects of fructo-oligosaccharides on performance of growing rabbits. *Proceedings*: 8th World Rabbit Congress, Puebla.

Mourao, J. L., V. Pinheiro, A. Alves, C. N. Guedes, L. Pinto, M. J. Saavedra, P. Spring, and A. Kocher. 2006. Effect of mannan oligosaccharides on the performance, intestinal morphology and cecal formation of fattening rabbits. *Anim. Feed Sci. and Technol.* 126(1–2): 107–120.

Nicodemus, N., J. Garcia, R. Carabano, and C. de Blas. 1999. Effect of the inclusion of soybean hulls in commercial feeds on rabbit digestion and performance at varying dietary lignin concentrations.

Pinheiro, V., C. N. Guedes, D. Outor-Monteiro, and J. L. Mourao. 2008. Effects of fibre level and dietary mannanoligosaccharides on digestibility, caecal volatile fatty acids and performance of growing rabbits. *Anim. Feed Sci.Technol.* 148(2–4): 288–300.

Rodriguez-Romero, N., L. Abecia, M. Fondevilla, and J. Balcells. 2011. Effects of levels of insoluble and soluble fibres in diets for growing rabbits on faecal digestibility, nitrogen recycling, and *in vitro* fermentation. *World Rabbit Sci.* 19: 85-94.

Sirotek, K., M. Marounek, V. Rada, and V. Benda. 2001. Isolation and Characterization of Rabbit Caecal Pectinolytic Bacteria. *Folia Microbiol.* 46(1): 79–82.

Trocino, A., J. G. Alonso, R. Carabano, and G. Xiccato. 2013. A meta-analysis on the role of soluble fibre in diets for growing rabbits. *World Rab. Sci.* 21(1): 145-160.

Trocino, A., M. Fragkiadakis, G. Radaelli, and G. Xiccato. 2010. Effect of dietary soluble fibre level and protein source on growth, digestion, caecal activity, and health of fattening rabbits. *World Rab. Sci.* 18(4):199-210.

V arga, Molly. 2014. *Textbook of Rabbit Medicine.* Second edition. Oxford: Butterworth Heinemann Elsevier.

Van Loo, Jan. 2007. How Chicory Fructans Contribute to Zootechnical Performanace and Well-Being in Livestock and Companion Animals. *J. Nutr.* 137: 25945–25975.

Volek, Z., M. Marounek, and V. Skrivanova. 2005. Replacing starch by pectin and inulin in diet of early-weaned rabbits: effect on performance, health and nutrient digestibility. *J. Anim. Feed Sci.* 14(2): 327–337.

Wang, X., M. Ma, L. Sun, C. Wang, Y Zhu, and F. Li. 2012. Effects of different protein, fibre and energy levels on growth performance and the development of digestive organs in growing meat rabbit. *Proceedings:* 10th World Rabbit Congress. Sharm El-Sheikh, Egypt.

Xiccato, G., A. Trocino, L. Carrara, M. Fragkiadakis, and O. Majolini. 2008. Digestible fibre to starch ratio and antibiotic treatment time in growing rabbits affected by epizootic rabbit enteropathy. *Proceedings:* 9th World Rabbit Congress, Veronametabolism in rabbits. *J Biol. Chem.* 42(3):491–506.

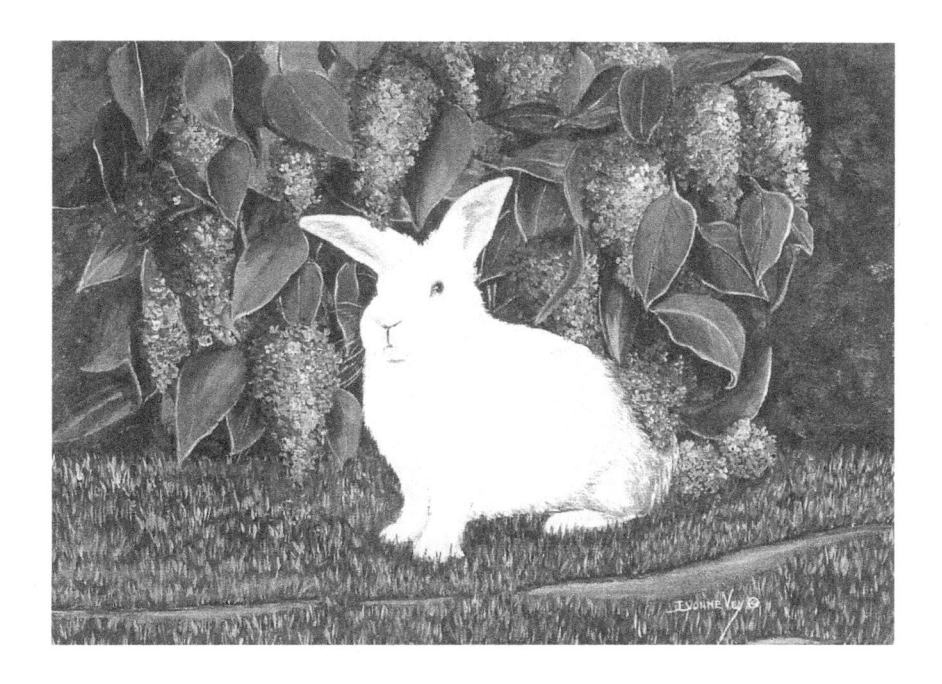

Chapter 4

FAT AND PROTEIN

When reading about the fat and protein content of rabbit diets, one is more likely to find warnings against feeding too much than cautions about feeding too little. Yet both fat and protein are necessary chemical compounds without which rabbits (and other mammals) cannot live, for they are needed for energy, growth, regeneration, and the structural integrity of the body and brain.

FAT

Fats, or *lipids*, are a group of chemical compounds that are usually insoluble in water but are soluble in alcohol. There are many lipids, including monoglycerides, diglycerides, triglycerides, sterols, terpenes, fatty alcohols, and fatty acids, among others. *Fatty acids* are simple fats consisting of carbon chains of differing lengths with hydrogen bound to the carbon atoms of the chain. At the beginning of the chain (the alpha end) is a -COOH acid (carboxyl group), and at the opposite (omega) end is a carbon atom with three hydrogens (methyl group). The carbon atoms constituting the chain are linked to each other either by single or double bonds. A fatty acid is *saturated* if all the bonds between carbons in the chain are single; *monounsaturated* if there is one double bond; and *polyunsaturated* if there are two or more double bonds. If the first double bond between carbons from the methyl end of the chain is at the third carbon, it is called an omega-3 fatty acid, and if at the sixth carbon it is called an omega-6 fatty acid. Fatty acids attach to other molecules to make more complex fats. For example, if fatty acids attach to a single glycerol molecule a monoglyceride is formed, if two are attached it a diglyceride, and if to three a triglyceride results.

Animal fats are saturated, while most plant fats, or oils, are unsaturated. Plant fatty acids are usually liquid at room temperature. Examples of unsaturated plant oils are canola, corn, cottonseed, safflower, soybean, and sunflower oil. However, tropical palm fatty acid (palmitrin) is an exception—it is saturated and contains sixteen carbons rather than the eighteen most plant fatty acids contain. Treating plant oils with heat and pressure in order to change their texture (as is done in making margarine) breaks the double bonds in the fatty acid and causes it to become saturated, producing what are termed *trans* fatty acids. In humans and several mammals it has been found that trans fatty acids can raise the level of the "bad" low density lipoproteins (LDLs) and lower the level of "good" high density lipoproteins (HDLs). Since LDLs carry cholesterol to various sites in the body, such as artery walls, and HDLs remove cholesterol from these sites and take it to the liver to be broken down, high levels of LDL may increase atherosclerosis (deposition of fat in blood vessels). Saturated animal fats and tropical palm oil, as well as trans fatty acids, can increase LDLs.

Cholesterol itself is a lipid, and is manufactured in the liver as well as being obtained through consumed dietary cholesterol. Cholesterol is necessary for the production of bile as well as vital sex hormones and vitamin D, which are needed for proper brain and nerve function.

When fat is consumed by a rabbit, the large fat molecules are emulsified to smaller ones by bile (primarily biliverdin in rabbits) from the gall bladder. The fats are then broken down to the component fatty acids and glycerol, which are used for energy by the rabbit. Most of the breakdown and absorption of fat occurs in the rabbit's small intestine with the aid of the enzyme *lipase*. Fats are highly digestible by rabbits, especially unsaturated fatty acids from plant oils. Plant fats still bound in structural plant material are a little less digestible, and saturated fats from animal sources are least digestible.

Fat is a necessary component of a rabbit's diet. Not only is fat a valuable source of energy for the rabbit's high metabolic rate, it's presence is necessary for the production of *motilin* (required for gut movement), it reduces the intestinal absorption of calcium (which may be important if conditions such as kidney or bladder problems exist), and is needed for the absorption of the vitamins A, D, E, and K, as well as the absorption of some therapeutic drugs. Fats are necessary for the production of many hormones and are involved in the control of blood pressure and cholesterol levels, aid in the prevention of arthritis, naturally reduce inflammation, add luster and gloss to a rabbit's coat, improve skin tone, and help reduce shedding.

Studies on the effects of differing levels of dietary fat on the microflora of the cecum have yielded inconclusive results. Some researchers have found that differing levels of dietary fat do not affect cecal fermentation; others have found the amount of VFAs to be higher in the cecum of rabbits consuming high-fat diets; still other researchers have found the amount of VFAs to be lower in rabbits on high-fat diets. (Volatile fatty acids, or VFAs, are produced in the hindgut as a result of microbial fermentation of carbohydrates, and are an important source of energy to the rabbit. Cecotrophs have high amounts of VFAs, which are partly responsible for their odor.) In an interesting study on rats (another hindgut-fermenter), researchers found that rats given a fat-supplemented diet had fewer intestinal pathogens and lower mortality than rats given a fat-free diet.

Fats may have effects on other physiological processes in rabbits. A group of rabbits was given a diet with no added fat while two other groups were given diets with added olive or sunflower oil. The groups that received the extra fat had less lipid oxidation in muscles than the group that received no extra fat (oxidation of lipids creates free radicals that can damage cells). Giving rabbits compounds from olive oil was found to help reverse the effects of atherogenic diets, and in another study adding plant oils to the diet of rabbit kits reduced mortality.

Fat causes foods to taste better to rabbits (as it does with many people!). A higher fat content not only helps bind commercial rabbit pellets and reduces dustiness; it also makes higher-fiber pellets more palatable to rabbits. Palatability of food can be critical, especially when dealing with older, ill, or anorexic rabbits.

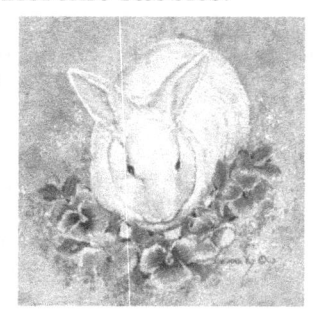

TABLE 4:1 **Fat content of selected foods,** expressed as grams fat per 100 grams of food. *Values compiled from multiple sources.*

Higher-fat foods	g/100g	Moderate to low-fat foods	g/100g	Very low-fat foods	g/100g
acorns	23.86	barley grain	2.3	banana	0.33
almonds	50.64	bread, rye	3.2	carrots	0.24
peanuts	46.0	bread, white	3.0	cherries	0.1
pumpkin seeds	48.50	bread, whole-wheat	2.95	dandelion greens	0.7
soybeans	19.0	crackers, saltine	9.0	dill, fresh	0.9
sunflower seeds	49.57	cranberries, dried	1.37	grapes	0.16
walnuts	59.0	hay, alfalfa	1.5	hay, Bermuda	0.9
		hay, timothy	2.0	kale	0.49
		oats, rolled	4.67	lettuce, Romaine	0.30
		wheat bran	2.1	nectarines	0.33
				parsley	0.80
				spinach	0.40

Excess and deficiency of fat in rabbit diets

A deficiency of fat in the diet of a rabbit can lead to gut motility problems, loss of hair, deficiencies of fat-soluble vitamins, slower repair after injury, lower sperm count in bucks, and retarded growth in young rabbits. Severe deficiencies can lead to brain and nerve problems.

Excessive dietary fat is not healthful for rabbits either, and can result in obesity, increase the risk of hepatic lipidosis (serious condition that occurs when stored fat is metabolized) if a rabbit becomes anorexic, and lead to atherosclerosis (deposition of fat in arteries), particularly in magnesium-deficient diets. Diets high in saturated fats may increase levels of blood cholesterol and its deposition in blood vessels, and cause hyperglycemia, insulin resistance, and cellular damage to the heart. High levels of unsaturated fats may also have negative effects: in one study on rabbits it was found that high levels of safflower oil in the diet increased the rabbits' blood pressure, although the effect was less if cellulose (a plant carbohydrate) was added to the diet. It should always be remembered that compounds do not act alone—there are many nutrient interactions.

Dietary fat recommendations

The amount of fat that is optimal for a rabbit's diet will depend upon many factors, including the age, breed, activity, and health of the rabbit. Long-haired, wool-producing rabbits such as American Fuzzy Lops, Jersey Woolies, and the angoras generally require higher levels of fat in their diets than shorter-haired rabbits. Rabbit does that are pregnant or lactating also require higher amounts of fat in their diet, as do rabbits that are very active. But in general, the fat in a rabbit's diet should comprise about 2.5–4% of the total diet. This translates into 25–40 grams of fat per kilogram (1 kilogram is about 2.4 pounds) of food.

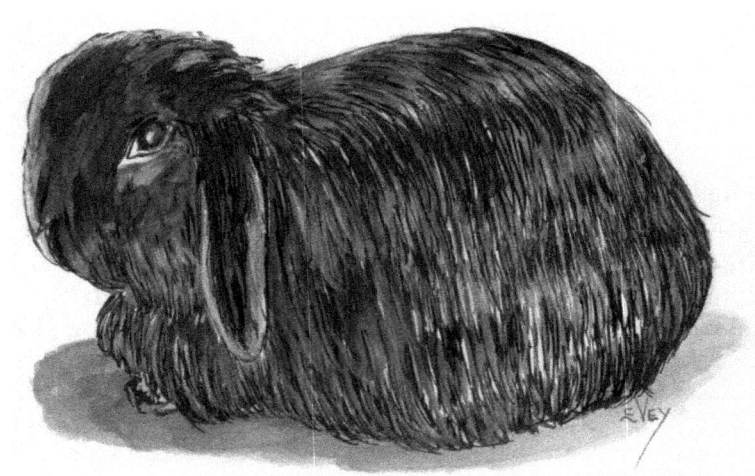

It is more healthful to consume unsaturated than saturated fats, both for humans and rabbits, although even unsaturated fats can be detrimental to health if eaten in excessive amounts. Mammals actually synthesize many fatty acids in their bodies. Those that are not synthesized by the body must be consumed, and are termed *essential fatty acids*, or EFAs (also called vitamin F). For rabbits, the essential fatty acids are linolenic acid and linoleic acid. EFAs are fragile compounds and are destroyed by rancidity.

Alpha linolenic acid, or ALA, is an essential fatty acid. One of the omega-3 fatty acids (the "good" fats that lower cholesterol), ALA is needed for the production of other essential omega-3 fatty acids. Adding dehydroepiandrosterone (DHEA)—another omega-3 fatty acid—to a rabbit's diet has been found to partially reduce the negative effects of a high-fat diet. Omega-3 fatty acids are found in fresh green grass, walnuts, flax seed, and rice bran. (The last two sources are often ingredients in commercial rabbit foods.)

Omega-6 fatty acids (e.g., linoleic, gamma-linolenic) are found in raw nuts, seeds, rice bran, molasses, and legumes. If a rabbit's diet contains alfalfa (lucerne) as an ingredient, the rabbit is most likely receiving adequate omega-6 fatty acids. Volatile fatty acids, or VFAs (see Chapter 2), are produced in the hindgut as a result of microbial fermentation of carbohydrates, and are another important energy source for rabbits.

The ratio of omega-3 to omega-6 fatty acids is also important in rabbit diets, for it has been found that inducing them in the proper proportions affects both the systemic immune system and intestinal immune response, leading to better health.

Nutritional healing

Rabbits with dry, scaly skin or poor coats may show improvement if a teaspoon of unsaturated plant oil (e.g., safflower) is added to their food. Rabbits with frequent GI hypomotility may also benefit from added fat. Most nuts are high in unsaturated fat (as well as vitamin E, potassium, magnesium, and arginine), and adding a couple of walnuts or almonds to a rabbit's diet can be a good way to increase fat. In some studies on people, eating nuts decreased the risk of heart disease by 30-50 percent.

If a rabbit has been found to have high cholesterol by a veterinarian, exercise and the inclusion of foods with high niacin and some vitamin C content (Chapter 5) may help lower it, as may ellagic acid, which is found in many fruits and nuts (Chapter 8). Adding selenium to the diet of rabbits may slow the onset and progression of aortic disease—researchers have found that both cholesterol and triglyceride levels in rabbits may be lowered by the addition of selenium to the diet. Fruits and vegetables containing the carotenoid *lycopene*, found in many red-or pink fruits (e.g., tomatoes) may also lower cholesterol and generally improve artery health. Fruits with high lycopene content include watermelon, tomatoes, pink grapefruit, and sweet red pepper. Other foods that may help lower cholesterol include carrots, apples, and bananas.

Rabbits that have been diagnosed with atherosclerosis may be helped by the addition of foods high in magnesium, zinc, selenium, and/or copper to the diet. It has been found in several studies that these minerals may be helpful in slowing the onset and progression of this disease. Iron may accelerate the process of atherosclerosis, and high dietary amounts of this mineral should be avoided. See Chapter 5 for more information on minerals.

PROTEIN

The primary role of protein is for the growth and repair of body structures. Excesses of protein in the diet can be used for energy, but the conversion of proteins for energy is not as efficient as is the conversion of carbohydrates and fats for energy. Proteins are large molecules composed of chains of amino acids (organic compounds with a nitrogen-containing amino group and an acid carboxyl group), the chains linked by peptide bonds. Each protein may contain from 400 to 500 amino acids. Some of the amino acids that compose the proteins are synthesized by the body, but the other amino acids must be consumed. These latter are called *essential amino acids*, and vary with the species of mammal. Humans have eight essential amino acids. The essential amino acids for rabbits are arginine, glycine, histidine, isoleucine, leucine, lysine, the aromatic amino acids phenylalanine plus tyrosine; the sulfur amino acids methionine plus cysteine (very important for fur growth); threonine, tryptophan, and valine.

Our rabbits primarily receive dietary proteins in commercial feeds, the seeds and leaves of plants, and cecotrophs. Plants are able to make all the amino acids, but the amounts present will depend upon the plant species, plant part, and age of the plant. The proteins in plant leaves are bound to cellulose, which reduces their

TABLE 4:2 Protein content of selected foods, expressed as grams protein per 100 grams of food. Note—protein content of hay in particular may vary depending on age when harvested. *Values compiled from multiple sources*

Higher-protein foods	g per 100g	Moderate protein foods	g per 100g	Low-protein foods	g per 100g
almonds	21.26	acorns	6.15	apricots	1.4
barley grain	12.48	alfalfa sprouts	3.96	banana	1.0
barleygrass, fresh	23.0	basil	2.5	carrots	1.0
carrot tops	13.0	bread, white	8.8	celery	0.8
hay, alfalfa	17.50	broccoli tops	3.0	cherries	0.87
hay, Bermuda grass	8.75	cilantro	2.0	cranberries, dried	0.06
hay, brome grass	11.0	dandelion greens	2.7	cucumber	0.7
hay, orchard grass	9.15	dates	2.45	grapes	0.67
hay, timothy	8.45	kale	2.94	lettuce, Romaine	1.6
oats, rolled	12.0	mustard greens	2.7	orange	0.9
pumpkin seeds	24.0	parsley	3.0	peaches	0.6
sunflower seeds	22.82	peas	5.42	pepper, sweet	0.9
walnuts	24.06	spinach	2.9	pineapple	0.54
wheat bran	13.2	straw, wheat	3.8	raspberries	1.2
wheatgrass, fresh	23.0	watercress	2.3	watermelon	0.64

availability to the rabbit. Older plants contain less protein than younger plants. Because of this variation, it is difficult to give a precise percentage of protein content for any plant unless an actual analysis is done. That said, grass hay often contains about 8–15% protein, alfalfa hay 17–23%, commercial pellets 13–21%, and grains such as oats or barley 10–18% protein.

Cecotrophs contain around 28–30% crude protein, about half of which is bacterial cells. Proteins not available to the rabbit during the first pass of the plant matter through the digestive system become available through this consumption of cecotrophs (see Chapter 2). For example, the digestibility of alfalfa protein increases from about 50% to 75–80% through cecotroph consumption. Cecotrophs are high in lysine, the sulfur amino acids, and threonine.

Dietary protein, except microbial protein, is mostly digested in the rabbit's stomach where it is broken down into the constituent amino acids. These are absorbed in the small intestine. In contrast, the majority of the microbial protein that is utilized by a rabbit is digested in the colon. A rabbit's digestive system is fairly effective at digesting plant protein. For example, the digestibility of the protein in alfalfa meal is less than 1% for pigs, about 65% for rats (another hindgut fermenter), and over 75% for rabbits.

Bacterial protein (made available though consumption of cecotrophs) includes the essential amino acids lysine, threonine, and the sulfur amino acids, methionine and cysteine. The necessity of cecotroph consumption is often emphasized in information on the care of rabbits. However, there is evidence that this consumption is not necessary for those rabbits fed a concentrate, such as a commercial pelleted food, for the rabbit receives enough of the essential amino acids and micronutrients in the pellets. Therefore, if a rabbit is unable to consume cecotrophs due to age or infirmity, the rabbit will be unlikely to suffer any dietary lack if the rabbit is consuming a quality commercial feed.

Excessive cecotroph production does not always signal a health problem in a rabbit. It has been found in various studies that rabbits on a low-carbohydrate/low-fat diet will consume more cecotrophs, as will rabbits on a low protein diet. Rabbits on these diets need to consume all their cecotrophs in order to try and consume adequate amounts of needed nutrients. Rabbits on a higher-protein diet will consume fewer of their cecotrophs, as they need less additional protein. In some cases where pet rabbits are not consuming all their cecotrophs and the excess is causing a sanitary problem, changing the feed to one with a lower percent of crude protein may reduce the amount of unconsumed cecotrophs while still providing adequate dietary protein for the rabbit.

One aspect of protein digestion that can result in health issues is the production of urea, which is a by-product of amino acid digestion. Urea is degraded by the enzyme urease (found primarily in the cecum) and converted to ammonia. In rabbits with diets low in carbohydrates, this ammonia may be absorbed in the gut and result in toxicity. For this reason, a high-protein low-carbohydrate diet would not be a healthy choice. Rabbits' sensitivity to ammonia is the reason non-dietary nitrogen (NDN) would not be a healthy ingredient to see on an ingredients list for a rabbit food. NDNs can lead to toxicity in the rabbit gut from the ammonia. Addition of 1% fructo-oligosaccharides to the diet may help reduce cecal ammonia.

Limiting proteins and protein food sources

Protein is necessary for proper body function. Proteins such as collagen provide structure; other proteins function as hormones (e.g., insulin); protein antibodies protect against bacteria and viruses; and still others function as the critical enzymes that catalyze biochemical reactions. The presence of proteins is also necessary for the absorption of many vitamins and minerals, and the proteins arginine, glutamine, and taurine play important roles in the immune system.

A mammal needs to consume all the essential amino acids not produced in its body, and needs to consume them each day since they are not stored by the body for future use. The balance of amino acids consumed is also important. Any amino acid that is lacking in a mammal's diet is termed *limiting*. In rabbits the amino acids lysine and methionine are most likely to be limiting and rabbits do better if they consume foods that provide these in adequate amounts. Both these amino acids are lacking in grains, although lysine is present in small amounts (0.1–0.2%) in grass leaves and stems.

Foods that contain relatively high amounts of lysine include parsley, spinach, watercress, walnuts, almonds, plums, alfalfa and other legumes, and seeds such as sunflower and pumpkin. It is also present in beet pulp, flax seed, and rice bran, which may be ingredients in some commercial feeds. High levels of methionine are found in alfalfa, turnip greens, spinach, raw zucchini, watercress, flax seed, sunflower and pumpkin seeds, and peanuts.

Excess and deficiency of protein in rabbit diets

A deficiency of protein in the diet can lead to poor tissue regeneration, restrict absorption of micronutrients, lead to changes in the appearance and amount of hair, and cause a reduction in the body's ability to eliminate some drugs and their metabolites. Peyer's patches reduce in size and number, possibly reducing resistance to enteritis.

One of the first signs of a lack of protein in the diet can be hair loss or a change in hair color. In human children with a protein deficiency (Kwashiorkor) hair takes on a reddish cast. This may also occur in rabbits. Fur may turn reddish and become thin, a phenomenon often seen in large rescues of malnourished rabbits. When dietary protein is returned to adequate levels, fur regains its normal hue and thickness.

Specific signs of diets low in the proteins most often limiting to rabbits are: methionine deficiency—creatinuria, muscle degeneration, weight loss, paralysis, and death; lysine deficiency—reduced growth and weight loss.

Excess protein puts a strain on the liver and kidneys, increases urine production, can alter the microflora and increase the pH of the cecum (possibly causing an imbalance leading to digestive upset), may increase urea production (if the diet is low in carbohydrates this can lead to urea toxicity), and may reduce gastrointestinal motility. Some commercial feeds contain extracts of yucca, which have been found to counterbalance the effects of excess urea.

Excess protein in the diet of young rabbits can be particularly harmful due to differences in the digestive system of young rabbits as compared to adult rabbits (see Chapter 2). In young rabbits on high-protein diets the protein is incompletely digested in the small intestine. It then enters the lower intestine where it causes severely detrimental changes to gut microflora (dysbiosis), potentially allowing pathogens such as *Clostridium* and *Escherichia coli* to proliferate. Death often follows. Reducing the protein content of the diet reduces populations of these pathogens and decreases mortality.

Gluten and rabbits diets

Gluten is a mixture of plant proteins, a gliadin and a glutanin, found only in the grain of some members of the grass family, including wheat, rye, and barley (rice and maize do not contain true gluten). About 0.5-1.0% of the human population has an abnormal immune reaction to partially digested gliadin, called celiac disease (not the same as gluten sensitivity or wheat allergy). Other animals, including Irish setter dogs, mice, macaques, and rats have also been found to have gluten-sensitive enteropathies similar to celiac disease. Some rabbits have been found to have high antigliadin IgG titers when fed a diet containing wheat. However, it is unclear whether the high titers reflected a pathology similar to celiac disease or were a nonpathological response to a frequently-consumed protein. Another researcher studying gluten-sensitive enteropathy in rabbits suggested a possible genetic factor.

Given that it is *possible* a gluten-sensitive enteropathy may exist in some rabbits, it might be helpful to try a gluten-free or reduced gluten diet in some cases of severe arthritis or other inflammatory disease since gluten-free diets have been found to be helpful in humans with celiac disease and gluten sensitivity. Giving such a diet to rabbits is not simple, however, since many rabbit foods include wheat, barley, and/or rye. Alfalfa pellets and hay could be tried in place of grass hay; and oats have less gluten than wheat, barley, and rye. Grass hay that has had grain heads removed could be fed, and fresh greens could also be part of a reduced-gluten diet.

Dietary recommendations for protein

As with all nutrients, the amount of protein an individual rabbit requires will depend upon many factors, including the age, health, gender, and breed of the rabbit. Angora rabbits and other wool rabbits need extra sulfur amino acids. Larger rabbits such as Flemish Giants may require more protein than smaller rabbits for proper development during their critical growth period between six months and eighteen months of age. Very young rabbits of any breed should be given lower-protein diets, while pregnant and lactating does need more protein. As is often the case in nutrition, the amounts of one nutrient affect another. It has been found that including digestible fiber and crude protein in a ratio over 1:3 improves the health of growing rabbits.

It is the level of crude protein that is most often given

on feed labels. Recommended levels of crude protein content in rabbit diets:

- 12–16% for pet rabbits
- 17–20% for long-haired rabbits and larger breeds (e.g., Flemish, Checkered Giant)
- 16-20% for pregnant does
- 18–21% for lactating does
- 12–14% for young rabbits (kittens) between 3–9 weeks of age

Due to the very large difference between recommended dietary protein amounts for lactating does and their kittens, it is recommended that precautions be taken to prevent consumption of the doe's food by rabbit kittens as they transition to solid food. Failure to do so may result in a high mortality rate among the rabbit kits.

It has also been found that growing rabbits have better health when the ratio of digestible fiber to crude protein is increased over 1.3 (DF>20% CP<16%).

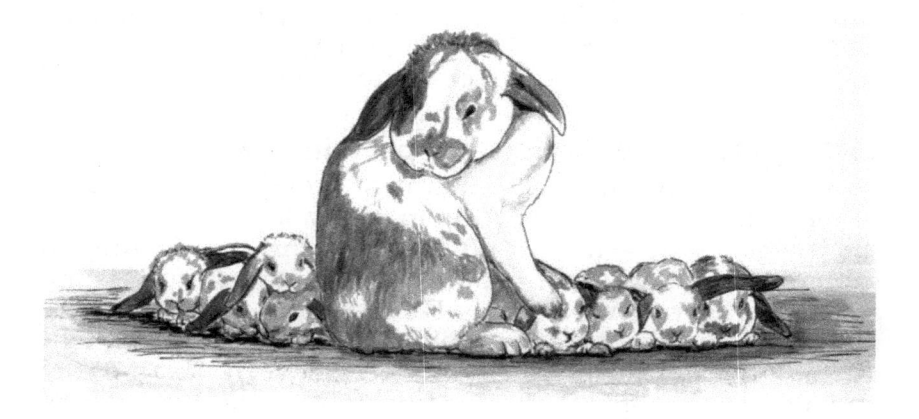

References

Abdelhalim, Mohamed Anwar K., Alhadlaq, Hisham A., Moussa, Sherif Abdelmottaleb. 2010. Elucidation of the effects of a high fat diet on trace element tissues using atomic absorption spectroscopy. Lipids in Health and Disease, Biomed Central Ltd. Accessed 2/25/10 @ http://www.lipidworld.com/content/9/1/2

Atkins, Laura, and Susan Smith. Protein. Accessed 2/28/10 at http://carrotcafe.com/n/protein.html

Aragno, M., G. Meineri, I. Vercellinatto, P. Bardini, S. Raimondo, P. G. Peiretti, A. Vercelli, G. Alloatti, C. E. Tomasinelli, O. Danni, and G. Boccuzzi. 2009. Cardiac impairment in rabbits fed a high-fat diet is counteracted by dehydroepiandrosterone supplementation. *Life Sci.* 85(1–2): 77–84.

Bethune, M. T., J. T. Borda, E. Ribka, and M-X Liu, K. Phillippi-Falkenstein, R. J. Jandacek, G. G. M. Doxiadis, G. M. Gray, C. Khosla, and K. Sestak. A Non-Human Primate Model for Gluten Sensitivity. Accessed on 2/20/13 at: http://www.phosone.org/article/info%Adoi%2F10.1371%2Fjournal.pone.0001614

Bovera, F., A. Lestingi, S. Marono, F. Jannaccone, S. Nizza, K. Mallardo, L. de Martino, and A. Tateo. 2012. Effect of dietary mannan-oligosaccharides on *in vivo* performance, nutrient digestibility, and caecal content characteristics of growing rabbits. *J. Anim. Phys. Anim. Nutr.* 96(1): 130-136.

Brosnan, J. T. and M. E. Brosnan. 2006. The sulfur-containing amino acids: an overview. *J. Nutr.* 136(6 Supp.): 1636S–1640S.

Bugaut, M. 1987. Occurrence, absorption, and metabolism of short chain fatty acids in the digestive tract of mammals. *Comp. Biochem. Phys. Part B* 86(3): 439-472.

Bullon, P., J. L. Quiles, J. M. Morillo, C. Rubini, G. Goteri, S. Ganados-Principal, M. Battino, and N. C. Ramirez-Tortosa. 2009. Gingival vascular damage in atherosclerotic rabbits: Hydroxytyrosol and squalene benefits. *Food Chem. Tox.* 47(9): 2327–2331.

Burstyn, P. G. and D. R. Husbands. 1980. Fat induced hypertension in rabbits. Effects of dietary fibre on blood pressure and blood lipid concentration. *Cardiovascular Res.* 14(4): 185–191.

Carabano, R., I. Badiola, S. Chamoro, J. Garcia, A. I. Garcia-Ruiz, P. Garcia-Rebollar, M. S. Gomez-Conde, I. Gutierrez, N. Nicodemus, M. J. Villamide, and J. C. de Blas. 2008. Review: New trends in rabbit feeding: influence of nutrition on intestinal health. *Span. J. Agri. Res.* 6(special issue): 15-25.

Casado, C., J. Moya, J. J. Pascual, E. Blas, and C. Cervere. 2013. Dietary fatty acid profile: effects on caecal fermentation and performance of young and fattening rabbits. *World Rab. Sci.* 21(4): 235-242.

Chrenkova, M., L. Chrastinova, M. Polacikova, Z. Formelova, A. Balazi, L. Ondruska, A. Sirotkin, and P. Chrenek. 2012. The effect of *Yucca schidigera* extract in diet of rabbits on nutrient digestibility and qualitative parameters in caecum. *Slovak. J. Anim. Sci.* 45(3): 83-88.

Coombs, R. R. A., M. Keiffer, D. R. Fraser, and P. J. Frazier. 1983. Naturally Developing antibodies to Wheat Gliadin Fractions and to Other Cereal Antigens in Rabbits, Rats, and Guinea Pigs on Normal Laboratory Diets. *Int. Arch. Allergy Immunol.* 70(3): 200-204.

Cusak, B. J., S. P. Young, V. L. Loseke, M. R. Hurty, L. Beals, and R. D. Olson. 1994. Effect of a low-protein diet on doxyrubicin pharmacokinectics in the rabbit. *Cancer Chemother. and Pharmacol.* 30(2): 145–148.

Daniels, Stephen. 2008. Lycopene as effective as statins for artery health: rabbit study. Nutra ingredients\.com accessed 2/24/10 at Http://www.nutraingredients.com/content/view/print/161800

Dass, N. B., J. Hill, A. Muir, T. Testa, A. Wise, and G. J. Sanger. 2003. The rabbit motilin receptor: molecular characterization and pharmacology. *Br. J. Pharma.* 140: 948-954.

Davidson, J. and D. Spreadbury. 1975. Nutrition of the New Zealand White Rabbit. *Proc. Nutr. Sci. 34: 75–83.*

Debray, Laurence, Isabelle Le Huerou-Luron, Thierry Gidenne, and Laurence Fortun-Lamothe. 2003. Digestive tract development in rabbit according to the dietary energetic source: correlation between whole tract digestion, pancreatic and intestinal enzymatic activities. *Comp. Biochem. Phys.* 135(3): 443–455.

Fraser, G. E. 2009. Nut consumption, lipids, and risk of a coronary event. *Clinical Cardiol.* 22(S3): 11-15.

Fortun-Lamothe, L. and S. Boullier. 2004. Interactions between gut microflora and digestive mucosal immunity, and strategies to improve digestive health in young rabbits. *Proceedings:* 8th World Rabbit Congress, Puebla.

Fraser, M. and S. J. Gerling. 2009. *Rabbit Medicine and Surgery for Veterinary Nurses.* Chichester: Wiley-Blackwell.

Glavin, G. B. 1983. Fat-supplemented diet protects against activity-stress ulcers in rats. *Cell. Molecular Life Sci.* 39(10): 1097–1099.

Goodrich, B. S., E. R. Hesterman, K. S. Shaw, and R. Mykytowycz. 1981. Identification of some volatile compounds in the odor of fecal pellets of the rabbit, *Oryctolagus cuniculus. J. Chem. Eco.* 7(5): 817-827.

Gu, Z.L., Y. F. Bai, B. J. Chen, G. C. Huo, and C. Zhao. 2004. Effect of protein level on lactating performance, daily gain and fur density in rex rabbits. *Proceedings*: 8th World Rabbit Congress, Puebla.

Hove, E. L., D. H. Copeland, J. F. Herndon, and W. D. Salmon. 1957. Further Studies on Choline Deficiency and Muscular Dystrophy in Rabbits. *J. Nutr.* 63(2): 289–299.

Karpati, S., M. Meurer, W. Stolz, A. Burgin-Wolff, O. Braun-Falco, and T. Krieg. 1992. Ultrastructural binding sites of endomysium antibodies from sera of patients with dermatitis herpetiformis and coeliac disease. *Gut* 33(2): 191-193.

Lebas, F. and G. Greppi. 1980. Water and food ingestion in the young rabbit given food deficient in methionine or lysine and drinking by free choice a solution of that amino acid or pure water. *Reprod. Nutr. Dev.* 20(5B): 1661–1665.

Leng, R. A. 2008. Digestion in the rabbit—a new look at the effects of their feeding and digestive strategies. *Proceedings*; MEKEARN Rabbit Conference: Organic rabbit production from forages (Eds: Reg Preston and Nguyen Van Thu), Cantho University, Vietnam.

Lopez-Bote, C. J., A. L. Rey, M. Sanz, J. I. Gray, and D. J. Buckley. 1987. Dietary vegetable oils and alpha-tocopherol reduce lipid oxidation in Rabbit Muscle. *J. Nutr.* 127 (6): 1176–1182.

Lowe, J. A. Pet Rabbit Feeding and Nutrition. In: *Nutrition of the Rabbit*. Carlos DeBlas and Julian Wiseman. 294-314.

Maertens, L. 1998. Fats in Rabbit Nutrition: A Review. *World Rab. Sci.* 6(3–4): 341–348

Mahfouz, M. M. Q. Zhou, and F. A. Kummerow. 1994. Cholesterol oxides in plasma and lipoproteins of magnesium- deficient rabbits and effects of their lipoproteins on endothelial barrier function. *Magnes. Res.* 7(3–4): 207–222.

March, J. B. 2003. High Antigliadin IgG Titers in Laboratory Rabbits Fed a Wheat-Containing Diet: A Model for Celiac Disease. *Digest. Dis. Sci.* 48(3): 608-610.

Mehta, U., B.P.S. Kang, R.S. Kukreja, and M. P. Bansai. 2002. Ultrastructural examination of rabbit aortic wall following high-fat diet feeding and selenium supplementation: a transmission electron microscopy study. *J. Ap. Tox.* 22(6): 405–413.

Morisse, J. P., G. le Gall, R. Maurice, J. P. Cotte, E. Boilletot. 1992. Effect of a fructo-oligosaccharides mixture on some intestinal and plasmatic parameters in young rabbits. *Rivista Zootecnia e Veterinaria*

20(1): 57-61.

Rabin, B. S. and S. J. Rogers. 1976. Nonpathogenicity of anti-intestinal antibody in the rabbit. *Am. J. Pathol.* 83(2): 269-282.

Raloff, J. 1990. Low-magnesium diet may clog heart arteries. Science News. Accessed 3/12/2110 at http://findarticles.com/p/articles/mi_m1200/is_n14_v137/ai_8921909?

Salma, U., A.G. Miah, Y. Akter, Z. H. Khandaker, and A. Reza. 2006. Effect of Different Levels of Protein Supplementation on Reproductive Performance of Rabbits. *Int. J. Agri. Biol.*6(5): 794–796.

Sidhu, S., S. Malhortra, and S. K. Garg. 2004. Influence of High Fat Diet (Butter) on the Pharmacokinetics of Phenytoin and Carbamazepine. *Exp. Clin. Pharmacol.* 26(8): 635–648.

Wang, X., M. Ma, L. Sun, C. Wang, Y. Zhu, and F. Li. 2012. Effects of different protein, fibre and energy levels on growth performance and the development of digestive organs in growing meat rabbit. *Proceedings:* 10th World Rabbit Congress, Sharm El-Sheikh, Egypt

Weigensberg, B. L., H. C. Stary, and G. C. McMillan. 1964. Effect of lysine deficiency on cholesterolatherosclerosis in rabbits. *Exp. Molec. Path.* 3(5): 444–454.

Yu, Y-M, W-C Chang, C-H Wu, and S-Y Chiang. 2005. Reduction of oxidative stress and apoptosis in hyperlipidemic rabbits by ellagic acid. *J. Nutri. Biochem.* 16(11): 675-681.

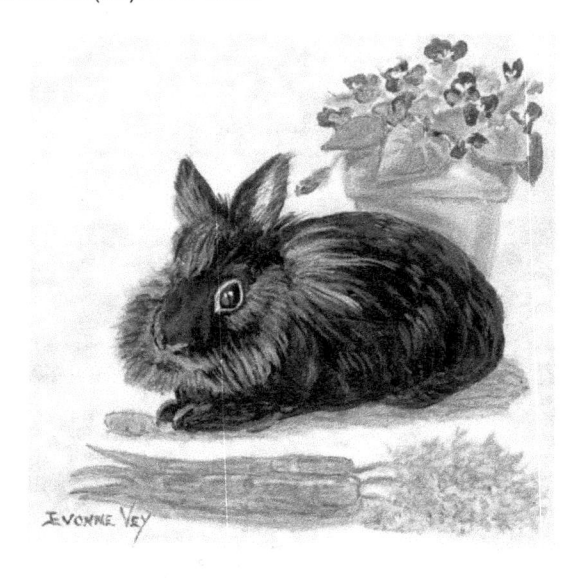

Chapter 5

VITAMINS AND MINERALS

Vitamins and minerals, sometimes called micronutrients, are as essential to biological life as are the macronutrients (carbohydrates, proteins, and fats), although the amounts required are much less. Among other roles, both vitamins and minerals function as coenzymes, working with enzymes to drive the chemical reactions that go on constantly within our bodies and those of our rabbits.

Vitamins are organic (compounds containing carbon atoms) micronutrients and minerals are inorganic (substances or compounds not having a carbon basis, although they may become incorporated into organic molecules) micronutrients. A few vitamins may be synthesized in the body; minerals are not synthesized. Vitamins have no common structural similarity as do the macronutrients; it is their biological activity – that of being necessary for metabolic processes – that they have in common. Some vitamins are water soluble and must be consumed every day because the body does not store them; others are fat-soluble and can be stored. Minerals are stored in the body and it is possible to accumulate excess amounts that may cause toxicity. Fat-soluble vitamins may also accumulate in toxic amounts.

Vitamins not synthesized within a mammal's body or not produced in needed amounts will have to be consumed, and all nutritional minerals must be consumed. Different mammals do not require the same micronutrients in the same amounts. For this reason, the micronutrients you and your rabbit require for optimum health will not be exactly the same. Vitamins that rabbits need to consume through their diets include A, B-complex, D, E, K, and to a lesser degree, C. Choline, a compound similar to vitamins and often included in the B-complex, is also necessary. Rabbits require the dietary minerals calcium, cobalt, copper, iodine, iron, magnesium, manganese, phosphorus, potassium, selenium, silicon, sodium, and zinc. Other minerals are also needed in varying amounts, but as they are rarely deficient in rabbits' diets they will not be addressed in this volume.

Before beginning the discussion on specific vitamins and minerals, it is necessary to define two terms that will be used frequently: "free radicals" and "antioxidants." *Free radicals* are unstable molecules formed from the chemical reactions continually occurring in our bodies. (They can also be formed as a result of outside factors such as exposure to radiation, pesticides, and smoke.) These unstable compounds need to either lose or gain another electron to become stable, so they are always "looking for" a molecule to attach to, thereby becoming stable. But when this happens, the state of the molecule the free radical attaches to is changed and it becomes a free radical. This can begin a chain reaction that ends in the death of the cell. Fat, one of the most chemically unstable compounds in the body, frequently undergoes free radical chain reactions, degrading important molecules such as proteins. *Antioxidants* are molecules with the ability to neutralize free radicals without becoming free radicals themselves because they are stable in both states. Many vitamins and vitamin precursors are antioxidants, and the mineral selenium is also a powerful antioxidant. It has been shown in multiple studies that consuming foods rich in antioxidants can lessen the risk of heart disease and some cancers in many mammals, including rabbits.

The food sources I list for the micronutrients are sources that would be good sources for rabbits. Therefore, many sources that humans might utilize are not mentioned. If you feel your rabbit requires more of a particular micronutrient than you can provide through foods high in that nutrient, there are supplements specifically formulated for small animals available from your veterinary practitioner.

When looking at the tables of vitamin and mineral content of foods, it should be remembered that the numbers only represent averages. Actual vitamin and mineral content in foodstuffs often varies widely depending upon a multitude of factors, including the soil in which plants were grown, conditions under which plants were harvested, time of year plants were harvested, the age of the plants, the conditions under which food is stored, length of time food is stored, and many other factors. The method of analysis also affects published values. Repeatedly I found published values for the same nutrient in the same plant species that varied several hundredfold. Due to its nature, nutrition is far from an exact science—values given must be taken as relatives, not absolutes.

VITAMINS
Vitamin A
Vitamin A (retinol, retinoic acid) is a fat-soluble organic alcohol that is formed from plant carotenoid pigments, alphacarotene, betacarotene, and betacryptoxanthin. Vitamin A is a good antioxidant, protecting against cell damage from free radicals. It is also necessary for successful reproduction, good vision, a healthy immune system, bones, good coat quality, and the maintenance of mucous membranes. Consuming retinol directly or consuming its precursors will fill dietary needs. Rabbits naturally consume the precursors found in plants, and are particularly good at using betacarotene, converting nearly 100% of the beta-carotene in their foods to retinol in their intestines. (However, the intestinal mucosa must be healthy for efficient conversion.) Good sources of vitamin A precursors include leafy greens, dark green vegetables, grasses, yellow to red fruits and vegetables, and legumes. Vitamin A is lost in the drying process, so hay is not a good source of this vitamin.

Vitamin A is often added to commercial rabbit feeds, but has a shelf life of only about three months and can be further degraded by heat and rancidity that can develop during storage. Most vitamin A content of plants is lost during the drying, storing, and processing of foods. The amounts of vitamin A in sun-cured grasses and alfalfa can vary widely since much is destroyed when the plants are dried. For example, the vitamin A in sun-dried alfalfa often ranges between 15,000–50,000 IU/kg (IU = international unit. For vitamin A, an IU equals 0.3 microgram (mcg) of retinol or 0.55 micrograms of retinyl acetate.)

A deficiency of vitamin A (hypovitaminosis) may occur at less than 2000 IU/kg, and can lead to low fertility, abortions, fetal malformations (including a high incidence of cleft palate), a high degree of enteritis in young rabbits, hydrocephalus (also in young rabbits), and/or a low survival rate of kits. Muscle weakness (ataxia), floppy rabbit syndrome, anorexia, and eye lesions and blindness

Table 5:1. Fat-soluble vitamin content of selected foods (per 100g of listed food). Due to its scarcity in natural foods, vitamin D content is not listed. Actual nutrient content of any food may vary greatly from listed values due to differing growth and storage conditions, as well as other fact ors. *Values compiled from multiple sources.*

Food	vit. A IU	vit. E mg	vit. K mcg	Food	vit A IU	vit. E mg	vit. K mcg
alfalfa sprouts	155.	0.02	30.3	lamb's quarter	9,744.	—	494.
almonds	1.0	19.1	0	lettuce	7,405.	0.29	173.6
apples	3.0	0.0002	2.0	lettuce, Romaine	290.	0.12	150.
apricots	96.0	0.0009	3.6	molasses*	0	0	—
arugula (rocket)	2,373.	0.43	108.6	mustard greens	10,500.	2.01	497.3
bananas	3.0	0.0001	0.50	oats, rolled	0	0.7	0
basil	5,275	0.80	414.8	oranges	295.	0.24	4.0
blueberries	3.0	0.0006	25.	parsley	8,424.	0.75	1,640.
brewer's yeast*	0	0	0	peaches	38.	0.002	7.8
broccoli	150.	0.78	100.	pineapple	3.0	0.00002	1.2
cabbage	153.	0.0001	76.	pumpkin, canned	15,563.	1.06	16.
cantaloupe	155.	0.05	2.5	pumpkin seeds	380.	0.48	51.4
carrot root	845.	0.001	0	purslane	1,320.	12.1	381.
carrot top	8,376	—	31.2	raisins	0	0.15	3.0
celery	449.	0.27	29.3	shepherd's purse	8,575.	0.1	330.
chicory	286.	0.002	297.6	soybeans*	22.	1.95	190.
cilantro	5,717	2.5	310.	spinach	9,377.	2.03	483.
dried cranberr	0	1.07	3.8	sunflower seeds	3.0	34.5	2.7
dandelion greens	247.	0.0048	830.	tomato	833.	0.54	7.9
dill	7,718	0	—	walnuts	20.	0.44	1.7
Kale	15,376	0	817.	wheatgrass	360	2.64	784.

* used as ingredient in some commercial rabbit foods

may occur in adults.

Since vitamin A is stored in the liver, toxicity (hypervitaminosis) can occur, and retinyl ester may be released into the blood. Vitamin A amounts in feeds of 190,000 IU or higher have caused vitamin A toxicity. Signs of vitamin A toxicity are the same as those of vitamin A deficiency, plus a low growth rate in rabbit kits. Supplementing B-complex vitamins may protect rabbits from some of the effects of vitamin A toxicity. Supplements of the vitamin A precursor beta carotene do not appear to be toxic in high doses.

Recommendations on the amount of vitamin A that a rabbit diet should contain vary. According to Lebas, 3,000 IU/kg meets the requirements. However, he notes that due to the sensitivity of vitamin A to oxidation, feeds often have extra vitamin A added, and suggests from 6,000–10,000 IU in a feed is likely to provide adequate vitamin A. Other sources recommend that rabbits have between 10,000–18,000 IU/kg of vitamin A per day plus 1,000 mg/kg beta carotene per day. Rabbit kits with coccidiosis require higher amounts of vitamin A since the disease interferes with vitamin A absorption.

B-complex vitamins
Vitamins usually included in the B-complex are: Vitamin B_1 (thiamin, thiamine), B_2 (riboflavin), B_3 (niacin), B_5 (pantothenic acid), B_6 (pyridoxine), biotin, B_9 (folate, folic acid), B_{12} (cyanocobalamine), and choline. Most of these vitamins are soluble in water and must be consumed every day since the body does not store them. They are also very heat-sensitive micronutrients and do not keep well in foods. The importance of consuming enough of them cannot be over-stated, as these vitamins are critical to the brain, nervous system, blood, cell membranes, skin, eyes, and intestinal tract. Deficiencies of some of the B-vitamins cause fewer antibodies to be produced.

Because cecotrophs are rich in several B-vitamins that are produced by cecal microflora, it is often stated in information about rabbits that no additional source of B-vitamins is necessary. However, this is not entirely true. There is evidence that rabbits do need additional dietary sources for B_6 (pyridoxine) and choline, and some sources list B_1 (thiamine), B_2 (riboflavin), B_3 (niacin) and/or biotin as requiring additional dietary sources as well. Even those

B-vitamins normally produced by cecal microflora in sufficient amounts may need to be supplemented if rabbits are on antibiotics.

Thiamine (also spelled thiamin), or vitamin B_1, is needed for brain function, muscle tone, and appetite. Legumes, parsley, cecotrophs (some sources specifically state cecotrophs do not provide adequate amounts of thiamine), chickweed, peppermint, raspberry leaf and whole grains are all rich courses of thiamine. Deficiencies of thiamine in rabbits can lead to a loss of appetite and mild ataxia (muscle weakness). The recommended dietary supplement for rabbits is 2 ppm.

Riboflavin, vitamin B_2, is a component of important coenzymes. It is necessary for red blood cell and antibody formation, and helps maintain mucous membranes in the digestive system. Good dietary sources include cecotrophs, legumes, spinach, whole grains, asparagus, broccoli, chickweed, leafy greens, peppermint, parsley, raspberry leaves, and nuts. Signs of riboflavin deficiency in other species include dermatitis and poor appetite. The recommended dietary supplement is 6 ppm for growing rabbits and 4 ppm for adults.

Niacin (nicotinic acid), vitamin B_3, is involved in the metabolism of fats and proteins, the secretion of biles, the synthesis of sex hormones, and is necessary for a healthy circulatory system and skin. Good dietary sources include alfalfa, broccoli, carrots, cecotrophs, chickweed, dandelion greens, dates, parsley, peanuts, peppermint, raspberry leaves, red clover, tomatoes, and wheat. A deficiency of niacin in a rabbit could cause loss of appetite, diarrhea, and weight loss. Recommended dietary supplement is 50 ppm for both growing and adult rabbits.

Pantothenic acid, or vitamin B_5, is needed by all the cells in the body. It is part of coenzyme A (CoA) which is necessary for many metabolic processes. It is found in brewer's yeast, cecotrophs, fresh vegetables, legumes, nuts, and whole grains. Deficiency of this B-vitamin in a rabbit would be extremely unlikely, although it could theoretically occur if a rabbit was on antibiotics. In other mammals, a sign of deficiency is fatigue. The recommended dietary supplement for rabbits is 20 ppm.

Pyridoxine (vitamin B_6) is needed for the production of hydrochloric acid, is involved in the absorption of fats and proteins, and is necessary for normal brain function and for the synthesis of DNA and RNA. It is found in alfalfa, banana, broccoli, cabbage, carrots, molasses, peas, soybeans, sunflower seeds, walnuts, and wheat germ. Deficiencies in rabbits can lead to dermatitis, neurological symptoms including convulsions, and weight loss. The recommended dietary supplement is 2 ppm for growing and adult rabbits.

Biotin has a role in the metabolism of carbohydrates, fats, and protein, and is needed for healthy skin, hair, nerve tissue, and bone marrow. Biotin is found in whole grains, brewer's yeast, and soybeans, and is produced by bacteria, so it is also found in cecotrophs. Signs of deficiencies in rabbits include alopecia and dermatitis. The recommended dietary supplement for both growing and adult rabbits is 0.10 ppm.

Folate (folic acid), vitamin B_9, is needed for the metabolism of amino acids and nucleic acids (DNA and RNA). It is found in asparagus, alfalfa and other legumes, brewer's yeast, dates, green leafy vegetables, oranges, root vegetables, and whole grains. This is another B-vitamin that would be extremely unlikely to be deficient in rabbits. Signs of deficiency in other mammals include anemia, digestive trouble, graying hair, lethargy, and a reddened, sore tongue. Recommended supplementation is 5 ppm for growing and adult rabbits.

Cyanocobalamine (cianocobal amine), vitamin B_{12}, is necessary for the proper digestion and absorption of nutrients and helps prevent nerve damage, among other roles. In one study rabbits given extra B_{12} had significantly less fat deposition in the aorta. There are not many food sources of this vitamin, but it is found in cecotrophs, brewer's yeast (it is added to the product), kelp, spirulina supplements, and the roots of legumes. Vitamin B_{12} deficiency in rabbits would be unlikely to occur unless the rabbit were on antibiotics. Some signs of deficiencies in other mammals are bone loss, lethargy, and neurological symptoms. The recommended dietary supplement is 0.01 ppm.

According to information on the website of the Linus Pauling Institute, **choline** is not a true vitamin, but a vitamin-like compound. It is needed for the transmission of nerve signals from the brain to the central nervous system, the regulation of gall bladder function, lecithin formation, liver function, the production of hormones, and fat metabolism. Choline is found in legumes such as alfalfa and soybeans, and in whole grains. A deficiency of choline in a rabbit's diet can lead to decreased growth, edema, liver damage, heart damage, ulcers, muscular weakness (possibly from the interruption of nerve impulse transmission to the musculature), paralysis, prolonged blood clotting, high creatine levels in blood and low in urine, and hemorrhagic kidney degradation. A deficiency may be one of the causes of "floppy rabbit" syndrome. Choline-deficient rabbits may also have increased retention of toxins, especially in the liver and lungs.

It is recommended that choline account for about 0.13% of the total rabbit diet since it has been found that levels of 0.12% or lower can lead to signs of deficiency. If B_{12} and folate are both deficient in a rabbit's diet, a choline deficiency may occur as well because of chemical reactions that take place. Recommended dietary supplementation is 200 ppm for rabbits up to 80 days old and 100 ppm for adults.

Vitamin C
Vitamin C (ascorbic acid) is another water soluble vitamin. It is one of the most powerful antioxidants known, increasing the life of immune cells and protecting cell membranes from free radicals, is necessary for healthy connective tissue, can possibly aid in ameliorating arthritic symptoms, and is used in over 300 metabolic processes in the body. Rabbits, like most mammals (humans and guinea pigs are two exceptions), synthesize vitamin C in the liver from glucose. For that reason, much literature on rabbits may state that additional dietary vitamin C is not necessary. However, it has been found that there are conditions under which rabbits do require additional vitamin C or have improved function with additional dietary vitamin C. During times of stress, including heat stress and illness, the plasma vitamin C drops significantly in rabbits, and supplementing the vitamin at these times can have beneficial effects. Supplementation of 25–30 mg per rabbit per day has been found to help with many of the above stress situations. Adding vitamin C to the diet also has positive effects on the health of pregnant, lactating, and growing rabbits.

Supplementation of vitamin C in rabbits has been found to reduce the severity of respiratory disorders in rabbits. It has been reported that when vitamin C is given daily in amounts of 50–100 mg/kg per rabbit, it may prevent enterotoxemia by inhibiting toxin production, and vitamin C may also be helpful in cases of lead toxicity in rabbits. In another studies, supplementation of 250 mg/liter in the drinking water reduced weaning stress for the two weeks after weaning of rabbit kits and reduced kit mortality. Supplementation of 25–30 mg per rabbit per day has been found to help with many stress situations, including heat stress. However, including as little as 1% vitamin C in the rabbit diet increases the need for copper. If the dietary copper is only 3 ppm, signs of copper deficiency could appear. If dietary copper is 5–15 ppm, copper deficiency will be unlikely to occur with vitamin C supplementation. The recommended dietary supplementation for vitamin C is 200–250 ppm.

There are no signs of vitamin C deficiency since the vitamin is synthesized in the rabbit's body, nor are there signs of excesses since even massive doses of the vitamin appear to be tolerated without toxicity.

There are many good plant sources of vitamin C, including fruits and green vegetables, especially leafy greens (Table 5:1). Vitamin C is chemically fragile and does not survive well in commercial feeds, especially if the feeds are exposed to heat. It is also lost during the drying process.

Vitamin D
Vitamin D is often called the sunshine vitamin because exposure to the sun causes it to be manufactured in the body. It plays a role in the secretion of insulin and glucose tolerance in rabbits. It is a fat-soluble vitamin (also a hormone) and excesses can be stored. The precursor ergocalciferol (in plants) may be consumed by rabbits, or vitamin D may be synthesized in the rabbit's skin when it is exposed to UV light. The precursors are converted in the liver and stored there.

In humans vitamin D is closely intertwined with calcium absorption, leading to fairly high requirements for the vitamin. However, in rabbits intestinal absorption of calcium is efficient in the absence of vitamin D, although it has been found that vitamin D does increase intestinal absorption of calcium if dietary levels of calcium are low. Vitamin D is also critcal to rabbit phosphorus metabolism.

Table 5:2. Water-soluble vitamin content of selected foods (per 100g listed food). Because of the rapid loss of vitamins during storage, vitamin contents of hays are not given. Actual nutrient content of any food may vary greatly from listed values due to differing growth and storage conditions, as well as other factors. *Values compiled from multiple sources*

	B_1 mg	B_2 mg	B_3 mg	B_5 mg	B_6 mg	biotin mcg	folate mcg	choline mg	C mg
alfalfa sprouts	0.06	0.12	0.60	0.54	0.03	0.2	35.7	14.	8.1
almonds	0.24	0.91	3.9	0.41	0.13	15.5	29.0	52.	0
apples	0.02	0.03	0.09	0.06	.004	0.02	3.0	3.4	5.1
apricots	0.03	0.04	0.60	0.24	0.05	----	9.0	2.9	10.
arugula	004	0.08	0.31	0.44	0.07	__	95.0	15.	15.
bananas	0.03	0.07	0.66	0.33	0.37	10.0	20.0	9.7	8.9
barley	0.65	0.28	4.6	0.28	0.32	0.9	19.0	37.	0
basil	0.03	0.07	0.90	0.21	0.15	----	68.0	11.	18.
blueberries	0.04	0.04	0.42	0.12	0.04	__	6.0	6.1	11.
brewer's yeast**	3.6	4.5	30.	1.8	2.4	115.	1800	240	0
broccoli	0.06	0.12	0.64	0.53	0.16	0.67	71.0	18.	93.
cabbage, raw	0.06	0.04	0.23	0.21	0.12	0.1	53.0	10.	41.
cantaloupe	0.02	0.03	0.73	0.10	0.07	__	21.0	6.9	36.
carrot root	0.06	0.04	0.84	0.23	0.15	0.6	8.1	8.7	9.3
carrot tops	—	—	—	—	—	—	—	—	95.
celery	0.02	0.67	0.32	0.24	0.07	0.1	36.0	6.2	7.0
cherries	0.02	0.04	0.18	0.11	0.04	0.3	8.0	5.5	4.6
chicory	0.06	0.10	0.5	1.2	0.11	----	110.	12.	24.
cilantro	0.07	0.16	1.1	0.57	0.15	----	62.0	13.	27.
cranberries, dried	0.01	0.02	0.99	0.22	0.04	__	0	4.4	0.2
dandelion greens	0.19	0.26	0.81	0.08	0.25	__	27.0	13.	35.
dill	0.06	0.29	1.5	0.39	0.18	----	150.	----	85.
endive/ escarole	0.08	0.07	0.40	0.9	0.02	__	142.	17.	6.5

	B₁ mg	B₂ mg	B₃ mg	B₅ mg	B₆ mg	biotin mcg	folate mcg	choline mg	C mg
kale	0.11	0.13	1.0	0.09	0.27	—	29.	0.4	120.
lamb's quarters	0.1	0.3	0.9	0.05	0.3	—	12.5	0.45	66.
lettuce, leaf	0.07	0.08	0.375	0.135	0.09	0.7	38.	8.5	18.
lettuce, romaine	0.072	0.067	0.313	0.142	0.074	0.7	136.	9.9	24.
molasses*	0.03	0	1.0	0.7	0.8	trace	0	13.3	0
mustard greens	0.080	0.110	0.80	0.210	0.180	—	187.	0.4	70.
oats, rolled	0.71	0.139	0.961	1.35	0.119	0.18	**151.**	18.	0.1
oranges	0.114	0.052	0.369	0.328	0.079	0.06	39.	8.4	53.2
papaya	0.032	0.041	0.41	0.28	0.022	—	49.	9.2	61.8
parsley	0.086	0.098	1.31	0.40	0.09	0.4	152.	13.	133.
peaches	0.012	0.026	0.641	0.23	0.019	0.2	3.0	6.1	3.8
pineapple	0.079	0.031	0.489	0.205	0.11	trace	15.	5.6	30.3
pumpkin, canned	0.024	0.056	0.367	0.40	0.056	0.4	12.	10.0	4.2
pumpkin seeds	0.21	0.32	1.75	0.339	0.224	—	58.	54.	1.9
purslane	0.047	0.112	0.48	0.036	0.073	—	12.	11.0	21.
shepherd's purse	0.15	0.27	0.5	1.1	0.32	—	180.	—	110.
soybeans*	0.874	0.87	1.62	0.79	0.38	160.0	375.	54.5	6.0
spinach	0.078	0.189	0.724	0.065	0.195	6.9	194.	22.	28.1
sunflower seeds	2.29	0.25	4.5	6.7	0.77	60.0	227.	52.8	1.4
tomato	0.037	0.021	0.594	0.10	0.080	0.90	15.5	6.7	13.
walnuts, English	0.341	0.14	1.07	1.26	0.583	34.	98.	33.1	1.4
water cress	0.090	0.120	0.20	0.310	0.129	—	9.0	9.0	43.
wheat bran	1.29	1.47	17.24	1.93	1.73	12.0	94.	74.5	0
wheat grass***	0.225	0.155	3.09	0.95	0.27	4.5	38.	28.0	3.0

* Used as ingredient in some commercial rabbit foods
** Contains B₁₂ if fortified..
*** Fresh grass is eaten without washing and therefore contains some B₁₂ from bacteria.

A deficiency can lead to a reduction of the intestinal absorption of phosphorus and affect bone calcification, leading to rickets in young rabbits and osteomalacia (softening of the bone) in adults. A diet of 1.0% Ca and 0.5% P, along with a deficiency of vitamin D, has been shown to lead to intestinal malabsorption of phosphorus and inadequate mineralization of the skeleton. Diets with less than 300 IU are considered deficient.

A vitamin D deficiency can occur if a rabbit does not have enough exposure to UV light and does not consume enough of the precursors in food. Hay may contain vitamin D, but the amount will depend on the curing process: sun-dried hay has higher content than hay that is dried artificially (the opposite of vitamin A, which has higher levels in artificially-dried hay). Many commercial feeds are supplemented with vitamin D, but the vitamin may have a shelf life of three months or less in these feeds.

Rabbits are extremely sensitive to vitamin D toxicity, adults more so than kits, and it has been demonstrated that amounts as low as 2300–3000 IU/kg in feeds can cause such toxicity. Signs of toxicity include high blood levels of calcium and phosphorus, high fetal mortality in pregnant does, anorexia, diarrhea, weakness, paralysis, calcification of tissues (especially the aorta and kidney), renal failure, and death. The risks of soft tissue calcification from excess vitamin D will increase if the rabbit is receiving a high-calcium diet.

The recommended amounts for vitamin D supplementation vary. Up to 300 IU/kg may provide insufficient vitamin D for a rabbit. For growing or breeding rabbits, 600–1000 IU/kg has been recommended; 800–1200 IU/kg of feed for adults. (An IU for vitamin D equals 0.025 microgram D_3/kg dry matter.)

Vitamin E

Vitamin E is another fat-soluble vitamin. It is an extremely powerful antioxidant, preventing the peroxides formed during metabolic processes from damaging cells. Vitamin E also improves circulation, is critical to the eyes, is necessary for tissue repair and healthy skin and hair, may help protect the heart and bladder from oxidative damage, and has been found to protect against atherosclerosis in rabbits. "Vitamin E" actually includes two groups of closely related compounds, *tocopherols* and *tocotrienols*. The latter group includes synthesized vitamin Es that are not nearly as active as tocopherols.

In humans vitamin E works synergistically with selenium. According to some studies there is not as much of a synergistic action between the two in rabbits, although it has been found that both selenium and vitamin E inhibit atherosclerosis in rabbits. In one study it was found that oxidative damage to fats and proteins in rabbits was more severe with deficiencies of both vitamin E and selenium than deficiencies of only one or the other. It has also been found that 40 mg of vitamin E/kg diet with selenium may reduce the effect of heat stress on sperm concentration and improve other reproductive processes.

Good sources of vitamin E include alfalfa and other legumes, cold-pressed vegetable oils, flaxseed oil, dark green vegetables, leafy greens including dandelion, nuts, young grass, raspberry leaves, and whole grains. Grass hay is not usually a good source of vitamin E since up to 90% may be lost in its production. Alfalfa hay has about 40mg/kg of vitamin E (not adequate), but dehydrated alfalfa has 120–200mg/kg and is a good source. Rabbit diets that contain 25% dehydrated alfalfa provide adequate vitamin E. The vitamin E content in cereal grains may also be lost if the grains are kept in moist conditions. Many supplements are from animal sources such as fish oil, but in one study fish oil vitamin E supplements were not adequate antioxidants for very long chain fatty acids in rabbits.

A deficiency of vitamin E (below 16 mg/kg per rabbit daily) can lead to infertility, abortions, still births, muscular weakness (including floppy rabbit syndrome and hind leg paralysis in young rabbits), a higher rate of coccidiosis in young rabbits, incoordination, fatty liver, and sudden death through damage to heart muscle. Rabbits have a tolerance for high vitamin E doses, and at the time of this writing, toxicity of this vitamin has not been described for rabbits.

Recommended amounts for vitamin E inclusion in rabbit diets vary. One source suggests 1 mg/kg of rabbit body weight or about 17 mg/kg of feed; another suggests 40–70 mg/kg of body weight or 50 mg/kg of feed, and others fall between these two recommendations.

Vitamin K

Vitamin K, sometimes called the "clotting factor," is needed for the clotting of blood, for bone formation and repair, and is also necessary for healthy kidneys, liver, and intestines. There are three forms of vitamin K, one from plants, one synthesized by bacteria, and a synthetic vitamin K. Since vitamin K is synthesized by rabbits' cecal microflora, a deficiency is unlikely to occur. However, if the rabbit is being given antibiotics, a deficiency could occur since the antibiotics will also kill the bacteria synthesizing vitamin K. Supplementation may also be necessary if the rabbit has coccidiosis or is not eating its cecotrophs. (Lebas described a vitamin K deficiency that developed in the absence of any digestive disorder, and resulted in high abortion rates and a decrease in the speed of coagulation in newborn kits.)

Grass is a good source of vitamin K, as are oats, cabbage, molasses, and dark green leafy vegetables. Alfalfa and most alfalfa-based feeds are also good sources of vitamin K, having about 20–25 mg/kg. Other feeds are not usually good sources, and often only contain about 1–2 mg/kg of feed. Vitamin K is lost during the drying process.

Signs of a vitamin K deficiency include muscle weakness, paralysis, and difficulty breathing. Insufficient vitamin K can also cause hemorrhagic abortions in deficient does. It is recommended that supplementation of vitamin K be considered if antibiotics are being given, if kits have coccidiosis, or if a rabbit is unable to eat its cecotrophs. The recommended supplementation is 2 ppm vitamin K or 1–2 mg/kg in diet. Since vitamin K is a fat-soluble vitamin and can be stored in the body, it can accumulate in excessive amounts. An excess of vitamin K (may possibly occur with levels of 8 g/kg feed) can cause nephritis (inflammation of the kidney).

CoQ10

CoQ10 (ubiquinone) is a fat-soluble vitamin-like compound with a structure similar to vitamin K. It is sometimes called "vitamin CoQ10," and its importance cannot be overstated. CoQ10 is involved in the transfer of energy throughout the body, and is essential for the health and proper function of all tissues and organs, including the heart and lungs. In order to function properly, CoQ10 requires the presence of adequate amounts of vitamins A, C and E and various phytonutrients. Although CoQ10 is produced by the mammalian body, the amounts decrease with age. Levels may also be low if cancer or other diseases are present.

The positive effects of CoQ10 on rabbits are numerous: it neutralizes free radicals, helps the immune system, and may help alleviate or prevent heart disease, some eye disease, bladder and kidney disease, and various conditions related to aging.

CoQ10 is found in whole grains, soy, and peanuts. Supplementing the diet of older rabbits (or those suffering from disease) with foods high in CoQ10 may be beneficial, as it has been found oral administration can increase tissue levels of the molecule.

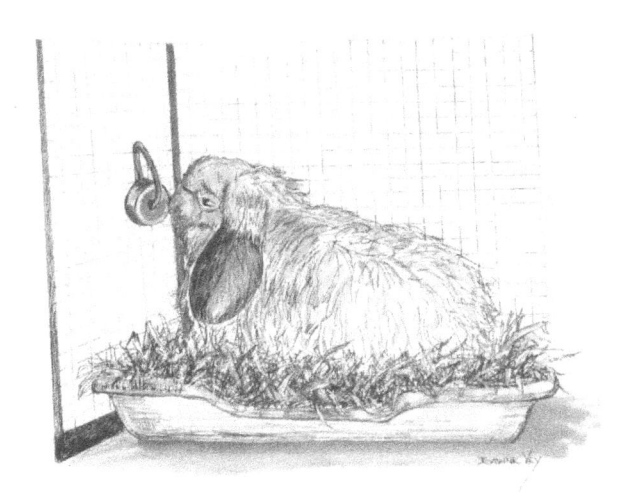

MINERALS

Calcium (Ca)

Calcium is necessary for the development and maintenance of healthy teeth and bones. It is also involved in nerve and muscle function, blood clotting, the permeability of membranes, enzyme activity, and the release of hormones. It is the most plentiful mineral in the mammalian body, and in rabbits, perhaps the most controversial one.

Calcium metabolism in the rabbit differs from that in other mammals. In most mammals, humans included, calcium levels are maintained within a narrow range by various regulatory mechanisms, one of the main ones of which involves vitamin D_3. In rabbits, calcium is absorbed in the intestine from consumed foods – regardless of metabolic needs – and the excess is excreted in the urine. Absorption is relatively independent of vitamin D_3, although according to Harcourt-Brown active vitamin D-dependent transport of calcium across intestinal mucosa is important if the dietary levels of vitamin D are low. Most mammals excrete less than 2% of dietary calcium in the urine, but rabbits commonly excrete about 44% in their urine. Levels of serum calcium vary widely both among and within rabbits. The parathyroid gland and parathyroid hormone (PTH) appear to be primarily responsible for maintaining the equilibrium of calcium in rabbits.

Rabbits are able to filter 45–60% calcium out of their blood (compared to 2% for most other mammals), but when the reabsorption capacity of the kidneys is reached, calcium precipitates out as crystals of calcium carbonate. This is what causes the cloudy and gritty qualities of rabbit urine. (Other crystals may also be found in rabbit urine, including phosphate, oxalate, and sulfadiazine – this last in rabbits taking sulphonamides). Jenkins suggests there is a difference between calciuria (calcium crytals in urine) and bladder "sludge," which Jenkins suggests be termed microurinary calculi, or MUC. Jenkins states that these tiny calculi (aggregates of crystals) form in response to cystitis (infection and inflammation of urinary bladder) or other conditions. Rabbits on low-calcium diets may actually have greater amounts of MUC.

Large aggregates are called stones, or uroliths, and may be found in the ureter (ureterolithiasis) as well as bladder (urolithiasis) and kidneys (nephrolithiasis). Predisposing factors to the formation of calculi include infections, arthritis, dehydration, nutritional imbalances, lack of exercise, and genetics.

Although in the past owners of rabbits with "sludge" and/or stones were often told to reduce the calcium in the rabbit's diet, many veterinary health professionals now recognize that fluid intake and exercise may be more important than the intake of calcium. Some researchers point out that rabbits have adapted to high calcium loads in their urine. In one study rabbits were put on several diets varying in calcium: alfalfa hay only, alfalfa and oats, grass hay only and grass hay and oats. None of the rabbits on any of the diets developed calculi and there was no significant difference in calcium deposits in the kidneys and aorta. The researchers concluded that water supply and exercise were more important factors in the development of urolithiasis than calcium content of the diet. Increased fluid intake reduces the concentration of the urine and keeps the urinary tract flushed out, and exercise helps keep particles from remaining in the bladder.

Deficiencies of calcium can lead to a loss of appetite, muscular tremors, osteomalacia, death in does in late gestation or early lactation, tooth problems such as ADD (acquired dental disease) and bone resorption. In one study, bone density was lower in rabbits receiving a low-calcium (0.15% Ca) diet than those on diets of 0.45 and 1.35 % calcium. Vitamin D deficiency may exacerbate Ca deficiency. Levels less than 0.2% can lead to spinal fractures.

When other physiologic or pathologic conditions exist, excessive dietary calcium can lead to urolithiasis and kidney disease. Prolonged high dietary calcium intake of more than 40 g/kg, or 4%, can lead to calcinosis, or the calcification of soft tissues (esp. aorta and kidneys) in rabbits, and this calcification is increased if vitamin D is supplemented in the diet. Rabbits with severe calcinosis may become anorexic and become emaciated. Prolonged excesses of dietary calcium also impair the absorption of zinc and phosphorus in the rabbit. If dietary phosphorus levels are already low, a phosphorus deficiency may be created. In one study it was found that giving an aqueous extract of cornsilk helped reduce calcium deposition in the kidneys of rabbits. Some veterinarians have found that giving potassium-magnesium citrate to rabbits with stones or MUC helps dissolve the calculi.

Foods that are high in calcium include parsley, spinach, carrot tops, mustard greens, borage, kale, dandelion greens, chicory, and lamb's quarters. However, it should be recognized that many of these greens, including alfalfa and spinach, have high levels of oxalate. This reduces the amount of calcium that is actually usable, or *bioavailable,* to the rabbit because much of it is bound as insoluble and indigestible calcium oxalate (see Chapter 7). For example, 60–70% of the calcium in alfalfa hay is bound in calcium oxalate. (Fiber content may also affect bioavailability of nutrients, including calcium.) This means that foods such as alfalfa and spinach that have high oxalate content will not provide as much calcium to a rabbit as would appear from the food's content of that mineral. Phytates and acetates (see Chapter 7) may also form complexes with calcium and reduce the bioavailability of calcium.

Recommended dietary calcium levels for rabbits are: 0.22 % for normal growth, 0.35–0.4% for maximum bone density in growing rabbits, 0.45–0.80 % for pregnant does, 0.75–1.10 % for lactating does, 0.4–0.8 % for non-lactating does, 0.5–1.0 % (500–1000mg) for pet rabbits. Does in late gestation or early lactation may have a drop in plasma calcium, phosphorus, and magnesium and develop milk fever (hypocalcemia). Signs include anorexia, tetany, muscle tremors, and ear flapping (see Chapter 10 for more information on milk fever).

Cobalt (Co)

Rabbits need only small amounts of this mineral in their diet, but it is essential since it is needed for the synthesis of vitamin B_{12} in the gut. Legumes usually have much higher cobalt content than grasses, and if the rabbit is receiving alfalfa hay or an alfalfa-based pellet a deficiency is unlikely. For rabbits not receiving alfalfa, giving a mineralized salt wheel with cobalt could ensure sufficient intake.

The signs of a cobalt deficiency are those of a B_{12} deficiency. A cobalt salt has been found to be an effective antidote to cyanide poisoning, increasing the oxygen uptake that is reduced by cyanide. Cobalt has also been found to have antiviral effects against herpes when applied to herpetic eye lesions.

Recommended level of cobalt in the rabbit diet is 0.1 ppm for young rabbits, adults, and lactating does.

Copper (Cu)

Copper easily accepts and donates electrons, and is therefore an important element in neutralizing free radicals and is also an important component of enzymes that catalyze the reduction of O_2 to water, beginning a process that eventually creates adenosine triphosphate,

Table 5:3. Oxalate, calcium, and phosphorus content of selected foods (per 100g of listed food). Actual nutrient values of foods may vary considerably from listed values due to differing growth and storage conditions, among other factors. *Values compiled from multiple sources.*

Food	oxalate mg	Ca mg	P mg	Food	oxalate mg	Ca mg	P mg
alfalfa sprouts	trace	31.8	69.3	lamb's quarter	1,430.	260.	60.6
almonds	370..	248.	474.	lettuce, leaf	17.4	36.	29.
apples	0.5	6.5	11.	lettuce, Romaine	trace	23.	37.
apricots	9.0	13.	10.	molasses*	trace	230.	31.
arugula (rocket)	18.7	160.	52.	mustard greens	10.7	103.	43.
bananas	2.2	5.5	21.	oats, rolled	18.	239.	523.
basil	115.	177.	69.	oranges	13.1	40.	14.
bell pepper,	7.1	9.0	19.	papaya	2.0	24.	5.0
blueberries	9.5	6.0	11.	parsley	900.	138.	56.
brewer's yeast*	84.	0	0	peaches	2.5	3.0	12.
broccoli	1.8	48.	66.	pineapple	2.6	13.	7.5
cabbage	3.0	105.	31.	pumpkin, canned	94.	29.	35.
cantaloupe	0.75	10.	17.	pumpkin seeds	32.	43.	1,174.
carrot root	15.7	27.5	37.	purslane	1.310.	60.	44.
carrot top	492.	1,940.	190.	raisins	6.3	49.	97.
celery	17.7	40.	24.	shepherd's purse	trace	290.	92.
chicory	27.3	100.	47.	soybeans*	1,500.	277.	704.
cilantro	10.	67.	48.	spinach	1,380.	99.	45.
cranberries, dried	6.2	12.	8.0	sunflower seeds	18.9	116.	705.
dandelion greens	24.6	187.	66.	tomato	44.5	10.	24.
dill	114.	208.	66.	walnuts	93.	81.	413.
endive/ escarole	60.	52.	28.	watercress	185.	120.	60.
kale	7.0	135.	56.	wheat/ barleygrass	—	28.	130.

*Used as ingredient in some commercial rabbit foods.

or ATP, which stores energy in the body. Copper also aids in the formation of bone and red blood cells, is involved in the healing of tissues, is necessary for healthy nerves and joints, is important to fetal growth and post-natal development, affects the coloring of skin and hair, and works with zinc and vitamin C to from elastin. The addition of copper to the diet of young rabbits reduces enteritis and diarrhea and increases weight gain. It was found in one study that the supplementation of 0.2% copper acetate to cholesterol-fed rabbits might inhibit the progression of aortic disease.

Signs of a copper deficiency include: anemia in recently weaned rabbit kits, bone abnormalities, decreased growth, dry scaly skin, the graying of genetically black hair, and hair loss. Copper primarily accumulates in the liver, but other tissues that may have high levels are brain, heart, and kidney. Excesses of copper can produce depression, irritability, nervousness and joint and muscular pain in some animals. Too much copper may also lead to low white blood cells.

Foods that contain copper include almonds, barley, beets, broccoli, green leafy vegetables, molasses, oats, oranges, radishes, and raisins.

It is recommended that rabbits have 2.7 mg of copper daily, or feed content of 5–20 ppm or 3 mg/kg of diet, the higher amounts recommended for rabbits between 4–12 weeks and lactating rabbits. Copper must be taken in balance with zinc and vitamin C.

Iodine (I)

Iodine is a non-metallic element. It is required for the synthesis of thyroid hormones and a deficiency can cause goiter and developmental abnormalities. In one study, the addition of potassium iodide to the diet helped prevent atherosclerosis in rabbits when it was given with the high-cholesterol diet. The researchers concluded this was from the iodide and not the potassium because other potassium salts did not have the same effect.

Deficiencies are not common in rabbits, although it has been shown that rabbits fed diets consisting exclusively of plants in the cabbage family develop simple goiter (see Chapter 6, glucosinolates). In rabbits the metabolism of sodium potassium, chlorine, and sulfur are little influenced by iodine deficiencies, but deficiencies do lead to decreases in calcium, magnesium, and phosphorus elimination. Excesses of iodine may be particularly dangerous for young rabbits; supplementation of 250–1000 ppm iodine for 2–5 days has resulted in increased mortality of newborn rabbit kits.

Iodine content is fairly high in green leafy vegetables, provided the vegetables were not grown in iodine-deficient soils. The recommended amount of dietary iodine for rabbits between 4–12 weeks and pregnant or lactating does is 0.2 ppm; for other rabbits it is 0.4–2.0 ppm.

Iron (Fe)
Iron is essential for many enzymes and is particularly important for the production of hemoglobin and myoglobin and the oxygenation of red blood cells. It is also critical to the immune system and protects against heart disease.

A rabbit's liver has a high iron storage capacity and a deficiency is unlikely, although it may occur in kits at weaning and will be evidenced by anemia. Excessive iron results in the production of free radicals and an increased need for vitamin E. In humans, excess iron may increase the incidence of heart disease and cancer, and it was found in one study on rabbits that iron may be more likely to play a role in the promotion of atherosclerosis in rabbits than copper.

Iron is found in many foods, including alfalfa, almonds, brewer's yeast, chickweed, dandelion, dates, green leafy vegetables, peaches, pears, prunes, pumpkin, peppermint, plantain, raisins, raspberry leaves, shepherd's purse, watercress, and whole grains.

It is recommended that adult rabbits receive 36 mg of iron daily, or 30-100 ppm in feed; 50 ppm for young rabbits and pregnant does, 100 ppm for lactating does.

Magnesium (Mg)
Magnesium is a major component of bone, is necessary to prevent the calcification of soft tissues, affects the immune system, is involved in the relaxation of muscles, and may help prevent cardiovascular disease and reduce cholesterol in rabbits. Magnesium is also a cofactor in many enzymes, and is involved in over 300 metabolic reactions. Magnesium is often deficient in diets where drinking water has had the minerals removed.

A deficiency of magnesium in rabbits can cause alopecia, a change in fur texture, fur chewing, loss of fur luster, blanching of ears, edema, poor growth, loss of weight, excitability, myocardial fibrosis, and convulsions. When a rabbit is eating a magnesium-deficient diet, bone apparently serves as a reservoir for the element and bone magnesium levels decrease. Any excess is excreted in urine so toxicity of this mineral does not occur in rabbits.

Magnesium is found in alfalfa, apples, apricots, bananas, brewer's yeast, cantaloupe, chickweed, dandelion, grapefruit, green leafy vegetables, molasses, nuts, parsley, peaches, peppermint, raspberry leaves, red clover, shepherd's purse, watercress, and whole grains. Note: foods high in oxalic acid (see Chapter 6) hinder the absorption of magnesium.

Recommended dieary magnesium for rabbits is 30–40 mg of magnesium sulfate/100 g diet or 5.6 mg/kg of diet.

Manganese (Mn)

Like magnesium, manganese is a constituent of many enzymes. It is also an activator of other enzymes. It is involved in the metabolism of carbohydrates, fat, and protein; is necessary for the synthesis of bone and the formation of cartilage, is involved in blood sugar regulation, is necessary for the utilization of many B-vitamins and vitamin E, and is involved in the healing of wounds. A deficiency of manganese in a rabbits diet (less than 0.3 mg/kg) can cause brittle bones and bone deformities in weanlings (including decreased weight, length, and ash content of bone). An excess of manganese can result in high mortality of newborn kits and abnormal skeletal development.

Manganese is found in blueberries, chickweed, dandelion, green leafy vegetables, legumes such as alfalfa, parsley, pineapple, peppermint, raspberries, red clover, nuts, seeds, and whole grains.

Recommended manganese is 2.5 mg/kg diet for adults and 8.5 mg/kg diet for growing rabbit kits. Other sources recommend 1 mg/day, 8.5 ppm for rabbits between 4–12 weeks, and 2.5 ppm for pregnant or lactating does.

Molybdenum (Mo)

The mineral molybdenum aids in activating some enzymes

and is necessary for nitrogen metabolism and normal cell function. Molybdenum deficiency can lead to mouth and gum disease and increased cancer incidence in some animals. Molybdenum accumulates in the kidneys, and excesses of molybdenum in rabbits induce copper deficiency and anemia, cause diarrhea, result in poor growth of kits, and may cause arthritis and joint and bone deformities. In one study rabbits fed 39 mg of Mo per kg of dry matter had apparent reduced digestibility of crude protein and fiber in the diet and increased free radical generation. In rabbits given a high Mo diet, over half the Mo ingested by a rabbit was excreted in the urine. Mo levels were highest in the kidneys and liver. Testes of rabbit bucks were more affected by high Mo than the female reproductive organs. However, both deficiencies and excesses of Mo are unlikely in rabbits.

Molybdenum is found in legumes such as alfalfa, dark green leafy vegetables, and whole grains

Phosphorus (P)

Phosphorus has an extremely important role in energy metabolism, and is found in phosphoproteins, nucleic acids (RNA and DNA), and phospholipids.

Calcium and phosphorus metabolism is interconnected. Low phosphous in the diet causes increased urinary excretion of calcium. In rabbits dietary P alone does not affect growth, but diets low in calcium *and* phosphorus lead to rickets in kits. In adults, low dietary calcium and phosphorus can cause a lack of fertility, abnormal behavior, and osteomalacia. Because of this interconnection, it is important that rabbits' dietary calcium and phosphorus be in the correct ratio. Ca: P ratios of 1:1–2:1 are recommended. Inverse ratios result in decreased bone density if the dietary P is over one percent.

Grass and hay are not good sources of phosphorus— they normally contain less than 0.4 % of the nutrient. Foods that are good sources of phosphorus include asparagus, wheat bran, brewer's yeast, dried fruits, alfalfa and other legumes, nuts, sunflower and pumpkin seeds, and whole grains. Growing parts of plants have higher phosphorus content than mature ones.

The amount of dietary phosphorus recommended for rabbits is 0.3 % for rabbits 4–12 weeks old, 0.5–0.8 % for lactating does, 0.37–0.5 % for pregnant does, and 0.4–

0.8% for pet rabbits. In one study increasing the phosphorus from 0.07% to 0.17 % resulted in improved calcification of bones.

Potassium (K)
Potassium is necessary for the nervous system, helps regulate heartbeats, helps prevent strokes, and has a role (with sodium) in controlling water balance. Low-potassium diets (less than 0.3%) in rabbits may lead to increased free radical generation, hypertension, and muscular dystrophy, or weakness. Potassium-depleted rabbits' heart muscle has less contractile force. Excessive potassium in the diet (0.8–1.0%) may lead to nephritis.

Good sources of potassium include: apricots, bananas, brewer's yeast, dates, legumes, molasses, nuts, ribwort plantain, raisins, spinach, and whole grains. Wheat straw has about 1% potassium content. Fall switchgrass has 0.95% and spring switchgrass (over-wintered) has 0.06%. As grasses mature the potassium content declines.

Recommended potassium in rabbit diets: 6–7g/kg (0.6–0.7%); higher for lactating does (0.9 %). Higher potassium (more than 0.8%) improves growth in rabbit kits.

Selenium (Se)
Selenium helps regulate the thyroid, is involved in antibody production, may help prevent some tumors, and is a constituent of many important (and several selenium-dependent) enzymes. One researcher concluded that selenium has the ability to retard the onset of progressive aortic disease in rabbits after they had been fed a high-fat diet. According to some sources, selenium does not have a role in the dispersal of peroxides (that is, it does not act as an antioxidant) in rabbits as it does in humans, but the results from some studies (see previous entry on vitamin E) can be interpreted as indicating such effects.

In other mammals a deficiency of selenium can cause sterility, increase the incidence of infections, and result in exhaustion. Excesses of this mineral are toxic and accumulate in the liver, kidneys, and heart.

Although plants do not require selenium, they sometimes absorb it. Good food sources of selenium include alfalfa, brewer's yeast, broccoli, chickweed, molasses, parsley, peppermint, raspberry leaves, and whole grains.

The dietary recommendation for selenium is 0.05 ppm for rabbits.

Silicon (Si)
Silicon is one of the most abundant elements on earth, but it does not occur in its pure form in nature. Instead, this non-metallic element usually occurs as silicates in rocks. Plants take monosilicic acid up from the soil and mammals consume silicon in the plant form of orthosilicic acid. The amount in plants will vary depending upon the type of soil in which they were grown; clays have higher amounts of silicates than sands.

In mammals, silicon is necessary for the formation of collagen in bone and the connective tissues in blood vessels, skin, cartilage, and hair. It also stimulates the immune system, has been found to counteract the effects of aluminum in the body, and has been found to help prevent osteoporosis in humans. In one study the blood vessels of rabbits given silicon were more elastic, and in another a silicon supplement given to rabbits protected against atherogenic plaques in blood vessels.

Silicon also helps wear teeth down properly. In nature the silica content of grasses—which gives them their abrasiveness—is actually a defense *against* being eaten by rabbits and other herbivores. In several studies it has been found that rabbits and other herbivores avoid higher-silica content grasses, and that grasses even increase their silica content in response to grazing by herbivores. In one study, a small increase in the amount of silica reduced consumption by rabbits over 50 percent.

Sodium (Na) and Chlorine (Cl)
Sodium regulates cellular pH (including blood pH), and water balance. The level of sodium affects the absorption of methioline, cysteine, and other amino acids in the gut. In one study on rabbit diets differing only in naCl content, researchers found that decreasing NaCl from 0.5% to 0.2% led to less protein absorbed in the gut.

TABLE 5:4 Mineral content of selected rabbit foods, expressed as mg or mcg per 100 grams of food. Because of the scarcity of published values, iodine content is not listed. Ca and P ar listed in Table 5:3. Actual nutrient contents of foods may vary considerably from listed values due to varying growing and storage conditions, among other factors. *Values compiled from multiple sources.*

	Co mcg	Cu mg	Fe mg	Mg mg	Mn mg	Mo mcg	K mg	Se mcg	Si mg	Zn mg
alfalfa sprouts	—	0.18	0.9	25.7	0.26	30.	78.3	0.6	—	0.9
almonds	6.3	1.11	4.3	275.	2.5	25.0	728.	2.8	3.11	3.36
apples	0.1	0.027	0.12	5.0	0.035	8.0	107.	0	1.21	0.04
apricots	3.46	0.078	0.39	10.	0.077	14.	259.	0.1	1.1	0.2
arugula	—	0.076	1.46	46.	0.321	—	309.	0.3	2.78	0.47
bananas	0.18	0.078	0.26	28.	0.27	0	358.	1.0	4.77	0.15
barley	—	0.498	3.6	133.	1.94	52.	452.	37.7	—	2.77
basil	—	0.385	3.17	64.	1.15	—	295.	0.3	1.4	0.81
blue-berries	—	0.057	0.28	5.5	0.336	0	77.	0.1	—	0.16
brewer's yeast*	54.7	3.0	3.3	96.	—	115.	1899.	189.	—	4.5
broccoli	10.1	0.045	0.88	25.0	0.229	53.	325.	3.0	0.78	0.4
cabbage, raw	—	0.021	0.67	14.5	0.16	56.	220.	0.5	0.53	0.18
canta-loupe	—	0.041	0.21	12.	0.041	16.	267.	0.3	1.82	0.18
carrot root	0.4	0.017	0.44	15.5	0.155	22.	235.	0.7	0.10	0.2
carrot tops	—	0.002	0.054	—	0.044	27.	407.	—	—	0.027
celery	—	0.35	0.20	11.	0.103	12.	260.	1.5	0.29	0.13
cherries	—	0.35	0.85	9.0	0.076	4.	127.	0	1.03	0.07
chicory	—	0.295	0.9	30.	0.429	—	420.	0.3	1.3	0.42
cilantro	—	0.225	1.77	26.	0.426	—	471.	0.09	8.42	0.50
dry cran-berries	—	0.08	0.53	5.0	0.265	0	40.	0.5	—	0.11
dande-lion leaf	—	0.171	3.1	36.0	0.342	—	397.	0.5	—	0.41
dates, dried	—	0.362	0.90	54.	0.286	—	696.	1.9	16.6	0.39
dill	—	0.146	6.59	55.	1.264	—	738.	—	2.4	0.91
endive/escarole	—	0.099	0.83	15.	0.42	22.	314.	0.2	—	0.79

	Co mcg	Cu mg	Fe mg	Mg mg	Mn mg	Mo mcg	K mg	Se mcg	Si mg	Zn mg
kale	__	0.29	1.7	34.	0.77	0	447.	0.9	__	0.4
lamb's quarters	0.4	0	0.9	28.5	0.6	__	381.	0.9	1.81	0.3
lettuce, leaf	1.03	0.029	0.86	13.	0.25	0	194.	0.6	1.1	0.18
lettuce, romaine	1.02	0.048	0.97	14.6	0.155	0	247.	0.4	0.58	0.23
molasses*	2.45	0.5	5.3	272.	1.7	15.	1644.	20.	3.0	0.33
mustard greens	__	0.147	1.46	32.	0.48	__	354.	0.9	1.3	0.20
oats, rolled	1.56	0.626	4.72	177.	4.9	115.	429.	0	11.39	3.97
oranges	0.15	0.059	0.13	10.	0.033	9.0	237.	0.7	0.2	0.09
papaya	__	0.017	0.12	10.	0.013	__	310.	0.6	__	0.08
parsley	__	0.149	6.2	50.	0.16	__	554.	0.1	0.64	1.07
peaches	0.26	0.063	0.27	5.5	0.09	0.1	190.	0.3	0.64	0.09
pineapple	0.3	0.099	0.28	13.	1.17	0	115.	0.1	3.93	0.1
pumpkin canned	2.55	0.107	1.39	23.	0.149	20.	206.	0.4	__	0.17
pumpkin seeds	__	1.38	14.97	53.5	3.3	__	807.	5.6	__	7.46
purslane	__	0.410	1.99	68.	0.303	__	494.	0.9	__	0.17
raisins	1.0	0.318	1.64	33.	0.26	13.	749.	0.6	8.91	0.2
soybeans*	__	1.7	15.7	280.	2.52	225.	1797.	17.8	2.49	4.9
spinach	__	0.130	2.71	79.	0.897	20.	558.	0.9	5.0	0.53
sunflr seeds	19.8	2.0	6.77	354.	2.02	__	689.	59.5	__	5.06
tomato	1.8	0.069	0.31	11.	0.15	6.0	237.	0.4	2.11	0.17
walnuts,	5.6	1.36	3.12	201.	3.89	0	491.	11.9	10.98	3.37
watercress	__	0.077	0.20	21.	0.241	0	330.	0.9	59.5	0.11
wheat bran	11.1	0.918	27.93	278.	9.03	127.	947.	8.0	17.	12.93
wheatgrass	3.3	0.261	2.14	53.0	1.858	42.	130.-146.	42.5	__	1.65

* Used as ingredient in some commercial rabbit foods.

Low levels of sodium chloride can also lead to decreased milk production in does and the possible loss of renal concentrating ability. Excess sodium consumed from the salt sodium chloride (NaCl) may stunt growth in young rabbits.

The recommended sodium in a rabbit's diet is 1.6–2.6 g/kg of dry matter or 0.2–0.25%. The recommended about of chlorine is 1.7–3.2g/kg or 0.17–0.32% of the rabbit's diet. If provided as the salt sodium chloride, 0.5–1.0% in feeds is recommended.

Zinc (Zn)

Zinc is yet another mineral that is involved in many enzymatic reactions. It is involved in the regulation of glands and the immune system; it helps protect the liver, is involved in the formation of collagen and the growth of reproductive organs, and helps wounds heal faster, including burns. In one study on rabbits it was found that supplemental zinc (1 g/kg) could potentially slow the development of atherosclerosis, although it did not significantly alter the total plasma cholesterol levels.

Deficiency of zinc in rabbit diets may result in reduced feed consumption, stunted growth, weight loss, graying of dark hair, loss of hair, dermatitis, sores around the mouth, wet matted hair on the jaw, frequent Pasteurella infections, smaller testes in bucks and a failure to ovulate in does. An excess can depress the immune system. Too much zinc also interferes with copper availability.

Zinc is found in alfalfa and other legumes, chickweed, dandelion, parsley, pumpkin, sunflower seeds, and whole grains. Plants with high phytic acid content may reduce zinc bioavailability.

Recommended dietary zinc for rabbits: 20-50 ppm for growing rabbits; 70-120 ppm for pregnant, lactating, and adult rabbits. Diets of 1.5 mcg/g diet have been shown to induce deficiency symptoms.

DRUG AND NUTRIENT INTERACTIONS
BY KATHY SMITH

Most people reading this book probably know that antibiotics can upset the balance of beneficial bacteria in the GI tract. But are you aware that most drugs we take (or give our animals) also rob the body of one or more essential nutrients? In fact, nutrient depletion may be the underlying explanation for many drug side effects. I first became aware of this fact three years ago when I picked up the book *Drug Muggers* by Suzy Cohen, RPh.

Drugs can create nutrient imbalances in a number of different ways. Medications can bind to specific nutrients in the GI tract, preventing them from being absorbed into the bloodstream. They may stimulate or inhibit enzymes, interfering with how these enzymes would normally activate nutrients, transport them around the body, and/or transform them into usable substances. Drugs can also change the acidity of the gastrointestinal or urinary tract and alter the body's ability to absorb, break down, and eliminate toxic compounds. Some medications require the presence of specific nutrients to work properly and/or to avoid toxicity while others become less effective when taken with certain minerals.

In addition to *Drug Muggers*, there are several great online resources (listed below) on the subject of drugs and nutrient depletion. Some talk broadly about classes of drugs like NSAIDs (e.g meloxicam) or fluoroquinolone antibiotics (Baytril® is one of these) while others list only the specific drugs like Levaquin® and Cipro® (both fluoroquinolone antibiotics like Baytril) where studies of nutrient depletion have been run and results documented. In the remainder of this section, I will list some of the medications I have personally given rabbits over the years and **possible** nutritional depletions that might be caused by them, based on these resources. While my list is derived from the resources listed below, it will **not** exactly match the information from any single resource.

I do not recommend giving supplements to a rabbit already taking medication(s) unless specifically instructed to do so by your veterinarian. Proper dosing would be difficult to determine and the added stress of giving more medicine would probably outweigh any benefits, even if dosing were perfect. What I do suggest is that if you are giving medications, check this section for possible nutritional deficiencies, offer a selection of foods rich in these nutrients, and see if your rabbit willingly eats them. You might also review this book's section on each nutrient to see what symptoms are associated with their deficiency and coax your rabbit a bit harder if you see any of these conditions start to develop.

Antibiotics

All antibiotics may deplete thiamine (B_1), riboflavin (B_2), niacin (B_3), pantothenic acid (B_5), pyridoxine (B_6), biotin (B_7), cyanocobalamine (B_{12}), and vitamin K.

Fluoroquinolones (all drugs whose generic name ends with "floxacin," including enrofloxacin, better known as Baytril) may also deplete calcium, iron, magnesium, and zinc. Levaquin and Cipro, potent human fluoroquinolones, have also been shown to deplete folate (B_9), potassium, Vitamins C and D, and CoQ10.

Tetracyclines (generic names ending in "cycline") may also deplete calcium and magnesium. Some drugs in this class also deplete folate (B_9), iron, potassium, Vitamins C and D, and CoQ10. In addition, humans are cautioned against taking calcium, iron, magnesium, or zinc supplements within an hour of taking tetracyclines as these minerals may bind to the drug, reducing its effectiveness. To be on the safe side, if your bunny is on a tetracycline antibiotic, avoid offering foods rich in these minerals within the one-hour window of giving your bunny his medicine.

Trimethoprim-containing antibiotics, including the trimethoprim sulfa often prescribed for bunnies, may also deplete folate (B_9). Some sulfa drugs also deplete calcium, iron, magnesium, potassium, Vitamins C and D, and CoQ10.

Penicillins (generic names ending in "cillin;" only injectable forms are safe for bunnies) may also deplete potassium. Some penicillins also deplete folate (B_9), calcium, iron, magnesium, Vitamins C and D, and CoQ10.

Aminoglycosides, such as gentamicin and amikacin, may cause imbalances of magnesium, calcium and potassium.

NSAIDs (non-steroidal anti-inflammatory drugs)

Metacam® (meloxicam), an NSAID, is the medication most commonly given our bunnies to relieve pain and inflammation. Other NSAIDs include Rimadyl® (carprofen), ibuprofen, and naproxen. Drugs in this class may deplete iron, zinc, all B-vitamins (especially folate or B_9), and Vitamin C. Some NSAIDs may also deplete calcium, magnesium, and potassium.

Heart Medications

Atenolol is a beta blocker which may deplete CoQ10. Avoid excessive potassium with this medication, so give banana to your rabbit sparingly.

Enalapril, an ACE inhibitor, can contribute to zinc deficiency. It can also deplete calcium, magnesium, and CoQ10. Iron can decrease absorption of this drug, reducing efficacy, so offer iron-rich foods between doses rather than as a reward for taking enalapril. Avoid excessive potassium with this medication, so give banana sparingly.

Lasix® (furosemide), a diuretic, may deplete potassium, magnesium, calcium, and, if used long term, Thiamine (B_1). It can also rob the body of folate (B_9), iron, niacin (B_3), and CoQ10

Acid Blockers

Either Pepcid® (famotidine) or Zantac® (ranitidine) will sometimes be recommended to help protect the GI tract during an extended bout of GI upset. Both drugs can deplete Thiamine (B_1), folate (B_9), Cyanocobalamine (B_{12}), calcium, iron, Vitamin D, and zinc.

Other GI Medications

Carafate® (sucralfate), is a potentially life-saving drug if ulcers are suspected. However, it can deplete calcium and phosphorus and can bind to both magnesium and calcium supplements. Calcium and magnesium-rich foods should be given between doses rather than as a reward for taking sucralfate.

Questran® (cholestyramine) is occasionally given to help remove toxins produced by an overgrowth of harmful bacteria in the GI tract. Questran must be given with large amounts of oral liquid and although it is considered safe because it is not absorbed by the body, it can deplete numerous nutrients includingfolate (B_9), Cyanocobalamine (B_{12}), calcium, iron, Vitamins A, D, E, and K, carotenoids, lycopene, omega-3 fatty acids, and CoQ10.

Reglan® (metoclopramide) is one of the two main GI motility drugs commonly prescribed for rabbits suffering GI stasis. In general, Reglan may interfere with absorption of nutrients in the intestines. No information is available on the second motility drug, cisapride, probably because it was withdrawn from the human market several years ago.

Simethicone, given to treat gas, is the only drug I researched and found the statement that it has "no known nutrient depletions." But there are other concerns with simethicone products. If you are giving simethicone and symptoms are not improving (or are worsening), try switching to a brand with **different** inactive ingredients.

Inactive Ingredients

Nearly all drugs contain "inactive ingredients" and not all inactive ingredients are benign. For example, most, if not all, brands of simethicone, both infant and adult formulations, will have one of the sugar alcohols (maltitol, xylitol, sorbitol, or another ingredient ending with "itol") or an artificial sweetener (aspartame, saccharin, sucralose, etc.) in its list of inactive ingredients. This is important because common reactions to sugar alcohols include abdominal pain, bloating, and gas. Armed with this knowledge and depending on how you feel about the safety of artificial sweeteners, as you read the labels for simethicone products you may have trouble finding one you are completely comfortable with. Ironically, I would be thrilled to find a formulation of simethicone sweetened with sugar! When choosing a brand of simethicone, read the labels and look for fewer inactive ingredients rather than the lowest price.

Both prescription and over the counter (OTC) medications contain inactive ingredients. Minimally, liquid medications will probably contain flavoring and/or sweeteners and tablets will contain binding agents. Compounded medications, including the flavored liquid Baytril that some veterinarians use and cisapride, may have even more inactive ingredients. If your rabbit is on a medication and you suspect he is having a **mild** reaction, it could be to inactive ingredients rather than the drug itself. If staying on the medication is important to your rabbit's health, discuss with your veterinarian trying a different formulation. If you are using a compounded or other liquid medication, ask if there is a tablet that you can dissolve in tap water just before dosing. If you are comfortable giving injections, the injectable form of many medications often has the fewest (and most benign) inactive ingredients.

For human OTC medications, inactive ingredients are printed on the box, but not the bottle inside the box. For human prescription medications, a Google search on the drug name along with the words "inactive ingredients" should lead you to at least one site (often the manufacturer's) that list those ingredients. Unfortunately, the same search for the veterinary-only medications Baytril and Metacam yielded the information, "No inactive ingredients found." If you have concerns about a veterinary-only medication's inactive ingredients, ask your veterinarian if he or she has (or can get) that information, or try contacting the manufacturer directly.

References:
http://www.nutritional-solutions.net/images/phocadownload/Rx_DepleteInteractions.pdf

http://pennstatehershey.adam.com/content.aspx?productId=107&pid=33&gid=000196

http://www.chiro.org/nutrition/ABSTRACTS/Nutrient_Depletion.shtml
http://www.lifeextension.com/magazine/2006/3/report_drugs/Page-01
http://naturaldatabase.therapeuticresearch.com

http://nutritionreview.org/2013/04/practical-guide-avoiding-drug-induced-nutrient-depletion/

Drug Muggers by Suzy Cohen, RPh, Rosedale Books, 2011

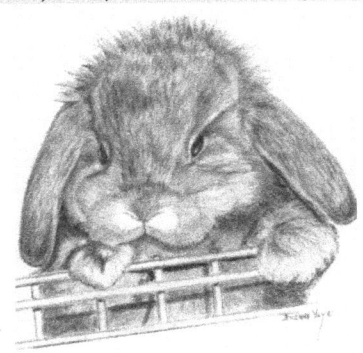

Chapter References

Abdel-Khalek, A. M., N. A. Selim, Sh. A. El-Medany, and S. A. Nada. 2008. Response of Doe Rabbits to Dietary Antioxidant Vitamins E and C During Pregnancy and Lactation. *Proceedings:* 9th World Rabbit Congress, Verona, Italy.

Abdel-Monem, H. Qar, and R. A. Attwa. 2012. Detoxification of Dietary Diazinon by Clay, Vitamin C and Vitamin E in Rabbits. *World App. Sci. J.* 19(1): 144-152.

Abou-Khalil, S., R. Poulson, M.B. Sternermen, S. Moore, and M.Z. Alavi. 1997. Vitamin B_{12} Inhibits Progression of Hypercholesterolemia and Atherosclerosis in Rabbits Fed a High Cholesterol Diet. *MJM* 3: 12-18.

Adu, O. A. and G. N. Egbunke. 2009. Enhancing Growing Rabbits Performance with Diets Supplemented with Copper. *Adv. Biol. Res.* 3(5): 179-184.

Aikawa, J. K., J. Z. Reardon, and D. R. Harms. 1962. Effect of a Magnesium-Deficient Diet on Magnesium Metabolism in Rabbits: A Study with Mg 281, 2. *J. Nutr.* 76: 90-93.

Al-Jawad, F. H., R. A. M. Al-Razzuqi, Z. A. Al-Ebady, and T. A. M. Al-Razzuqi. 2012. Nephroprotective effect of Corn Silk extract on oxalic acid-induced nehprocalcinois in rabbit model. *J. Intercult. Ethnopharmacol.* 1(2): 75-78.

Al-Sayer, H., H. M. Dashti, A. A. Al-Bader, R. L. Bang, and A. B. Mattappallil. 2007. Serum zinc, selenium, manganese and magnesium in zinc-altered diet and burn wound healing. *Trace Elements and Electrolytes.* Accessed March 12, 2010 at: http://www.britannica.com/bps/additionalcontent/18/25762654/Serum-zinc-selenium-manganese-and-magnesium

Arrington, L.R., R.N. Taylor, Jr., C.B. Ammerman and R.L. Shirley. 1965. Effects of Excess Dietary Iodine upon Rabbits, Hamsters, Rats, and Swine. *J. Nutr.* 87:394-398.

Baumann, E. J., S. Kurland, and N. Metzger. 1931. Mineral metabolism during involution of simple goiter. *J. Biol. Chem.* 94(2): 383-391.

Bayo, N. O., O. D. Eyarefe, and R. O. A. Arowolo. 2010. Effects of Tahitian Noni Juice on Ketamine Anaesthesia in Some Local Rabbits. *Br. J. Pharmacol. Toxicol.* 1(2): 81-84.

Bentley, P. J. and B. R. Grubb. 1991. Effects of a zinc-deficient diet on tissue zinc concentration in rabbits. *J. Anim. Sci.* 69: 4876-4882.

Bersenyi, A., E. Berta, I. Kadar, R. Glavits, M. Szilagyi, and S.G. Fekete. 2009. Effects of high dietary molybdenum in rabbits. *Acta Veterin. Hung.* 56(1): 1588-2705.

Bersenyi, A., S. Fekete, I. Hullar, I. Kadar, M. Szliagy, R. Glavits, M. kulcsar, L. Zoldag, and M. Mezes. 1999. Study of the soil-plant (carrot)-animal cycle of nutritive and hazardous minerals in a rabbit model. *Acta Veterin. Hungar.* 47(2): 181-190.

Broadhurst, L. C. Silicon's Elemental Benefits. Accessed 7/31/10 at: http://prolithic.com/hpages/ref_cocs/orthosil.html

Brommage, R., S. Miller, C. Langman, R. Bouillon, R. Smith, and J. Bourdeau. 1988. The effects of chronic vitamin D deficiency on the skeleton in the adult rabbit. *Bone* 9(3): 131–139.

BSAVA Manual of Rabbit Medicine and Surgery. Second edition. 2006. Edited by Anna Meredith and Paul Flecknell. Glouster: British Small Animal Veterinary Association.

Burke, D. S., C. R. Smidt, and L. T. Vuong. 2005. *Momordica cochinchinensis, Rosa roxburghii,* wolfberry, and sea buckthorn- highly nutritional fruits supported by tradition and science. *Current Topics Nutraceut. Res.* 3(4): 259-266.

Chamorro, S., M. S. Gomez-Conde, C. Centeno, R. Carabano, and J. C. DeBlas. 2007. Effect of dietary sodium on digestibility of nutrients and performance in growing rabbits. *World Rab. Sci.* 15: 141–146.

Cheeke, Peter R. 2010. Nutritional Management of Rabbits and Principles of Rabbit Nutrition. Notes, 2010 ARBA National Convention

Cheeke, Peter R. 1987. *Rabbit Feeding and Nutrition.* Orlando: Academic Press.

Clauss, M., B. Burger, A. Liesegang, F. del Chicca, M. Kaufmann-Bart, B. Riond, M. Hassig, J. M. Hatt. 2012. Influence of diet on calcium metabolism, tissue calcification and urinary sludge in rabbits (*Oryctolagus cuniculus*). *J. Anim. Phys. Anim. Nutr.* 96(5): 798-807.

Cotterill, J. V., R. W. Watkins, C.B. Brennan, and D.P. Cowan. 2006. Boosting silica levels in wheat leaves reduces grazing by rabbits. *Pest Manage. Sci.* 63(3): 247–253.

DalleZotte, A., M. Culleve, A. Sartori, A. DalBosco, Z. Gerencser, Z. Matica, M. Kovas, and Z. Szendro. 2014. Effect of dietary supplementation of spirulina (Arthrospira platensis) and thyme (Thymus vulgaris) on carcass composition, meat physical traits, and vitamin B12 content in growing rabbits. *World Rab. Sci.* 22(1).

Dr. Duke's phytochemical and Ethnobotanical Databases. Http://www.ars-grin.gov/duke/

Eckermann-Ross, C. 2008. Hormonal Regulation and Calcium Metabolism in the Rabbit. *N. Am. Exotic An. Pract.* 11(1): 139–152.

Ellis, G. H., S. E. Smith, and E. M. Gates. 1947. Further studies of manganese deficiency in the rabbit. *J. Nutr.* 34:21–31.

Epstein, S. P., Y. Y. Pashinsky, D. Gershon, I. Winicov, C. Srivilasa, K. J. Kristic, and P. A. Asbell. 2006. Efficacy of topical cobalt chelate CTC-96 against adenovirus in a cell culture model and against adenovirus kertoconjunctivitis in a rabbit model. *BMC Opthal.* 6(22): 1471-2415.

Evans, C. L. 1964. Cobalt compounds as antidotes for hydrocyanic acid. *Br. J. Pharmacol. Chemother.* 23(3): 455-475.

Fortun-Lamothe, L. and S. Boullier. 2004. Interactions between gut microflora and digestive mucosal immunity, and strategies to improve digestive health in young rabbits. *Proceedings:* 8th World Rabbit Congress, Puebla.

Fortun-Lamothe, L. and F. Drouet-Viard. 2002.Review: II—Diet and Immunity: Current State of Knowledge and Research Prospects for the Rabbit. *World Rab. Sci.* 10(1): 25-39.

Fraser, G. E. 2009. Nut consumption, lipids, and risk of a coronary event. *Clinical Cardiol.* 22(S3): 11-15.

Fraser, M. and S. J. Gerling. 2009. *Rabbit Medicine and Surgery for Veterinary Nurses.* Chichester: Wiley-Blackwell.

Garrido-Maraver, M. D. Cordero, M. Oropesa-Avila, A. F. Vega, M. de la Mata, A. D. Pavon, M. deMiguel, C. P. Calero, M. V. Paz, D. Cotan, and J. A. Sanchez—Alcazar. 2014. Coenzyme Q10 Therapy. *Mol. Syndromol.* 5(3-4): 1-68. Accessed 3/24/16 at www.ncbi.nlm,nih.gov./pmc/articles/p

Gilsanz, V., T. F. Roc, J. Antunes, M. Carlson, M. L. Duarte and W. G. Goodman. 1991. Effect of dietary calcium on bone density in growing rabbits. *Am. J. Physiol. Endocrinol. Metab.* 260(3): E471–E476.

Harbers, L. H., S. L. Callahan, and G. M. Ward. 1980. Release of calcium oxalate crystals from alfalfa in the digestive tracts of domestic and zoo animals. *J. Zoo An. Med.* 11(2): 52–56.

Harcourt-Brown, F. M. 1996. Calcium deficiency, diet and dental disease in pet rabbits. *Vet. Record* 139(23): 567–571.

Harcourt Brown, Frances. 2002. *Textbook of Rabbit Medicine.* Oxford: Butterworth Heinemann.

Harkness, John E., Patricia V. Turner, Susan VandeWoude, and Colette L. Wheler. 2010. *The Biology of Rabbits and Rodents.* Singapore: Blackwell Publishing.

Hokin, B., M. Adams, J. Ashton, and H. Louie. 2004. Analysis of cobalt in Australian foods. *Asia Pac. J. Clin. Nutr.* 13(3): 284–288.

Hove, E. L. and D. H. Copeland. 1954. Progressive muscular dystrophy in rabbits as a result of chronic choline deficiency. *J. Nutr.* 57(3): 391–405.

Hove, E. L., D. H. Copeland, J. F. Herndon, and W. D. Salmon. 1957. Further studies on choline deficiency and muscular dystrophy in rabbits. *J. Nutr.* 63(2): 289–299.

Howe, J. C., J. R. Williams, and J. M. Holden. 2004. USDA Database for the Choline Content of Common Foods. Nutrient Data Laboratory, Agricultural Research Service, USDA.

Hunt, J. W., A. P. Dean, R. E. Webster, G. N. Johnson, and A. R. Ennos. 2008. A Novel Mechanism by which Silica Defends Grasses against Herbivory. *Ann. Bot.* 102(4): 653–656.

Hydery, T., J. C. Schuler, R. E. Leggett, and R. Levin. 2009. Treatment of Obstructive Bladder Dysfunction in Rabbits with Coenzyme Q10 and Alpha Lipoic Acid. *LUTS: Lower Urinary Tract Sympt.* 1(2): 98-102.

Jenkins, J. R. 2010. Evaluation of the Rabbit Urinary Tract. *J. Exo. Pet Med.* 19(4): 271-279.

Jenner, A., R. Minqin, R. Rajendran, N. Pan, B. T. K. Huat, F. Watt, and B. Halliwell. 2007. Zinc supplementation inhibits lipid peroxidation and the development of atherosclerosis in rabbits fed a high cholesterol diet. *Free Rad. Biol. Med.* 42(4): 559–566.

Johnson, Dam. 2009. Rabbit calcium metabolism, "bladder sludge," and urolithiasis (Proceedings). Accessed 8/21/10 http://veteromarycalendar.dvm360.com/avhc/content/printContentPo pup.jsp?id=648133

Joseph, C. E., S. H. Ashrafi, and J. P. Waterhouse. 1981. Structural Changes in Rabbit Oral Epithelium Caused by Zinc Deficiency. *J. Nutr.* 111: 53–57.

Joythi, B. A., K. Venkatesh, P. Chakrapani, and A. R. Rani. 2011. Phytochemical and Pharmacological Potential of *Annona cherimola*—A Review. *Int. J. Phytomed.* 3: 439-447.

Juan, Y-S., T. Hydery, and A. Manjkaro. 2008. Coenzyme Q10 protects against ischemia/reperfusion induced biochemical and functional changes in rabbit urinary bladder. *J. Mole. And Cell. Biochem.* 311(1-2): 73-80.

King, J. L., R. J. Miller, J. P. Blue, Jr., W. D. O'Brien, Jr., and J. W. Erdman, Jr. 2009. Inadequate dietary magnesium intake increases atherosclerotic plaque development in rabbits. *Nutr. Res.* 29(5): 343–349.

Kubola, J. and S. Siriamornpun. 2011. Phytochemicals and antioxidant activity of different fruit factions (peel, pulp, aril and seed) of thai gac (*Momordica cochinchinensis* Spreng.). *Food Chem.* 127: 1138-1145

Lamb, D. J., G. L. Reeves, A. Taylor, and G. A. Ferns. 1999. Dietary copper supplementation reduces atherosclerosis in the cholesterol-fed rabbit. *Athero.* 146(1): 33–43.

Lebas, F. 2004. Reflections on Rabbit Nutrition with a Special emphasis on Feed Ingredients Utilization. *Proceedings*: 8th World Rabbit Congress, Puebla.

Lebas, F. 2000. Vitamins in Rabbit Nutrition: Literature review and recommendations. *World Rab. Sci.*8(4): 185–192.

Lee, J. C., V. A. Rowe, C. D. Thatcher, D. P. Sponenberg, and G. K. Saunders. 1988. High dietary NaCl increases cholesterol and coronary atherosclerosis in cholesterol-fed rabbits. *Nutr. Res.* 8(4): 413–419.

Libert, B. and V. R. Franceschi. 1987. Oxalate in crop plants. *J. Agri. Food Chem.* 35(6): 926–938.

Linus Pauling Institute at Oregon State University. Website: http://lpi.oregonstate.edu/

Loeper, J., J. Goy-Loeper, L. Rozensztajn, and M. Fragny. 1979. The antiatheroscleromatous action of silicon. *Athero.* 33(4): 397–408.

Lowe, J. A. 2010. Pet Rabbit Feeding and Nutrition. In: *Nutrition of the Rabbit*. Second edition. Eds., Carlos DeBlas and Julian Wiseman. Wallingford: CABI Publishing.

McWilliams, D. A. 2001. Nutritional Pathology in Rabbits: Current and Future Perspectives. Paper: Ontario Commercial Rabbit Growers Asso. Congress.

Mahfouz, M. M., Q. Zhou, and F. A. Kummerow. 1994. Cholesterol oxides in plasma and lipoproteins of magnesium-deficient rabbits and effects of their lipoproteins on endothelial barrier function. *Magnes. Res.* 7(3-4): 207-222.

Martorelli, J., D. Bailon, N. Majo, and A. Andaluz. 2012. Lateral approach to nephrotomy in the management of unilateral renal calculi in a rabbit (*Oryctolagus cuniculus*). *AVMA* 240(7): 863-868.

Massey, F. P. and S. E. Hartley. 2006. Experimental demonstration of the antiherbivore effects of silica in grasses: impacts on foliage digestibility and vole growth rates. *Proc. Biol. Sci.* 273: 2299–2304.

Massey, F. P., M. J. Smith, X. Lambin, and S. E. Hartley. 2009. Are silica defenses in grasses driving vole population cycles? *Biol. Lett.* 4(4): 419–422.

Mateos, G. G., P. G. Rebollar, and C. de Blas. 2010. Minerals, Vitamins, and Additives. *In: Nutrition of the Rabbit.* Second edition. C. De Blas and J. Wiseman, eds. Wallingford: CABI Publishing.

Matsumoto, S., R. E. Leggett, and R. Levin. 2003. The effect of vitamin E on the response of rabbit bladder smooth muscle to hydrogen peroxide. *Molec. Cell. Biochem* 254(1–2): 347–351.

Mehta, U., B. P. S. Kang, R. S. Kukreja, and M. P. Bansai. 2002. Ultrastructural examination of rabbit aortic wall following high-fat diet feeding and selenium supplementation: a transmission electron microscopy study. *J. Ap. Toxicol.* 22(6): 405–413.

Muller, A., J. Pallauf, and E. Most. 2002. Parameters of dietary selenium and vitamin E deficiency in growing rabbits. *J. Trace El. Med. Biol.* 16(1): 47–55.

Nutrient Requirements of Rabbits. Second revised edition. 1977. National Academy of Science, Washington.

The Nutrition of the Rabbit. 1998. Edited by de Blas and Wiseman. Wallingford: CABI Publishing.

Pitcairn, Richard H. and Susan Hubble Pitcairn. 2005. *Dr. Pitcairn's Complete Guide to Natural Health for Dogs and Cats.* Third edition. Emmaus: Rodale, Inc.

Pitt, M. A. 1976. Molybdenum toxicity: Interactions between copper, molybdenum, and sulphate. *Inflamm. Res.* 6(6): 758–769.

Powell, J. J., S. A. McNaughton, R. Jugdaohsingh, S. H. C. Anderson, J. Dear, F. Khor, L. Mowatt, K. L. Gleason, M. Sykes, R. P. H. Thompson, C. Bolton-Smith, and M. J. Hodson. 2005. A provisional database for the silicon content of foods in the United Kingdom. *Br. J. Nutr.* 94: 804–812.

Raafat, B. M. M. W. Shafaa, R. A. Rizk, A. A. Elgohary, and A. Saleh. 2009. Ameliorating Effects of Vitamin C against Acute Lead Toxicity in Albino Rabbits. *Austrl. J. Bas. App. Sci.* 3(4): 3597–3608.

Rajendran, R., Ren, P. Ning, B. T. K. Huat, B. Halliwell, and F. West. 2006. Promotion of atherogenesis by copper or iron—which is more likely? *Biochem Biophys. Res. Comm.* 353(1): 6–10.

Raloff, J. 1990. Low-magnesium diet may clog heart arteries. *Science News.* Accessed 3/12/2010 at: http://findarticles.com/p/articles/mi_m1200/is_v137/ai_8921909/

Rosell, J. M., R. Garriga, J. Martinez, M. Domingo, and L. F. de la Fuente. 2012. Calcinois in Female Rabbits. *Proceedings:* 10th World Rabbit Congress, Sharm El-Sheikh, Egypt.

Rosenkrantz, H. 1955. Studies in Vitamin E Deficiency I. The oxygen consumption of various tissues from the rabbit. *J. Biol Chem* 214: 789–797.

Saini, R. 2011. Coenzyme Q10: The essential nutrient. *J. Pharmacy &*

Bioallied Sci. 3(3): 466-467.

Samson, R. and B. Mehdi. 1998. Strategies to reduce the ash content in perennial grasses. R.E.A.P. Research Report.

Saunders, Richard A. and Ron Rees Davies. 2005. *Notes on Rabbit Internal Medicine.* Oxford: Blackwell Publishing.

Schwenke, D.C. and S. R. Behr. 1998. Vitamin E combined with selenium inhibits atherosclerosis in hypercholesterolemic rabbits independently of effects on plasma cholesterol concentrations. *Circ. Res.* 83(4): 366–377.

Selim, N. A., A. M. Abdel-Khalek, S. A. Nada, Sh. A. El-Medany. 2008. Response of growing Rabbits to Dietary Antioxidant Vitamins E and C. 1. Effect on Performance. *Proceedings:* 9th World Rabbit Congress, Verona, Italy.

Setiawan, B., A. Sulaeman, G. W. Giraud, and J. A. Driskell. 2001. Carotenoid Content of Selected Indonesian Fruits. *J. Food Comp. Anal.* 14(2): 169-176.

Simnett, K. I. and G. H. Spray. 1965. The effect of a low-cobalt diet on rabbits. *Brit. J. Nutr.* 19: 119–123.

Singh, R. B., N. Shindey, R. K. Chopra, M. K. Niaz, A. S. Thayer, and Z. On. 2000. Effect of coenzyme Q10 on experiemental atherosclerosis and chemical composition and quality of atheroma in rabbit. *Atheroscler.* 148(2): 275-82.

Staggs, C. G., W. M. Sealey, B. J. McCabe, A. M. Teague, and D. M. Mock. 2004. Determination of the biotin content of select foods using accurate and sensitive HPLC/avidin binding. *J. Food Comp. Anal.* 17(6): 767–776.

Stevens, C. E. and I. D. Hume. 1998. Contributions of Microbes in Vertebrate Gastrointestinal Tract to Production and Conservation of Nutrients. *Phys. Rev.* 78(2): 393–427.

Torrey, George. Zeaxanthin May Decrease Your Risk of Macular Degeneration. American Macular Degeneration Foundation. Accessed 9/7/2010 at: http://www.macular.org/nutrition/zeaxan.html

Turner, K.B. 1933. Studies on the prevention of cholesterol atherosclerosis in rabbits. *J. Exp. Med.* 58(1): 115–126.

Umar, K. J., L. G. Hassan, S. M. Dangoggo, and M. J. Ladan. 2007. Nutritional Composition of Water Spinach Leaves. *J. Appl. Sci.* 7: 803-809.

Vahtaer, M. and E. Marafante. 1987. Effects of low dietary intake of methionine, choline, or proteins on the biotransformation of arsenite in rabbits. *Tox. Let.* 37(1): 41–46.

Verma, D. D., W. Hartner, T. Levchenko, and V. Torchilin. 2007. Coenzyme Q10-loaded liposomes effectively protect the myocardium in rabbits with an acute experimental myocardial infarction. *J. Mole. & Cell. Card.* 42: 190-218.

Vreman, H. J., D. Thorning, and M. W. Weiner. 1980. Effects of dietary acetate and bicarbonate on experimental atherosclerosis in rabbits. *Athero.* 35(2): 145–153.

Vuong, L. T., A. A. Franke, L. J. Custer and S. P. Murphy. 2006. *Momordica cochinchinensis* Spreng. (gac) fruit carotenoids reevaluated. *J. Food Comp. Anal.* 19(6-7): 664-668.

Wang, M-Y, B. J. West, C. J. Jensen, D. Nowicki, C. Su, AfaK Palu and G. Anderson. 2002. *Morinda citrifolia* (noni): A literature review and recent advances in Noni research. *Acta Pharmacol. Sin.* 12: 1127-1141.

Ward, J. P. T. 1990. Cardiac muscle function following chronic dietary potassium depletion in the rabbit. *Cardiovas. Res.* 24: 647–652.

Westerfelde, W. W. and D. A. Richert. 1953. Distribution of the xanthine oxidase factor (molybdenum) in foods. *J. Nutr.* 51: 85–95.

White, R. N. 2001. Management of calcium ureterolithiasis in a French lop rabbit. *J. Sm. Anim. Pract.* 42(12): 595-598.

Wiggert, B., D. L.Van Horn, and B. L. Fish. 1982. Effects of vitamin A deficiency on [3H] retinoid-binding proteins in rabbit cornea and conjunctiva. *Exp. Eye Res.* 34(5): 695-702.

Yang, B. C., D. Y. Li, Y. F. Weng, J. Lynch, C. S. Wingo, and J. L. Mehta. 1998. Increased superoxide aninon generation and altered vasoreactivity in rabbits on low-potassium diet. *Am. J. Phys.* 43(6): H1955–H1961.

Yousef, M., G. A. Abdallah, and Kl. Kamel. 2003. Effect of ascorbic acid and Vitamin E supplementation on semen quality and biochemical parameters of male rabbits. *Anim. Repro. Sci.* 76(1): 99-111.

Yousef, M. I., M. H. Salem, K. I. Kamel, G. A. Hassan, and F. D. El-Nouty. 2003. Influence of Ascorbic Acid Supplementation on the Haematological and Clinical Biochemistry Parameters of Male Rabbits Exposed to Aflatoxin B1. *J. Env. Sci. Health Part B* 38(2): 193-209.

Zerrouki, N., F. Lebas, C. Davoust, and E. Corrent. 2008. Effect of mineral blocks addition on fattening rabbit performance. *Proceedings*: 9th World Rabbit Congress, Verona.

Chapter 6

PELLETS, HAY, GRASS, AND MYCOTOXINS

Commercial pelleted feed and hay are arguably the most important components of your rabbit's diet. Pellets provide the concentrated source of nutrition that the rabbit's digestive system needs and hay is an excellent source of the fiber that keeps the rabbit gut functioning. A diet in which either of these two foods is lacking is unlikely to be healthy for your bunny. Small quantities of fresh grass, although not necessary, can add variety and nutrition to a healthy adult rabbit's diet.

Domestic rabbits have different energy needs than their wild cousins, yet researchers who have studied rabbit diet suggest that the proportions of the different nutrients required by wild *Oryctolagus cuniculus* are similar to those required by domestic rabbits. Moreover, it has been found that the health of wild rabbits forced to eat high amounts of less-nutritious high-fiber foods declines and mortality increases. Rabbits, being concentrate selectors, have evolved to need both lower-fiber nutrient-dense foods and less nutritious high-fiber foods.

Rabbits like variety in their diet. There is a biological basis for this preference, and rabbits do best on diets that include a variety of foodstuffs. Even when it comes to fiber, it has been found that the botanical origin of the fiber can influence digestion and the activity of the cecal microflora and that supplying fiber from a single botanical source is not as healthy as supplying it from several sources. There have also been several interesting studies where rabbits were found to have the ability to adjust their diets to consume needed fiber, nutrients, and water. However, rabbits cannot adjust their diet in this manner if they are not provided a variety of feedstuffs that will allow them to make such dietary choices. It should also be noted that some companion rabbits develop strong food preferences and will selectively eat certain foods. These rabbits must sometimes be coaxed to eat a variety of foods by only providing one at a time.

For most domestic rabbits, a diet composed of a good-quality commercial rabbit feed, grass hay, greens, and small amounts of fruit, nuts, seeds, and grains will fulfill their digestive and nutritional needs. The amount of each that should be provided will vary according to the age, sex, breed, environment, and health of the individual rabbit.

Mycotoxins are a danger in nearly all the foods a rabbit might eat, and it is important for those with rabbits to learn the signs of mycotoxin poisoning and what steps they can take to reduce the chances any of their rabbits will consume dangerous amounts of these prevalent toxins.

PELLETS

There are many excellent pelleted rabbit feeds on the market today that provide nutritionally balanced diets for rabbits. The claim by some persons that commercial pellets are made for fattening short-lived production rabbits and are unhealthy for longer-lived rabbits is dated and simply untrue. Note that "Do," a Jersey Wooly rabbit who held the title for oldest living rabbit (2010-2012) in *Guinness World Records*, was fed a diet that consisted exclusively of hay and pellets; no other foods or treats. (He died at 17 years old.) Clearly the diet did not harm Do!

Many commercial pelleted rabbit feeds are specifically created to fulfill the nutritional needs of "companion," "pet," or "show" rabbits. Nor is it true that a pellet-based diet will necessarily lead to overweight rabbits – many show rabbits receive a pellet-based diet, and an overweight show rabbit would not receive any awards! In fact, the judge would most likely disqualify an overweight rabbit and have it removed from the competition.

While it is *theoretically* possible to feed a rabbit a nutritionally complete diet without giving any commercial pellets, it is extremely difficult to do so. It has been estimated by some experts that it would take a precise combination of about 14–17 different vegetables fed in specific amounts in addition to grass hay to provide a rabbit a nutritionally complete diet composed of fresh vegetables and hay alone. Not all of us have time and money to find and purchase such vegetables, nor may they be available in all geographical areas. Not to mention that—rabbits being the selective eaters they are—it would be very difficult, if not impossible, to persuade any one rabbit to consume all 14–17 vegetables every day in the precise amounts required for the rabbit to receive all the necessary nutrients! For most of us, limited by time, money, living place, or a combination of the three, compounded pelleted rabbit feeds provide an easy, relatively inexpensive way to ensure our rabbits receive adequate nutrition.

However, the quality of pelleted feeds does vary. Rabbits may pick out favored items in a feed mix, and usually do better if fed a uniform forage-based pellet with no added grains, dried fruits, or seeds. Such uniform pellets may be produced by pressure or by extrusion. Most compounded pellets on the market are manufactured by compressing the feed ingredient mix at fairly low temperatures. With extruded feeds, the ingredient mixture is cooked and pasteurized, resulting in a feed that is more easily digested and of more uniform nutritional content. Theoretically, the low temperatures at which compressed feeds are manufactured could possibly allow more fungal/bacterial growth than heat-treated extruded feeds. However, most compressed feeds are perfectly safe, and as extruded feeds are usually more expensive, many persons with limited budgets and/or or multiple rabbits may prefer to rely upon compressed feeds.

Kathy Smith, author of *Rabbit Health in the 21st Century*, often uses extruded foods. She explains why she prefers these pellets for many of her rabbits:

Extruded rabbit foods
by Kathy Smith.

Extruded feeds are pasteurized at a high temperature (whereas pellets are compressed at a relatively low temperature). Because of King Murray, years ago I spoke to a nutritionist at Kaytee Products who explained that extruded food (like their Rainbow Exact) is easier to digest than pellets, a statement confirmed in Harcourt-Brown's *Textbook of Rabbit Medicine*. Harcourt-Brown also specifically mentions *extruded* complete food for nutritional support during recovery from GI disorders. Extruded rabbit food has a less brittle texture than pellets and most (though not all) rabbits will eagerly eat it, often considering it a "treat."

Many caregivers have reported improvement in their rabbits with chronic GI problems after switching to an extruded food and it softens nicely if syringe feeding becomes necessary. Some caregivers have also observed that feeding Kaytee Rainbow Exact has helped their rabbits with chronic molar spurs extend the time between dental filings. A few caregivers have reported problems maintaining weight on larger breed rabbits with some extruded food brands, raising the question whether food created using higher heat may destroy some nutrients; other caregivers feel their rabbits gain weight on such a diet. If switching from pellets to an extruded diet, check the label for nutritional analysis and ingredients and compare to what you are currently feeding. Make the change gradually, monitoring your rabbit for changes (good or bad) in appetite, weight, fecal output, and/or cecal production.

Kaytee Rainbow Exact is the only extruded food widely available in the United States. Several brands of extruded food are available in the UK and Canada, and Blue Seal also makes an extruded food that is available in the Eastern US. While most extruded foods are alfalfa based, Martin Mills in Ontario, Canada now offers an extruded timothy-based food.

Resources:
Martin Mills (www.martinmills.com)
Nutritionist at Kaytee (personal communication, 2002)
Harcourt-Brown's *Textbook of Rabbit Medicine*

Should your rabbits have become accustomed to eating feed mixes with items such as seeds and dried fruits, persuading them to accept pellets without such additions may be difficult. Try starting by giving a 50/50 mixture of the accustomed feed with a new uniform pelleted feed. Then resist giving in if the rabbit picks out favorite "bits" and does not want to eat the other food. As the rabbit begins to eat more of the uniform pellets, reduce the amounts of the mixed feed. This process can take considerable time and may end up being a contest between your will and that of your bunny!

Some researchers have found that rabbits do better if concentrate foods are provided twice daily, morning and evening, as this more closely mimics a wild rabbit's eating patterns and is more natural to a rabbit's "gut cycle." For this reason you may wish to give half the pellets in the morning and half in the evening. If you prefer to give the pellets at one time, other nutrient-dense foods such as fresh vegetables can be given at the other end of the day. (For the amounts to feed, see *Free-feeding vs. limited pellets* at the end of this section.)

Finally, any changes in the kind of pellet you give your bunny should be made gradually, mixing a little of the new pellet with the old, gradually adding more and more of the new pellet. This allows rabbit's microflora to adjust to the diet without digestive upset and the rabbit will also be more likely to accept the new pellet. Some rabbits will starve themselves rather than accept abrupt changes in their accustomed diet.

Grass-based vs alfalfa-based pellets

The debate between grass-based feed pellets and alfalfa-based pellets is long-standing and occasionally acrimonious. While some in the rabbit community prefer to feed their rabbits grass-based pellets because of the fat and calcium levels present in alfalfa, many other persons feeds their rabbits alfalfa-based pellets for years with no adverse outcomes. And it should be noted that some grass-based pellets actually have *higher* levels of calcium (and even fat) than some alfalfa-based pellets. It depends upon the specific pellet and is one of the reasons reading feed labels is a must.

There is another issue in the alfalfa versus grass-based pellet debate. While I am aware of no studies that have been done on the subject, some experienced rabbit caretakers have reported that their rabbits are more often affected by mycotoxins (see section on mycotoxins later in this chapter) from grass-based pellets than alfalfa-based pellets. It is my *personal opinion*, based on my personal experiences and anecdotal evidence from others, that there *may* be something to this idea. Yet many rabbit owners feed their rabbits grass-based pellets for years without any of their rabbits becoming affected by symptoms of mycotoxin poisoning. Until the proper studies are carried out to determine whether this difference does in fact exist, and why, it can only be mentioned as a possibility.

While the thought of mycotoxin poisoning is very frightening, a person should realize that the number of rabbits that suffer from mycotoxin poisoning from either grass-based or alfalfa-based pellets is quite small. Although it is necessary to be aware of the risk and to recognize the symptoms of potentially fatal mycotoxin poisoning, most people will be unlikely to see it in their rabbits whether they feed them grass-based or alfalfa-based pellets. It should also be understood that mycotoxins may be present in hay and other foods as well as pelleted feeds, so it is not possible to avoid such poisoning by avoiding giving rabbits commercial feeds.

Reading labels and choosing a pellet

There are many good grass-based and alfalfa-based pellets available on the market, and more expensive does not necessarily mean "better." Nor is it necessary to buy widely known brands—many brands with more limited distribution can be quality products. There are several tips to select a good pellet. First look at the pellet (if you can – some packaging may prevent this). Pellets should be of a uniform green, with no yellowish, brownish, or blackish areas. Pellets should also be firm, not crumbly. Size is important as well; pellets that are larger will be likely to have longer fiber particles. Large amounts of fines and dust are undesirable as well, as the fine particles can potentially cause respiratory problems or be a means of introducing mycotoxins into the rabbit's body. Check the packaging as well—you do not wish to buy any bags that are torn or have evidence of having been wet.

Whether you prefer to feed your rabbits grass-based or alfalfa-based pellets read the label and be sure you are buying a fresh, high-quality product. The first item that should be checked is the date because pellets only maintain optimal nutrition for about 3-6 months. (The fat-soluble vitamins A, D, and E may have a shelf-life of only 3 months.) Smaller sacks may move faster and have better dates. The date may be located on the ingredient label or be found elsewhere on bag.

After the date, the next thing that should be examined is the *guaranteed analysis* on the feed tag. This part of the feed tag tells you how much of various critical nutrients are in the feed, usually by percentage. The *crude protein* (total protein calculated from the total nitrogen present) minimum is often listed first, and should be between 13–17% for most rabbits (too much protein for rabbits not needing it can lead to excessive cecotroph production and high ammonia in the cecum and urine. These last could possibly result in toxic body levels and respiratory problems. Long-haired rabbits, large rabbits, rabbits kept outside, and lactating does need higher protein, from 17–20 percent. It is recommended that young rabbit kits (between 3–9 weeks) be given pellets with a crude protein content of 12–13% to help prevent potentially fatal digestive disorders.

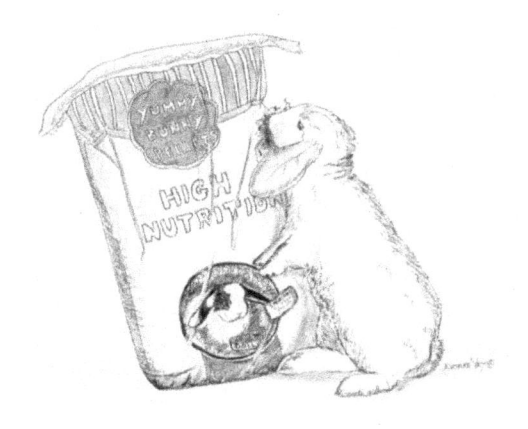

    Fat content is often listed as crude fat minimum (meaning it might have more fat but not less). Many experts cite values of 1–5 % is acceptable for crude fat, and levels as high as 8% can be acceptable for angora and large breeds. Fat also increases the palatability of pellets, especially of high-fiber pellets, and helps reduce their dustiness. Crude fiber (indigestible plant material) is often listed by both minimum and maximum. The minimum in a good feed should be at least 16–18%; 20% is best for the maximum. It is often recommended that very young rabbit kits (between 3 and 9 weeks of age) be given pellets containing 20–25% crude fiber. Calcium is often also listed with both minimum and maximum amounts. A minimum of around 0.6%, and a maximum of about 1.1% is acceptable unless the rabbit has a special need for a low-calcium feed. Phosphorus is usually listed as minimum (0.4% is acceptable). Salt as may be listed with both minimum (0.5%) and maximum (1.0%) content. Vitamin A, an important vitamin added most feeds, may be listed in the guaranteed analysis and will likely be about 4500–5000 international units (IU) per pound of feed. Vitamin D should not be supplemented in amounts over 2000 IU (see Chapter 5).

After the guaranteed analysis, the actual *ingredients* of the pellet will be listed in order with the ingredient present in the highest amount listed first. If the pellet is alfalfa-based, you might expect the ingredient list to start with "dehydrated alfalfa meal," but may be surprised to find the term "forage products." Feed manufacturers are allowed to use what are called "collective" or "group" terms. It has been claimed that only lesser-quality feeds list group terms, and that this is done as a cost cutting measure so manufacturers can use lower-quality ingredients. This is not necessarily true; many reputable feed manufacturers use the terms in order to be able to produce a nutritionally consistent product. The nutritional quality of any feed ingredient can vary greatly, depending upon multiple factors, and using the group terms allows manufacturers to keep the nutrition of the product the same without having to constantly re-label (and raise the price).

Although these group terms are more often seen on the ingredient tags for other livestock feeds, some rabbit feeds may also use these terms, and it is a good idea to familiarize yourself with them. Following is a list of several collective terms and what food products may be included (in varying quantities) in that group:

- *Forage products*: alfalfa meal, grass hay, soybean hay, lespedeza (legume related to clover) meal, dehydrated silages.

- *Grain products*: barley, oats, wheat, corn, rice, and/or rye.

- *Processed grain by-products*: wheat millings, corn gluten feed, rice bran, wheat bran, brewers and distillers dried grains.

- *Plant protein products*: cottonseed meal, soybean meal, canola meal, peanut meal, sunflower meal, linseed meal, soybean, and cultured yeast.

- *Animal protein products*: hydrolyzed poultry feathers, fish meal, milk products, and other items not natural to the rabbit digestive tract. (If this term is listed on the tag for a rabbit food, you may wish to think before using that particular feed for rabbits.)
- *Animal products*: bone meal, meal, blood meal, fish meal, and feathers. (Another term best not seen on a tag for rabbit food.)
- *Roughage products*: apple products, beet and citrus pulp, and the hulls of cottonseed, soybeans, oats, peanuts, and rice.
- *Molasses products*: beet or sugar cane molasses and beet pulp. (These may be added to give some sweetness and palatability to the feed.)

If the label has more specific terms, most likely the first listing under ingredients will be "dehydrated alfalfa meal," followed by ingredients such as "wheat middlings" (granular by-product of grain milling), soybean hulls and/or meal, molasses, wheat flour, "oat mill by-product" (brans or middlings). After these forage and grain products, ingredients added for palatability may be listed: molasses or cane molasses, corn gluten meal, safflower oil.

Any micronutrients and preservatives that were added to the pellet will also be listed on the ingredients tag, and may include calcium carbonate, iron oxide, DL-methionine, vitamin E, choline chloride, riboflavin, niacin, calcium pantothenate, vitamin B_{12}, manganese sulfate, vitamin D, ferrous sulfate, cobalt carbonate, calcium iodate, copper sulfate, zinc sulfate, magnesium oxide sodium selenite. One added nutrient you would not wish to see on an ingredients list for a rabbit food is NDN, or non-dietary nitrogen, as rabbit do not utilize NDNs well and they can cause toxicity.

Additional listed ingredients on rabbit tags may include yucca (helps control ammonia in rabbit waste), papaya (to aid digestion), and any probiotics or prebiotics, such as *Lactobacillus, Streptococcus, and Saccharomyces*. Mold inhibitors such as proprionic acid or calcium propionate may also be added. At the bottom of the tag (or elsewhere on the feed packaging) other pertinent information about that specific pellet may be added, such as "Ruminant meat and bone meal free."

Feeding guidelines will also be given on the bag or tag. These should not be ignored, for although the best amount to give a particular rabbit may vary depending upon its age, health, breed, and other factors, it should be remembered that feeds are specifically formulated to fulfill a rabbit's nutritional needs. If the feed is formulated to give the rabbit enough protein if ¼ cup is fed per 5-pound rabbit but the amount of feed is cut in half for a rabbit of that weight, the rabbit will not be receiving recommended amounts of the included nutrients.

Table 6:1 on page 127 lists the guaranteed analysis and ingredients for two compressed pellet feeds and one extruded rabbit feed. Despite the small differences in maximum and minimum contents, the ingredients of the pellets are probably quite similar despite the use of the group feed terms in pellet #1. All have several added vitamins and minerals; pellets #2 and #3 have more probiotics and prebiotics added.

Free-feeding vs. providing limited pellets

As with almost every diet/nutrition topic, determining the best amount of pellets to give your particular rabbit(s) is not simple. The answer may be different for each rabbit you have, depending upon its age, health, breed, activity, and other factors. A good place to start is with the tag guidelines or ¼ cup pellets per kilogram (approximately 2.4 pounds) of rabbit. If he or she maintains a healthy weight, continue feeding that amount. If the rabbit appears hungry or loses weight add another two tablespoons per day, and repeat the process until the rabbits maintains a good weight.

Remember that our domestic rabbits are not naturally lean/slender animals, but mammals of a moderate build. Look at your rabbit: are his sides caved in? If so, he/she is too thin. Feel his or her back and sides. You should be able to just barely feel the backbone and ribs. If you have difficulty feeling them, the rabbit is too fat; if the bones are easily felt, the rabbit is probably too thin. Remember that in general both young rabbits and older rabbits need to eat more food to meet their nutritional and energy needs.

Table 6:1 Comparison of three rabbit pellet ingredients tags.

RABBIT PELLET #1
Guaranteed analysis:
Crude protein (min) 16.0000%, Crude fat (min) 1.5000%, Crude fiber (min) 17.0000%, Crude fiber (max) 20.0000%, Calcium (min) 0.6000%, Calcium (max) 1.1000%, Phosphorus (min) 0.4000%, Salt (NaCl) (min) 0.5000%, Salt (NaCl) (max) 1.0000%, Vitamin A (min) 4600.00 IU/LB
Ingredients:
Forage products, processed grain by-products, grain products, plant protein products, roughage products, molasses products, calcium carbonate, salt, iron oxide, DL-methionine, vitamin E supplement, choline chloride, riboflavin supplement, calcium pantothenate, vitamin B12 supplement, vitamin A supplement, manganese sulfate, vitamin D supplement, ferrous sulfate, cobalt carbonate, calcium iodate, copper sulfate, zinc sulfate, magnesium oxide, sodium selenite. **RUMINANT AND BONE MEAL FREE**

RABBIT PELLET #2
Guaranteed analysis:
Crude protein, Min 16.0% Crude fat, Min 2.5% Crude fiber, Min 14.0% Crude fiber, Max 18.0% Calcium, Min 0.75% Calcium, Max 1.05% Phosphorus, Min 0.60% Salt, Min. 0.25% Salt, Max 0.75% Vitamin A, Min 5,000 IU/lb
Ingredients:
Dehydrated alfalfa meal, wheat middlings, wheat flour, soybean hulls, dehulled soybean meal, can molasses, salt, oat mill by-product, calcium carbonate, monocalcium phosphate, manganese sulfate, manganese proteinate, riboflavin, B12 supplement, folic acid, biotin, thiamine mononitrate, pyridoxine hydrochloride, vitamin a supplement, vitamin D3 supplement, vitamin E supplement, L-ascorbyl-2-polyphosphate (source of vitamin C), DL-methionine, choline chloride, menadione sodium bisulfite complex (source of vitamin K activity), brewers dried yeast, dried streptococcus faecium fermentation product, dried lactobacillus acidophilus product, dried saccharomyces cerevisiae fermentation solubles, yucca schidigera extract.

RABBIT PELLET #3 (EXTRUDED)
Guaranteed analysis:
Crude protein (min) 14.0 % Crude fat (min) 1.0 % Crude fiber (min) 16.0 %Crude fiber (max) 20.0 % Moisture (max) 12.0% Calcium (min) 0.4 % Calcium (max) 0.6 % Phosphorus (min) 0.35 % Salt (min) 0.25 % Salt (max) 0.75 % Vitamin A (min) 3000 IU/lb Omega-3 fatty acids (min) 0.5 % Docosahexaenoic acid (DHA) (min) 0.5 % L-Carnitine (min) 25mg/kg
Ingredients:
Sun-cured alfalfa meal, wheat middlings, ground oats, soy hulls, ground wheat, ground flax seed, soybean meal, dried cane molasses, salt, whole cell algae meal (source of DHA), fructooligosaccharide, soy oil, DL-methionine, L-lysine, mixed tocopherols (a preservative), yeast extract, dicalcium phosphate, yucca schidigera extract, vitamin A supplement, choline chloride, vitamin E supplement, riboflavin supplement, manganese proteinate, copper proteinate, copper sulfate, ferrous sulfate, zinc oxide, manganous oxide, vitamin B12 supplement, niacin, calcium pantothenate, menadione sodium bisulfite complex (source of vitamin K activity), rosemary extract, citric acid, cholecalciferol (source of vitamin D3), L-carnitine, pyridoxine chloride, thiamine mononitrate, folic acid, biotin, calcium iodate, dried A. oryzae fermentation extract (source of protease), dried bacillus subtillus fermentation extract, dried Bacillus lichenformin fermentation product, dried Bacillus subtillus fermentation product, cobalt carbonate, sodium selenite, artificial color.

Many rabbits can actually be allowed free access to pellets and will self-regulate the amount they eat after the first 2–4 weeks, although it is not unusual for them to eat a bit too much the first few days. Kathy Smith suggests that rabbits receiving high-quality hay they like to eat will be better candidates for the free-feeding of pellets. This method of feeding also appears to work especially well with those rabbits that get adequate exercise. It has the advantage that rabbits can adjust their own intake, eating more when they are more active or the temperature is colder, and less when they are inactive or weather is warm. In a study where young rabbits were allowed access to feed at all times they were no less healthy and had no higher a mortality rate than those rabbits receiving rationed feed. However, not all rabbits will self-regulate and some will become overweight if allowed free access to pellets. Rabbits that do not get much exercise and/or bored rabbits that may eat as a form of recreation are not good candidates for free-feeding pellets.

HOMEMADE TREATS

Most of us do not have the time, knowledge, equipment, or money to make our own pellets. However, most of us *do* have the time to make a special treat for our rabbits. Lisa Hodgson, editor and publisher of the British rabbit magazine *Bunny Mad!* generously gave permission to reprint her article on making a great bunny treat:

Homemade Bunny Biscuits
by Lisa Hodgson[2]

We all love to spoil our bunnies but some of the shop bought treats can be loaded with sugar and other things that may not always be good for our bunnies. That's what makes these treats perfect as you know exactly what ingredients go into them and can alter the recipe to your rabbit's taste and dieatary

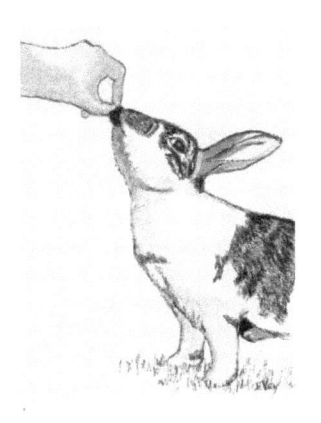

---

[2] Hodgson, Lisa. 2012. Homemade Bunny Biscuits. *Bunny Mad!* Issue 14. Reprinted with permission.

needs. As with any treat please remember to slowly introduce them into your rabbit's diet and feed sparingly, as you don't want to risk upsetting their tummies. Hoppy baking!

Ingredients you will need:

To make the dry mix –
  1 cup of rolled oats
  ½ cup of your rabbit's usual rabbit pellets

To make wet mix –
  ¼ cup of basil leaves (or any other favourite herb)
  ½ carrot
  ¼ of a banana
  1 tablespoon of water

Other items needed:
  A blender or coffee grinder
  Greaseproof paper

How to make:

- Preheat oven to gas mark, 180 degrees Celcius (350 degrees F)
- To make your dry mix, use a blender or coffee grinder to grind the rolled oats and rabbit pellets and put in a bowl to one side.
- To make your wet mix, puree all the wet ingredients together in a blender until smooth.
- Now add the wet puree to the bowl of prepared dry ingredients and mix to form a sticky dough. If your dough is looking a bit dry then add a splash more water and knead.
- Place your dough between two sheets of greaseproof paper/wax paper (this will stop the dough from sticking to everything!) and roll to about ¼ inch.
- Remove the top sheet of paper and score the dough with a knife to form small squares. It

is easier to do this now as when baked the biscuits will be very hard.

- Bake in an oven for 25 minutes but check after 15 minutes and cover with foil if they are looking brown. For a crunchier, longer lasting treat, turn off the oven after 25 minutes and leave biscuits to sit in the cooling oven.

- Allow to cool before feeding to bunnies then sit back and watch them enjoy your hard work! Store in an airtight container.

Buntastic ideas:

Use different cookie cutters to make fun shaped biscuits.

Pop biscuits into a gift bag to make the perfect gift for a bunny friend or rescue.

Play about with ingredients to make your own special recipe. Try other fruits and herbs such as cranberries, strawberries, raspberries, parsley, dill, coriander, fennel and mint.

Hide biscuits in toys for added fun!

Author note: I love this recipe from *Bunny Mad!* (and so do my rabbits!) because it is so versatile. You may have to adjust the wet mix proportions depending on the water content of the herbs and fruits you use. I prefer to bake the buscuits slowly at 300 degrees Fahrenheit until they are thoroughly dried and just turning golden brown. That way they keep a long time if stored in an airtight container.

HAY

Unquestionably hay is an important part of a domestic rabbit's diet. Rabbit digestive systems require fiber for proper function and hay is a good source of fiber. It should be remembered, however, that although rabbits need fiber for the proper motility and function of their digestive system, *rabbits receive very little nutrition from fibrous foods such as hay* because they pass so rapidly through the gut. In addition to hay, rabbits require more easily-digested foods from which to obtain the nutrition necessary to maintain their bodies. If a rabbit were fed *only* hay it would *very slowly* (over a period of months or years depending upon the age and health of the rabbit) become malnourished and eventually die, either from malnutrition or related digestive and other illnesses. That said, hay *is* an important constituent of rabbit's diet.

Hay is not necessarily grass. Any dried leaf matter may be called hay; alfalfa hay and clover hay are two other examples. Alfalfa hay has less fiber and more nutrients, fat, and calcium than does grass hay. For this reason it is not generally recommended for overweight rabbits, rabbits with sludgy urine or other signs of a high-calcium diet, or very young rabbits if they are being given an alfalfa-based pellet. However, for growing rabbits over six months of age, undernourished adult rabbits, and older rabbits with no signs of excess dietary calcium, alfalfa hay can be a valuable feed. It can also be helpful when it is necessary to coax an anorexic rabbit to eat, since many rabbits prefer alfalfa hay to grass hay.

Most often, grass hay is fed to domestic rabbits. It is widely available, generally inexpensive, contains silicates and other minerals that help tooth wear, and provides necessary fiber. But grass hays are not all the same—the nutritional quality of grass hay depends on the specific species of grass, at what age it was harvested (older plants have more lignin), how is was dried (sun-dried hay has more vitamin D), and how it was stored (loss of nutrients, especially of vitamins A, D, and E, occurs if hay is stored at high temperatures or for extended lengths of time), among other factors. Hay is the most variable-quality feed crop in the United States. So in actuality it is very difficult to tell the precise nutritional content of a bag of hay unless you have it analyzed, which most of us have neither the money nor time to do! Therefore the nutritional content values of hays given in charts in this book are only averages and any particular bag may have a great deal more or less. Vitamin content is not listed since so much is lost during storage.

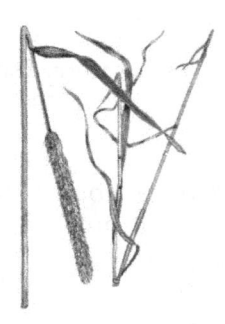

In the US timothy is often recommended as a good hay for domestic rabbits, but there are many other good grass hays, including slender wheatgrass (common in the western US), Bermuda grass (common in the south and east), orchard grass, meadow fescue grass, and oatgrass. Brome grass and ryegrass are less common, but may be purchased in some areas. Legume hay such as clover hay, which is often richer in food value, can be given to rabbits in small amounts. Like grass hay, legume hay should be carefully checked for any discoloration or other sign of mold.

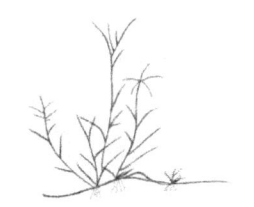

If hay is bought in small sacks produced for pet rabbits, the quality is generally uniform and there are few, if any, weeds. Hay purchased in these small sacks can be quite expensive though, particularly if you have multiple rabbits. Buying hay by the bale, either loose or compressed (compressed bales weigh the same but take up less space) is considerably less expensive. However, if you buy hay in bales the quality is unlikely to be uniform throughout the bale and there may be weeds and/or insect parts that will need to be taken out before feeding the hay to the rabbit.

Whatever you purchase hay by the bag or bale, try to select hay that has few, if any, blades with yellowish or blackish discoloration. This may be almost impossible to do when buying hay by the bale since you cannot see the quality of the entire bale from the outside, so inspect the hay frequently as you use the bale.

Heat that is created in bales destroys nutrient content. In a study on bales of Bermudagrass it was found that the density of the bale did not affect heat production but that moisture content of the grass when it was baled did (increasing moisture content leading to more heat and destruction of nutrients).

Feeding a rabbit a variety of hays is not necessary, particularly since hay is fed more for its fiber than its nutrients. So if good orchard grass hay is available in your area, it is fine to feed that hay alone; it is not necessary to always feed timothy hay. (That said, I do recommend giving a healthy adult rabbit that is being given alfalfa hay some grass hay as well.) If you change types of hay depending upon what is available at your feed store (as I do), be sure to add the new hay gradually so the rabbit's intestinal microflora has time to adapt.

Table 6:1 Typical nutrient content of selected hays. Nutritional values of hay vary widely depending upon various factors, including soil in which grown, age at which h harvested, and storage. *Values compiled from multiple sources.*

Hay	% crude protein	% fiber	% Mg	% Ca	% P	Ca:P ratio
alfalfa	17.50	30.0	0.30	1.23	0.24	5.1 1
Bermuda grass	9.1	32.0	0.16	0.38	0.16	2.4: 1
bluegrass, Kentucky	8.8	20.0	0.19	0.34	0.27	1.4: 1
brome grass	9.7	32.0	0.36	0.32	0.16	1.8: 1
clover, red	15.1	21.8	0.34	1.22	0.22	5.5: 1
clover, white	18.92	26.9	0.32	1.50	0.29	5.2: 1
fescue, meadow	9.0	31.0	1.61	0.33	0.25	1.3: 1
oatgrass	8.6	42.4	0.26	0.29	0.23	1.3: 1
orchard grass	8.15	31.0	0.16	0.28	0.23	1.2: 1
ryegrass	7.9	26.0	0.12	0.42	0.18	2.3: 1
timothy	8.25	28.0	0.11	0.36	0.17	2.1: 1
wheatgrass, slender	8.0	36.4	0.22	0.23	0.23	1: 1
wheat straw	3.5	40.7	0.11	0.19	0.14	1.4: 1

Hay may be "first cutting," "second cutting," "third cutting," or even fourth or fifth cuttings depending upon your geographical area. Hay from a first cutting may be coarser and have more stems (and often more weeds if you buy hay in bales). Protein content is usually lower, although the lignin and fiber content is higher. Second cutting hay is often softer, greener, and more palatable to most rabbits. It often has higher overall nutritional content but has less lignin content. This generalization does not always hold however, as second- or third-cutting hay that is harvested later than it should be may also be stemmy and coarse and lower in nutrition. Unless a rabbit has a specific need due to a health issue, the reality is that it makes little difference whether a healthy rabbit is fed first, second or third-cutting hay. If your rabbit prefers one over the other, it is unlikely to hurt to indulge the rabbit's preference.

Some rabbit owners may also feed straw to their rabbits. Straw is mostly the dry coarse stems of cereal grasses that is used primarily for livestock bedding and for packing. Since it is fully mature when harvested, it has very high lignin content and very little other nutrition. Although it is safe to feed straw to rabbits provided their nutritional needs are being met with other foods, many rabbits do not like it and it has little value beyond the high fiber content. However, it may be beneficial to feed young growing rabbits small amounts of straw; lignin has been found to help prevent diarrhea and other digestive ills in very young rabbits.

Hay should be of a fairly uniform color, smell sweet, not musty, and not have too much dust. Hay with a bright uniform green color has the most beta-carotene and is the best, but sun-bleached hay (a light golden-yellow) is also acceptable (the interior of such a bale may often be green). However, hay that was harvested at too late a stage and is a uniform yellowish brown is not of the best quality, and hay that is brown is unacceptable. All hay (and straw) should be kept in a place that is dry and cool and out of the reach of insects, rodents, and other mammals (e.g., raccoons). Keeping hay and feed in airtight containers or sacks is not advisable since this can increase the chances of deterioration, but keep it protected from excess moisture and sun. Unless you have specific knowledge that a particular weed found in a hay bale is safe for rabbits, discard it. Also remove any discolored and/or moldy-looking pieces of hay, even if they are dry.

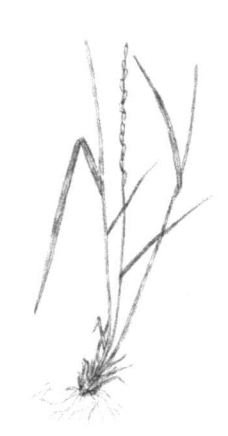

Although it is often recommended that rabbits be provided unlimited hay, the research does not in fact support that this is necessary. Different rabbits will have different needs for hay depending upon their age, health, and other factors. But for most healthy adult rabbits, a small amount of hay (about what will stuff into a large empty tissue box) given daily provides enough fiber. However, giving more hay is unlikely to harm a rabbit (provided the rabbit is receiving enough pellets and other food to meet its nutritional needs) and may help alleviate boredom for rabbits, *so by all means give unlimited hay to your healthy adult rabbit if you wish, as long as the rabbit is also receiving other foods.* Remember that a diet *too* high in indigestible fiber can lead to irritation of the gut and impaction of the cecum.

Grass-hay-only diets

I am strongly against feeding grass-hay-only diets to domestic rabbits under most circumstances. Not only does a grass-hay-only diet fail to provide fiber from multiple botanical origins, but it can also cause health problems. A grass-hay-only diet may not provide adequate digestible energy for body maintenance (eventually leading to hepatic lipidosis and death if there is no intervention), can lead to nutrient deficiencies and their corresponding negative effects on health, and predispose the rabbit to mucoid enteropathy and cecal impaction, both a possibility in diets with crude fiber content of more than 20-22 percent.

Another risk is that when the digestible energy to protein proportion of the diet is out of balance there can be an increase in ammonia (see protein section in Chapter 4) and imbalances in the microflora of the gastrointestinal tract may develop, often leading to more serious disorders of the digestive tract. Rabbits digest protein far better than fiber. When they consume excessive dietary fiber it can result in a dietary protein level that is higher than the digestible energy of the diet, causing a protein surplus and energy deficit. This promotes growth of proteolytic microflora that produce ammonia and cause imbalances of the microflora that can cause severe digestive ills.

Many studies have shown that rabbits digest grasses less well than equines and ruminants, and researchers have concluded that rabbits evolved a concentrate-selector feeding strategy along with the rapid passage of lignified and other indigestible fibrous material in order to allow them to obtain enough energy to meet their high metabolic needs.

It has also been found that the amount of indigestible fiber in the diet of rabbits affects the intestinal mucosa, an important part of the immune system. The mucosa protects the intestinal epithelium from physical and chemical damge and helps keep bacteria from adhering to the intestinal wall. Too much insoluble fiber may negatively affect the integrity of the gut mucosa. In responses to the first edition, I also heard of rabbits diagnosed with "thickened bowel loops," a condition similar to infiltrative colonic disease in horses. The affected rabbits improved after having the amount of hay in their diet reduced.

Common sense as well would appear to show that a grass-hay-only diet would not be good for most rabbits. Hay is not a particularly nutritious food, and rabbits require both nutrient-dense low-fiber *and* lower-nutrition high fiber foods. Neither does it provide the proper balance of indigestible to digestible fiber that is necessary for optimal digestive health. How can a rabbit be expected to do well if one component is removed from their diet? Humans have evolved to eat a variety of foods as well, yet if put on a meat-only diet for long periods will develop multiple health problems. Why would one expect a rabbit to thrive if forced to subsist on a hay-only diet when they also have evolved to eat a variety of foods?

BALANCED DIETS

Many researchers in the area of rabbit nutrition have stressed the importance of balance in rabbit diets: balance between the types of fiber and balances between fiber and other nutrients. I could not agree more. If I had to pick out the one single aspect of rabbit diet that I believe to be the most important, it would be *balance*. Rabbits need both low-fiber nutrient-packed foods and high-fiber foods of less nutrition. They need succulent foods to balance dried ones, they need a balance of soluble and insoluble fiber for their digestive systems to function optimally, and they need foods that provides nutrition from a balanced variety of botanical origins.

On a personal note, I give my rabbits a diet that is extremely varied and includes food items such as commercial pellets, various grass hays, fresh grass, fresh vegetables (including a variety of lettuces), herbs such as celery, parsley, cilantro, and carrot tops, fruit (including occasional small amounts of grapefruit and tomato in addition to apples, grapes, and berries), grains such as oatmeal, and occasional seeds and nuts. Yet I can count on the fingers of one hand (one time) the number of occasions all my rabbits put together have ever had an episode of gastro-intestinal hypomotility (stasis), and they almost never have any other digestive or dental-related illnesses. I believe a good part of the reason I have been so fortunate is that my rabbits' diets are both varied and balanced.

FRESH GRASS

Rabbits love to eat fresh grass as well as grass hay. Although giving large amounts of fresh grass is not recommended for rabbits under six months of age, small amounts of fresh grass can be a nutritious addition to a healthy adult rabbit's diet, and even young rabbits can usually be given a blade or two (and this may actually help the rabbit's digestive system become accustomed to the food). However, as with any food in a rabbit's diet—introduce grass slowly into a rabbit's feeding program.

It is not a good idea to feed your rabbit grass clippings from mown lawns (they ferment rapidly and the lawn may have been treated pesticides and other chemicals), but there are safe ways to give your rabbit this vitamin and mineral-rich treat. If you live where you have grass that has not been treated with any chemicals and can make your rabbit safe from dogs, cats, hawks, and other predators, you may consider allowing your rabbit to go outside and graze on fresh grass. Some people enclose small areas with chicken wire walls and ceiling (and stay with the rabbit to be sure he/she does not dig out or predators dig their way in). The rabbits usually love such outings, and the fresh air, exercise, and vitamin D from sunshine are additional benefits. Christine Carter, author of *The Wonderful World of Pet Rabbits,* describes how to make a grazing pen for your rabbit:

> The ultimate way to provide the freshest vegetation is to let your rabbit have a mobile hutch or playpen. When grazing naturally, your bunny can consume plants while they are still living. You may choose either a permanent hutch structure or a temporary pen used for several hours during the day.
>
> The pen itself can be constructed similar to a child's playpen, with a roof for shade and wire around the sidewalls. Affix wire at the base, taking care to use a gauge that is an appropriate size. It must not be so small to restrict access to foliage or have holes large enough to enable digging of an

escape tunnel—something that generally only the females are prone to do. Typically, the lawn would be used for a grazing pasture, however if you have one make the most of a vegetable plot growing grass and weeds.

Grazing pens must be secure against predators and protect bunnies from exposure to harsh weather conditions. Lawns growing lush areas of clover are not suitable for grazing, as clover should not be eaten in excess. Do not allow bunnies to graze on recently fertilized pasture, pasture sprayed with weedicide or where dog droppings are present. Be sure to provide a container of water and move the grazing pen as appropriate.

However, there are risks to taking your rabbit outdoors, even in an enclosed/protected area, and these should be considered before making your final decision. Bacteria and/or fungi may be present and parasite eggs may adhere to grass blades if you live in an area frequented by wildlife or even cats and dogs. Myiasis and/or warbles can be a danger to rabbits while outside if flies are present. Predators can break into or dig into enclosed areas if rabbits are left unattended, even for short times. Because I live in an area with many predators and a large fly population, I choose not to allow my rabbits outdoors; Evonne Vey, the illustrator of this book, lives in a different geographical area and feels the benefits of allowing her rabbits outside outweigh the risks.

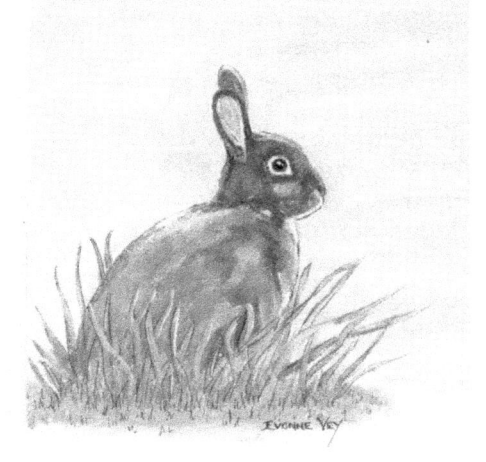

For those who like the idea of giving fresh grass to their rabbit but are not comfortable with taking their rabbit outside, growing grass indoors can be the answer. Growing fresh wheatgrass, barleygrass, buckwheat, or oat- grass is easy and the fresh grasses are very nutritious. Barleygrass and wheatgrass are extremely high in beta-carotene, high in the B-complex vitamins, vitamins E and K, phosphorus, magnesium, potassium, protein, and other nutrients. They also contain large amounts of silicates that will help wear a rabbit's teeth. Fresh-grown wheatgrass, if it is not washed before giving it to the rabbit, also provides a source of vitamin B_{12}, which is produced by bacteria that adheres to the grass blades.

Wheatgrass is not just for rabbits: some people enjoy sharing the nutritional benefits of wheatgrass with their rabbit by pressing some of the grass and drinking the juice. Pet rabbit owner Elizabeth Sharp explains how to grow your own wheatgrass:

Growing wheatgrass for your rabbit

by Elizabeth A. Sharp and Serendipity

My nine-year-old rabbit Serendipity (Sara) and I have personally enjoyed the benefits of consuming wheatgrass for over four years. It is fun, simple, and rewarding to grow.

There are several wheat "berries," or seeds, you can use; I use organic hard red winter wheat berries which can be purchased at any health food store. The first step is to germinate the berries in a glass jar with cheesecloth over the top (or you can use a sprouting lid, available at most health food stores). Pour in ½ cup of berries and fill the jar with spring or distilled water to double the volume of the seeds. Allow to soak overnight.

In the morning, pour the water out and let the jar drain at a 45 degree angle for an hour or so. Lay the jar on its side and leave it in a warm spot out of the sun's light (you can place it in a brown paper bag). Leave the jar for about 1–2 days, rotating it occasionally, until the seeds pop (germinate) and you can see white hairs on them. Now they are ready to plant!

The next step is to prepare the planting trays. I use 12" plastic plant saucers with no holes in the bottom, although you can use low-sided cat litter pans or any other shallow container. Fill your chosen tray with about an inch of dirt. I use organic potting soil, but you can use any good garden or natural soil. Moisten the dirt well before spreading the berries (seeds) on top of the dirt. Spray the filled trays lightly with water and cover with another 12" plant saucer (or a second of whatever container you are using).

Place the planting trays in an area away from direct sunlight. Check daily until you see the grass growing (1–3 days), then remove the top and let the grass get a little sunlight to stimulate chlorophyll production. Keep the trays moist, but not soaked. There is always the possibility of mold, depending upon growing location, so it is better to under-water than over-water. (Should mold develop on the bottom of your grass mat throw it away and start over, keeping it less moist.)

The grass usually grows to about 5–6 inches in a week, at which time it is ready for the first harvest. You can put the tray down on the floor and let your bunny graze to his heart's content! Or, if you wish to harvest the grass and prepare wheatgrass juice for your own or your rabbit's consumption, you can now cut the grass down to just above the soil surface. Extract the wheat grass juice in a macerating juicer or a hydraulic press, as a centrifugal juicer will not work. Place a few drops of the extracted juice in your rabbit's water. If you wish to try drinking some as well, I recommend that you only consume ½ oz or less at first. You can also freeze the juice in ice cube trays for easy consumption.

After harvesting the grass the first time, you can place the tray back in the growing area, and after a few days the grass mat will be ready for a second harvest, and even a third. After you are done you can compost your leftover wheatgrass mat or plant it outside, where it may even come up once again.

Enjoy!

OTHER FRESH FOODS
Vegetables and herbs
Most adult rabbits can eat one cup of greens and/or root vegetables per 2.3 kg (5 pounds) of body weight per day without problems, although some may have sensitivities to

particular vegetables (see Chapters 7 and 10). Introduce new greens and vegetables in small amounts. Fresh vegetables, especially dark leafy greens (which contain iodine) provide many needed nutrients.

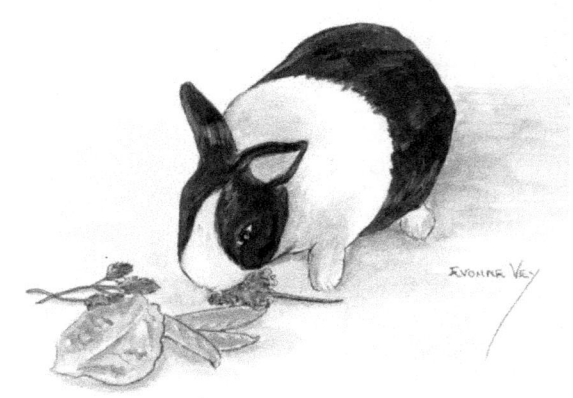

There is some disagreement among experts as to whether fresh vegetables and herbs are safe for very young rabbits. While I acknowledge there is a massive amount of evidence that shows a high-protein diet is not good for very young rabbits, and I recognize that giving young rabbits large amounts of vegetables with high-protein content might well be deleterious, there are also arguments in favor of giving *very small amounts* of some fresh vegetables to young rabbits. It is during this critical time that the digestive systems of young rabbits become populated with the flora that help digest foods properly, and giving tiny amounts of a variety of fresh vegetables could potentially help accustom the rabbit to eating that food and ensure a healthy and varied population of gut microflora. The key is *tiny amounts*. If you are unable to restrain yourself from giving into a rabbit's begging for more of a favored food it is best not to give any items that could cause problems if given in large amounts.

Fruit

Although high in some sugars, such as fructose, fruits are also high in hemi-cellulose and pectins, which can be beneficial to digestion (see Chapter 3), as well being high in many flavonoids and other compounds (Chapter 7). Papaya contains the enzyme papain, which can aid digestion, and fresh or unpasteurized frozen pineapple contains bromelain, a protein-digesting enzyme. Pineapple is also very high in manganese (good for bones and connective tissue), may help prevent blod clot formation, is an anti-inflammatory, may help reduce tumor growth, and has an exterminative effect on intestinal worms. Noni (*Morinda citrifolia*) has been found to have a calming and relaxing effect on rabbits. It also stimulates the immune system and is very high in vitamin C. Acai, the fruit from a South American palm tree (*Euterpe oleracea*), is a popular "health food" at the time of this writing. The fruits of *Lycium barbarum* and *L. chinense* (aka goji, wolfberry) are also popular. These members of the Solanaceae family have fruit that contains compounds that lower fever, reduce inflammation, and protect the liver and kidneys. However, many other more easily-obtained berries, such as cranberries and blueberries, contain compounds that have the same effects, so it not necessary to buy expensive imported fruits to provide potentially helpful nutrients and phytonutrients.

Given in relatively small amounts, fruit can be a valuable addition to a rabbit's diet. Most rabbits like fruit, and it can also be of use in persuading anorexic rabbits to eat. Many times I have been able to persuade a severely ill rabbit to eat a little fruit when it would eat nothing else on its own. Although caution should be observed in giving dried fruits, which do have higher levels of sugar and may contain preservatives, small amounts can be given safely, as many of us who give dried cranberry "treats" to our rabbits know.

Some experts on rabbit diet suggest giving fruit in amounts of 1–2 tablespoons per 2.3 kg body weight/day. I would recommend starting with just a bite or two and slowly working up to 2 tablespoons if there are no negative reactions to the particular fruit being fed. There have been many studies on the effects of adding fairly high amounts of various fruits, including dates, to the diets of rabbits, and as with those studies on vegetables, adding the fruits in moderate amounts usually causes no significant negative effects and may have some positive effects (Chapter 3). I give my rabbits fruit daily, in amounts ranging from a tablespoon to ¼ cup, depending upon the fruit and the size of the rabbit. As with fresh vegetables and other new foods, fruit should be introduced gradually into the diet of a rabbit, giving very tiny amounts at first and slowly adding more. The more unusual fruits that are now available in many areas (e.g. mangosteen) can also be fed to rabbits provided they are introduced into the diet slowly and seeds are removed (or the juice or pulp given).

Nuts, seeds and grains

I often read articles on rabbit care in which the author states that nuts, seeds, and grains should never be given to rabbits, even as a treat. I disagree strongly. Unless a rabbit is obese or has another medical problem that contraindicates their consumption, some nuts (e.g., almonds, walnuts), seeds (e.g., pumpkin, sunflower) and grains (rolled oats), *given in small amounts,* can add valuable nutrients such as CoQ10 to a rabbit's diet. In fact, fats and protein are necessary in a rabbit's diet. The wild rabbits from which domestic rabbits descended evolved eating small amounts of nutrient and energy-dense foods along with low-energy high-fiber foods such as grass, and there is no reason a healthy adult domestic rabbit cannot eat these foods—if introduced slowly into the diet—without experiencing unduly negative effects. (See Chapter 4 for more information on fat and protein.)

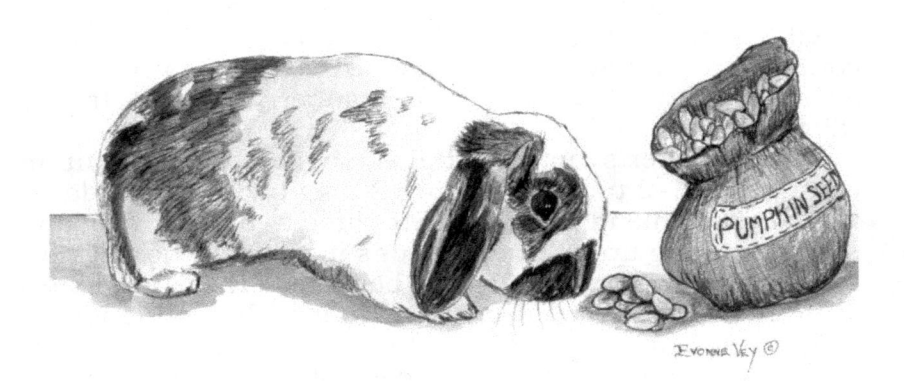

Nuts, seeds and grains can be particularly valuable sources of energy for large rabbits such as the giant breeds, wool rabbits such as angoras, fur rabbits such as Rex, and any rabbit living where ambient temperatures are low. These rabbits need more protein and energy, and nuts, seeds and grains can provide both. A couple of walnuts or almonds or a few pine nuts can markedly improve the condition of skin and fur in long haried rabbits. Pine nuts contain a high percent (85%) of unsaturated fatty acids and have been found to have antimicrobial effects and to improve cardiovascular health (as may walnuts and almonds). However, very small seeds (e.g., milo) *can* be a danger to rabbits because of the possibility a rabbit might swallow them whole. Swallowed whole, small seeds could become stuck in the pylorus and cause a serious blockage. Give your rabbit only larger seeds such as sunflower seeds and pumpkin seeds.

Most healthy adult rabbits will suffer no harm and may benefit from the addition of about one tablespoon of a grain such as rolled oats, a tablespoon of seeds such as raw pumpkin seeds, a teaspoon or less of nut meats such as almonds or walnuts, or a fourth-teaspoon of pine nuts. This is for rabbits between 4–6 pounds; decrease the amount slightly for smaller rabbits and increase it slightly for larger rabbits, wool or fur rabbits, and rabbits living in cooler temperatures.

FORAGING

There are other aspects to feeding rabbits than nutrition in and of itself. As I mentioned earlier in this chapter, giving a confined rabbit hay can help alleviate boredom. Just as a person may receive benefits other than the food itself from a meal depending upon how it is presented (think of a meal in a fine restaurant or one at a large family gathering), so can rabbits. Debby Widolf explains some of the ways your rabbit's life can be enriched by the way in which the food is presented.

Foraging, or Hide and Seek for Rabbits
by Debby Widolf

Hopping, stretching, reaching, smelling, tasting, digging, tunneling, exploring are all behaviors seen when the cautious but curious wild rabbit forages for their daily food. As relatives of the European wild rabbit, our domestic rabbits have these same innate skills that are not actively used, due to a sedentary lifestyle where food is placed in a bowl in the same spot day after day. Although it is reassuring to know food is forthcoming, we can add a bit of fun, exercise and mental stimulation when feeding our rabbits by having them forage for their meals.

There are many creative ways to add foraging to a rabbit's daily routine. Use your imagination and creativity and you will be surprised at what can be added to the rabbit's environment, whether they live in a cage/condo, pen or have free roam of a room or the house. When rabbits are living in a shelter or a small cage space, foraging will add needed environmental stimulation. I am listing some foraging tips that I have used or seen used by people that have rabbits as companions or are their caregivers at shelters and sanctuary:

- Grow grass seeds or sod from your yard in a wide pot. After the rabbits have eaten the grass down, remove the pot and let it re-grow.

- Hide a spoonful of oats under a light weight flower pot or bowl.

- Hanging food/hay balls can be purchased commercially in stores that specialize in rabbit toys and equipment.

- Hay boxes can be made out of clear file boxes. The lids keep the hay secure and can easily be refilled. Near the bottom cut a slit the length of the box by 2.5 or 3 inches high rectangle for the rabbits to pull out the hay. Mount it high enough on a pen or house, held in place by a bungee cord so that the rabbits have to stretch to get the hay.

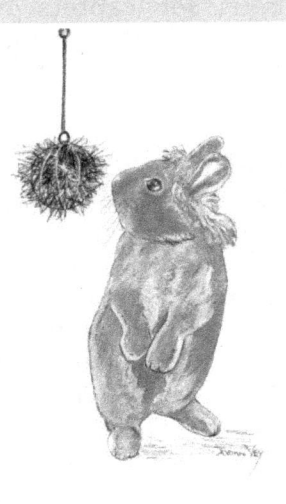

- Make a hanging sock from a plain white cotton men's sock tied with rabbit safe twine or rope and hang from the side of a pen or top of their condo/cage. Fill the sock with barley or oat hay as a treat.

- Fill a toilet paper roll with a mixture of hay and pellets. You can also add a small piece of fruit to the mix.

- Tie a string or rope across the top of a pen and use wooden clothespins to hang herbs or pieces of fresh greens. A variation is to clip greens to the side of the pen.

- Lunch-size plain paper bags can be filled with hay and other nutritious food. Roll the top of the bag tight and have fun watching your rabbit explore.

- Hide a special treat under a loose blanket or towel to encourage foraging.

This volume on rabbit nutrition will provide many healthy food suggestions to keep your rabbit excited about foraging. As always, keep safety in mind when adding new materials such as string, clips, shelving etc. to your rabbit's home. Have fun keeping the rabbits happy!

WATER

Water is necessary for almost every bodily process in all mammals, including rabbits. It is the primary means by which nutrients are transported throughout the body, it carries oxygen to cells through blood, carries toxins away from cells and removes wastes from the body, helps regulate body temperature, lubricates joints, and is needed by lung tissue to replace water lost through exhalation.

It is easier for most mammals to go for short times without food than without water, but, amazingly, this is apparently untrue for rabbits. Rabbits' digestive systems require more frequent food than many mammals, and although a rabbit could theoretically survive a short time by consuming its cecotrophs, without any additional food it would not be long before it would go into hepatic lipidosis and die. But rabbits are able to go long periods without water, provided they are consuming some food. Brewer reports that wild rabbits have been found to survive two months on vegetation containing only 7–10% water, although they may lose almost 50% of their body weight—an amazing tolerance of dehydration considering that camels can't tolerate a water loss of more than 40% of their body weight.

For domestic rabbits water intake is extremely variable, depending upon food intake, activity, housing, and many other factors, and domestic rabbits may not be able to tolerate the same percent of water loss from their bodies that their wild cousins can. Some sources report domestic rabbits drink approximately 50–120 ml/kg of body weight in a 24-hour period, which is about twice as much by volume as the amount of food they consume. Rabbits given a dry diet or one high in fiber or protein will increase their consumption of water, about 200ml/day or more. Rabbits not getting enough food will also drink more. High ambient temperatures cause a large increase in water consumption (around 450ml/kg at 86 degrees F), and lactating does may require up to 10 times their normal amount of water. Some diseases (e.g. kidney failure) may also cause increased water consumption in rabbits. Interestingly, in a study on New Zealand White rabbits, boredom was a cause of increased water consumption.

Rabbits eating lots of fresh green vegetables may drink little water or none at all, depending upon fiber and protein content of the diet. Rabbits that do not have enough water available will reduce their food consumption in order to keep the food/water consumption ratio near normal. And although an increase in ambient temperature will cause an increase in water consumption, rabbits suffering from the physical condition of heat stress may drink little water.

A drop in water consumption causes a decrease in the blood volume, and it is this which triggers the sensation of thirst. Although rabbits can tolerate great dehydration, it can still have very serious consequences in rabbits because their digestive systems require the constant absorption and excretion of water along the tract. For this reason, dehydration is common in rabbits with digestive disorders. Giving the rabbit fluids is often critical for recovery in rabbits with digestion-related illnesses.

However, dehydration is not always easy to spot in a rabbit. Rabbits store about half of the water they drink (that is not immediately excreted) in their skin. According to some experts, "tenting" the skin as one might do with a cat to test for dehydration will not work with rabbits because the rabbit's body may redistribute water. Signs of dehydration in a rabbit may include a reduction in appetite or refusal to eat (conversely, a rabbit not receiving enough food may drink more), dry mucous membranes, loose wrinkled skin around the perineum, and a rapid loss of weight. Dehydrated rabbits produce less urine with a high urea content. (Normal urine output is about 130ml/kg/day.)

It is important that rabbits drink water, especially if they eat a diet with lots of hay and/or commercial pellets, both of which require plenty of water to digest. Sometimes adding a few drops of fruit juice to the water will persuade rabbits to drink more. The container in which water is provided may also affect water consumption; it has been found that rabbits drink more from open bowls than from nipple waterers.

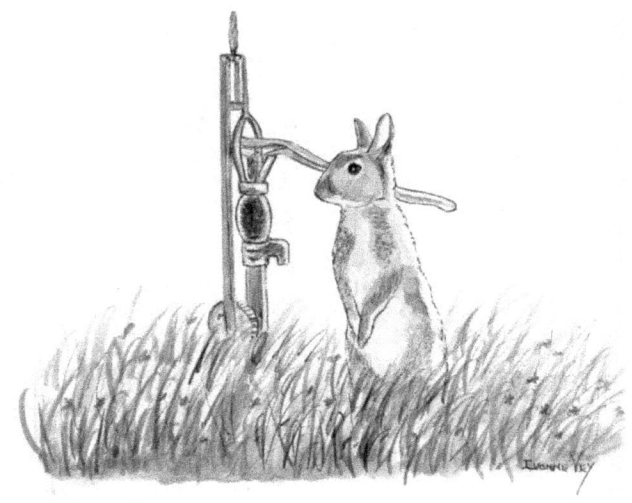

Nutritional healing

Drinking enough water could possibly prevent and/or improve several medical conditions, including arteriosclerosis, arthritis, cataracts, constipation, gastrointestinal hypomotility (stasis), kidney stones, and obesity. Dehydrated rabbits are not able to remove urea from the body efficiently and may develop prerenal azotemia (kidney toxicity).

However, drinking very hard water may *contribute* to the creation of kidney stones and to arteriosclerosis through mineralization of the arteries. If you are on well water or live in an area with abnormally hard water you may wish to filter or soften your rabbit's water before use or purchase bottled water. Kathy Smith discusses different kinds of water:

Tap Versus Bottled Water
by Kathy Smith

Tap water supplied by public utilities is regulated by the EPA. In addition to using processes that remove both biological and chemical contaminants, municipal water treatment plants in many areas put additives in their water—most notably fluorine to prevent cavities and/or chlorine to kill germs. Recent investigations have shown some large city water supplies may contain measurable amounts of caffeine and other drugs (both over the counter and prescription).

Once it leaves the water treatment plant, tap water can be re-contaminated by decaying (but not yet broken) water mains or by interaction with the pipes in your house. Water can be boiled to eliminate microbial contamination; however, since boiling can actually increase the concentration of chemical contaminants such as nitrates, it is important to know the nature of suspected contamination before attempting to compensate for it.

Water from private wells is not regulated by the government. However, since most owners of private wells are using the water for themselves and their families, there is no reason to assume well water is less safe as long as the well is properly maintained and water is tested on a regular basis. Well water often contains a higher concentration of minerals which *may* contribute to damaging arteries and kidneys.

Bottled water is an increasingly popular alternative to tap water, but it is not the failsafe solution some believe it to be. Bottled water is regulated by the FDA. The FDA's website states that it "establishes allowable levels for contaminants in bottled water." It is important to understand that these are *different* guidelines than the

EPA uses for tap water. Analysis of which set of guidelines provides safer, healthier drinking water is far beyond the scope of this book. It is important to note that just as tap water may (or may not) pick up contaminants from its "containers" (water lines both outside and inside the home), bottled water may (or may not) pick up toxins from the plastic containers in which it is stored.

There are several different kinds of bottled water defined by their original source and how they are processed. A large part of the FDA's responsibility is ensuring accurate labeling. The main types of bottled water available are:

- **Artesian** water is distinguished by the fact that it flows down to the (natural) aquifer that contains it, yet is under sufficient pressure to come to the surface without mechanical pumping. It is considered by some to be the purest and best water and is usually priced accordingly.

- **Distilled** water is a form of purified water that has been boiled, evaporated, and condensed back into liquid form. The distillation process removes all types of microbes—along with all trace minerals, both harmful and helpful.

- **Mineral** water comes from a physically and geologically protected underground source that *naturally* contains a minimum of 250 ppm of "dissolved solids." Mineral water from any given source has a consistent level and proportion of these minerals and trace elements. Minerals cannot be added to a product with this label.

- **Spring** water originates underground and flows naturally to the earth's surface at identified location(s). Like artesian water, spring water is considered superior—and priced accordingly.

A variety of water filter systems are an option for those who are not 100% comfortable with their tap water but wish to avoid bottled water. Some are designed to work for your entire house while others work at the individual faucet level. Not all systems filter all contaminants, so it is important to know what most needs to be filtered before shopping for a system.

References
http://www.ehso.com/ehshome/DrWater/_drinkingwater.php
http://www.epa.gov/water/
http://www.fda.gov/water/
http://www.waterfiltercomparisons.com/

MYCOTOXINS

The existence of specific mycotoxins, although suspected, was not proven until the mid-1900s. Since that time their prevalence and negative effects on animals (including humans) has become of greater and greater concern. Technically, mycotoxins are secondary metabolites of microfungi called molds. Just as some plants produce compounds that discourage other organisms from eating them (e.g., tannins), so do some fungi, although not *all* fungi produce mycotoxins. Since fungi grow mainly upon plant matter, mycotoxins can be found on hay and in many forage-based and grain-based manufactured feeds, including rabbit feeds. Mycotoxins are usually very stable compounds that resist heat and cold, moisture and dry conditions, and the effects of sunlight. Therefore, they tend to persist once they are produced by the molds.

Mycotoxins present a concern for rabbit owners for several reasons:

- The mycotoxin can persist after the mold itself has died, leaving no obvious signs of its presence

- Rabbits are more sensitive to many mycotoxins than other animals

- Signs of mycotoxin poisoning (mycotoxicosis) are similar to signs of many other medical conditions in rabbits and may be misdiagnosed

- Poisoning from mycotoxins in food can affect a single rabbit or a whole household of rabbits, taking lives with frightening rapidity.

Given that the molds that produce mycotoxins are not always present on all plant matter, how do they get introduced into our rabbit's hay or feed? The answer lies in the mold spore. Mold spores are extremely resistant to environmental extremes and other conditions that would kill the mold itself. One can think of these spores as "lying in wait" on almost all plant matter, waiting for conditions to be right for them to germinate. Moisture, oxygen, and heat are key. The proper conditions may occur almost anywhere in the chain of production of rabbit feeds and hay, from the farmer to the rabbit owner. For example, if the weather is particularly wet a certain year, mold populations in the farmer's fields will be much higher. Contamination may also occur while feeds are in the hand of the middlemen, through improperly cleaned storage and processing areas and equipment. At the other end of the chain, if a rabbit owner stores pellets where they can absorb moisture or leaves wet pellets in a feeding dish on a warm day, toxin-producing mold may appear.

While it is true that in some tests of rabbit feeds certain manufacturers have feeds that have consistently tested positive for mycotoxins at a higher rate than other feeds, almost all manufacturers of rabbit feeds will have mycotoxins show up in their feed at one time or another. Ethical/reputable manufacturers of feeds are aware of the danger and will store feed ingredients properly and have a frequent testing program for the presence of mycotoxins. If you prefer a particular rabbit feed brand, contact a representative of the company and question them about their practices to lower the risk of mycotoxins. Reputable manufacturers will have employees willing to take the time to address your concerns; if a particular company does not take such time you might think again about using their product!

Some manufacturers may add proprionic acid derivatives or calcium propionate to the feeds to help prevent mold growth. It has been shown that the yeast *Saccharomyces cerevisiae* and lactic acid bacteria (e.g., *Lactobacillus*) have the ability to bind several mycotoxins, including aflatoxins and ochratoxins, and these probiotics may be added to some feeds for this reason. Other bacteria of various genera (e.g., *Leuconostoc, Propionibacterium, Streptoccuocus, Enterococcus, Eubacterium*) have also been found to have the ability to bind some mycotoxins. Activated charcoal absorbs mycotoxins, but different types of activated charcoal have varying abilities to bind the poisons, so are not widely used. Hydrated calcium aluminosilicates (e.g., zeolites) are also able to bind mycotoxins in the gut and prevent their absorption into the body. Zeolites and other clays such as montmorillonite and bentonite may be added to feeds for their mycotoxin-binding properties, although the manufacturer will not be able to make claims based on the addition since the toxin-binding effects are variable.

Another factor that most likely affects the frequency of mycotoxin poisoning in rabbits is the governmentally allowed levels of the mycotoxins in commercial feeds. These levels are set by law, and – given rabbits' extreme sensitivity to many mycotoxins – there is some validly to the argument that the levels may be set too high for rabbits' safety. For example, rabbits are more sensitive to aflatoxin B_1 than ducklings, which are considered to be one of the most sensitive animals to mycotoxins. Rabbits are about twice as sensitive to aflatoxin B_1 than are cats and pigs, 2 ½ times more sensitive than rainbow trout and dogs, 3 times more sensitive than sheep, 6 times more than guinea pigs, 21 times more than chickens, 30 times more than mice, 34 times more than hamsters, and 60 times more sensitive than female rats.

Should one of your rabbits become ill from mycotoxins and subsequent testing shows mycotoxins present in the feed used, it is recommended the manufacturer be notified. It is best to do this in a non-combative manner, keeping in mind that—given the prevalence of mold spores on nearly all plant matter—it is essentially impossible to keep mycotoxins out of all feeds all the time (and hay is essentially *never* free of mold spores). Hopefully the manufacturer will respond in a helpful manner, but the sad truth is that this does not always happen. Some persons have even claimed to have been the recipient of threats from persons employed at producers of rabbit feeds and hay after informing the company their feed tested positive for mycotoxins.

Should you experience helpfulness or obstruction, share your experience with other rabbit owners. A manufacturer whose representative responds in a helpful manner should be rewarded, and it is good to warn other rabbit owners by spreading the word about those whose representatives are not helpful. As an attorney once told me, you have a legal right to share your personal opinions and your personal experiences; just remember to qualify them as such! Try to avoid making blanket statements.

Lessening the chances of mycotoxin poisoning

There are several actions a person can take to help reduce the chance that one of their rabbits will become poisoned by mycotoxins. Select your rabbit's pellets, hay, and vegetables carefully. Do not feed pellets, hay or vegetables that have obvious mold growing on them or that are discolored (although the presence of mold and/or spores does not necessarily mean mycotoxins are present). Store hay and pellets where they will remain cool and dry, but not in airtight containers. Remove uneaten pellets, hay, and water each day and replace with fresh. Keep the rabbit's dishes clean and dry. If possible, wash and dry the rabbit's food containers each day or wipe out with white vinegar. Keep the area around the feeding containers clean and free of spilled food. Older rabbits, smaller rabbits, and rabbits that are ill are the most likely to be severely affected by mycotoxins, and extra care should be taken in keeping the containers and feeding area of these rabbits clean.

Christine Carter, in her book *The Wonderful World of Pet Rabbits,* suggests that feeding a rabbit a variety of foods may lessen the effects of any mycotoxins present in a particular food. I found this an interesting suggestion, and believe there could be some validity to it, since the more of a mycotoxin that is consumed, the more likely negative effects will express in the rabbit. Certainly feeding a variety of foods might reduce the amount of mycotoxins consumed from any one food.

Mycotoxin distribution in feeds and hays is often patchy; that is, it often occurs in small areas in a large amount of feed or hay. It is for this reason that smaller rabbits are more likely to be affected by acute mycotoxin poisoning: For example, if six pellets are contaminated with mycotoxins, it is likely that one rabbit will be given and will consume all six pellets. If the rabbit is large, signs of mycotoxin poisoning may be minor or even go unnoticed by the owner; if the rabbit is smaller, the amount per body weight ingested is larger and signs may be severe. I have had personal experience with this phenomenon—the one rabbit I have had that suffered from mycotoxin poisoning was my smallest rabbit, a little Polish (she recovered after intensive treatment and nursing). None of my other rabbits showed any sign of such poisoning, although all had consumed the same grass-based pellet. For this reason, it is sometimes suggested that feeds be well-mixed before giving to the rabbit; this can break up any patches and lessen the chance of a rabbit receiving a large amount of mycotoxins.

Remember, however, that there will not always be obvious signs that pellets, hay, or other foods have mycotoxins in them. Should your rabbit(s) refuse to eat a food he/she has always eaten before, be open to the possibility the rabbit may be responding to the presence of mycotoxins and consider dumping the whole bag (especially if you have other rabbits who are also reluctant to eat the food). It is much better to sacrifice a bag of food or hay on the possibility of mycotoxins than to continue using the food and possibly having signs of mycotoxin poisoning appear in your rabbit!

Common mycotoxins

There are many different mycotoxins, and a rabbit's sensitivity to them will vary. This list does not contain all possible mycotoxins that may affect rabbits, but only a few of the most common ones.

aflatoxin B_1

Aflatoxin was the first-described mycotoxin and it is one of those most likely to contaminate food. It is produced by the molds *Aspergillus flavens* and *A. parasiticus*. Rabbits may become affected both by consuming it in food and by breathing contaminated dust, such as pellet or hay dust. It may affect airways and lungs as well as the liver and is a carcinogen. Aflatoxin B_1 is especially common on corn (maize) and peanuts, although it may also occur on soybeans, cottonseeds, rice, sorghum, and other cereals. Aflatoxins bind to macromolecules such as nucleic acids and nucleoproteins, resulting in reduced protein synthesis in the affected animal's body. Acute poisoning by afltaoxins may result in death after a short time of reduced appetite. Less acute poisoning in rabbits may result in decreased immune function, changes to blood profile, slow growth and eventual lung and liver damage.

citrinin
This mycotoxin is produced by *Penicillium* and some *Aspergillus* molds. In rabbits it often causes swelling of the kidneys, followed by necrosis. Citrinin is often found with OTA (see entry for ochratoxin A) in cereals such as wheat and barley. Rabbits exposed to smaller amounts of this mycotoxin may have lowered reproduction.

ergot alkaloids
Ergot is found in many grain seedheads, especially rye. The alkaloids are produced by the fungus *Claviceps purpurea*, found in more temperate to cold climates. The alkaloids cause vasoconstriction, which reduces blood flow and can lead to gangrene of the extremities in colder climates. They may also delay the start of lactation in does.

fumosin B_1
This mycotoxin is produced by *Fusarium* molds and may be found growing on corn, beans, rice, and wheat, among other plants. It is toxic to kidneys (nephrotoxic) and livers (hepatotoxic) in rabbits and may affect the reproductive abilities of bucks and the development of the embryos in pregnant does. Fumosin B_1 is extremely toxic to horses, causing swelling and eventual liquefaction of brain matter after earlier signs of dwindling appetite and lethargy. Fumosin B_1 may also have detrimental effects on the brains of rabbits; researchers have reported brain hemorrhaging in rabbits affected by fumosin B_1.

ochratoxin A (OTA)
Produced by *Aspergillus ochraceus*, other *Aspergillus* molds, *Penicillium viricatum* and *P. citrinum*, OTA is particularly widespread in temperate regions of the world. It is particularly common on barley, corn, and wheat, but may be found in sun-dried and/or vine-dried fruits as well. OTA is extremely toxic to cells, disrupting cellular processes, and may cause destruction of red blood cells in rabbits. It is also a carcinogen and is particularly toxic to the kidneys. As OTA is resistant to both high and low temperatures, this mycotoxin survives most processing. It is also very difficult to remove from the rabbit's body once

it has been absorbed because it is not water soluble. It may suppress the immune system, result in enlarged kidneys, and cause excessive liquid consumption and excessive urination.

trichothecenes (including T-2 and HT-2)
These mycotoxins are found in cereal crops and are mainly produced by *Fusarium* molds, although some trichothecenes are produced by other species of mold. These toxins may be found in many cereal crops, but are especially common in oats. Trichothecenes inhibit cellular protein synthesis, and a deficiency or excess of vitamins A and E may increase the toxic effects. At the time of this writing trichothecenes are not proven carcinogens. They inhibit protein synthesis and often affect the skin and digestive system. Affected rabbits may be sleepy, eat less or refuse to eat, salivate excessively, have dermatitis, bleed from the large intestine, exhibit incoordination, and become emaciated.

Vomitoxin/deoynivalenol (DON) is a mycotoxin included in the trochothecenes. Although toxic effects of this particular mycotoxin (produced by *F. graminearum*) are rare in rabbits, it's presence in feedstuffs is of import because where DON is found, there are often other mycotoxins present. Pregnant does consuming DON may lose weight.

Signs of mycotoxin poisoning
Poisoning by mycotoxins is called *mycotoxicosis* (plural mycotoxicoses). Mycotoxin poisoning can be chronic or acute, and signs will differ between the two, as well as depend upon the specific mycotoxin involved. If more than one mycotoxin is present, signs may be particularly severe. Signs of acute mycotoxicoses often involve the gut and/or liver and kidneys and may include any combination of the following:

- refusal to eat and/or drink
- fever
- icterus (jaundice)
- bloating
- gastrointestinal hypomotility (stasis)

- impaction
- bleeding from the large intestine
- brownish-yellow discharge from the anus
- mucus in the feces
- low body temperature
- incoordination
- twitching of limbs
- odd mouth movements (caused by ulcers in mouth and/or esophagus)
- head tilt
- severe pain
- convulsions.

Other signs in rabbits may include corneal ulcers, kidney problems, severe liver damage, a low red blood cell (RBC) count and high blood urea nitrogen (BUN). Mycotoxins may also suppress the immune system, cause cancer, result in genetic mutations, cause bone marrow problems, and damage the brain, lungs, spleen, heart, and reproductive organs. In acute poisoning there may be sudden failure of major organs such as kidneys, liver, and heart; chronic poisoning may cause a slow deterioration as these organs are gradually affected. The severity of signs will also depend upon the age, breed, length of exposure, and any existing stress from illness, heat, or other factors.

Treatment of mycotoxicosis

If mycotoxin poisoning (mycotoxicosis) is suspected, your vet may take a history, and take into account such factors as season of the year (mycotoxin poisoning can be more common in hot, humid weather) and possible routes of exposure. It is not necessary to consume all mycotoxins in order to be affected by them; exposure can also occur through contaminated bedding or inhalation of contaminated hay or feed dust. Bloodwork may also be done, and possibly radiographs. The latter can be helpful in diagnosing mycotoxicoses since a common finding is bloat without blockage.

Treatment of mycotoxicosis will differ depending upon the specific rabbits and signs present. Because of the ulcers that are often present in the digestive system with mycotoxin poisoning, treatment will often include giving sucralfate (Carafate), which acts by binding to the surface of ulcers and creating a protective coating that shields the open wounds in the digestive tract from bacteria which can cause blood poisoning (septicemia). Although sucralfate can be very effective in treating ulcers, it is not recommended that it be given in conjunction with cimetidine, phenytoin, tetracycline, or digoxin due to potential interactions. (It is suggested it be given at different times than other drugs, preferably with several hours between administration.) Prilosec (opmeprazole) or Zantac (ranitidine) may also be prescribed for ulcers.

Rabbits do not tolerate pain well, and because mycotoxin poisoning can cause severe pain a pain medication is often advisable. The NSAID Banamine has been found to be good for soft tissue pain, including that of the digestive tract. A narcotic painkiller such as butorphanol may also be prescribed, depending upon the specific case. Antibiotics may also be prescribed to help protect the rabbit from bacterial infection in the wounded intestinal tract, and fluids will almost always be given to help flush toxins from the body.

If the rabbit refuses to eat, syringe feeding may be necessary for a time, but always have fresh water and food available for when the rabbit recovers enough to eat on his/her own. Cristina Forbes, PhD, who has an excellent article on mycotoxin poisoning online, suggests feeding the rabbit wheat bran (with a little wheat germ and oatmeal added for taste) soaked in warm water and then drained and cooled, once a day to provide needed nutrition and promote healing of the digestive tract. The digestive system is likely to be sensitive for a long time after recovery starts, and Dr. Forbes suggests that fresh vegetables may be one of the most easily tolerated foods.

Because body temperature is often depressed with mycotoxin poisoning it should be monitored closely. If the temperature drops below normal, *slowly* warm the rabbit with hot water bottles or a pillow that can be heated in a microwave.

Having nursed a rabbit through mycotoxin poisoning, I know how difficult and stressful it can be for both the rabbit and owner. It often is truly a fight for life, but it can be successful. My little Polish rabbit lived many years after her bout with mycotoxicosis.

NUTRITIONAL HEALING

It has been found that giving supplements of large neutral amino acids (e.g., tryptophan), and antioxidants such as vitamin E, selenium, coenzyme Q10, or omega-3 fatty acids (see Chapter 4) can help lessen the effects of mycotoxin poisoning. If the mycotoxin is known to be one of the trichothecenes, giving vitamins A and E may help reduce toxic effects; although excesses of these same vitamins will *increase* the same toxic effects (see Chapter 5 for recommeneded vitamin amounts). Aloe vera can be given orally to help heal ulcers in the mouth and digestive tract. (If you harvest your own, peel leaves and remove the reddish portion along the vein.)

Clays such as bentonite have been found to absorb toxins, and may be helpful in treatment of mycotoxicosis as well as reducing the toxicity of dietary diazinon, although giving excessive amounts of clay should be avoided. Clays or clay-based products can accumulate in the cecum and lead to impaction if given in large doses or over long periods of time.

Nutrition can play an even larger role in preventing serious mycotoxin poisoning, given the evidence that some probiotics (e.g., *Lactobacillus, Saccharomyces*) can bind many mycotoxins in the gut before they do their damage (see Chapter Nine).

References

Abdel-Monem, H. Qar, and R. A. Attwa. 2012. Detoxification of Dietary Diazinon by Clay, Vitamin C and Vitamin E in Rabbits. *World App. Sci. J.* 19(1): 144-152.

Abdelhamid, A. M. 1990. Effect of feeding rabbits on naturally moulded and mycotoxin-contaminated diet. *Arch-Tierernahr* 40(1–2): 55–63.

Adams, T. 2009. Reading and understanding feed labels. Accessed 4/18/2010 ay http://www.farmandranchguide.co m/articles/2009/12/31/ag_news/livestock_news/live2.txt

Amr, A. R. and E. E-K Abeer. 2011. Hypolipidemic and hypocholestermic effect of pine nuts in rats fed high fat cholesterol diet. *World App. Sci. J* 15(12): 1667-1677.

Bayo, N. O., O. D. Eyarefe, and R. O. A. Arowolo. 2010. Effects of Tahitian Noni Juice on Ketamine Anaesthesia in some local rabbits. *Br. J. Pharmacol. Toxicol.* 1(2): 81-84.

Bommakanti, A .S. and F. Waliyar. 2000. Importance of aflatoxins in human and livestock health. Accessed 3/12/2010 at http://www.aflatoxin.info/health.asp

Brewer, N. R. 2006. Biology of the Rabbit. *J. Am. Asso. Lab. An. Sci.* 45(1): 8–24.

BSAVA Manual of Rabbit Medicine and Surgery, 2nd. edition. 2006. Edited by Anna Meredith and Paul Flecknell. Glouster: British Small Animal Veterinary Association.

Bucci, T .J, D. K. Hansen, and J. B. LaBorde. 1996. Leukoencephalomalacia and hemorrhage in the brain of rabbits gavaged with mycotoxin fumosin B_1. *Nat. Toxins:* 4(1): 51–52.

Carabano, R., I. Badiola, S. Chamoro, J. Garcia, A. I. Garcia-Ruiz, P. Garcia-Rebollar, M. S. Gomez-Conde, I. Gutierrez, N. Nicodemus, M. J. Villamide, and J. C. de Blas. 2008. Review New trends in rabbit feeding: influence of nutrition on intestinal health. *Span. J. Agri. Res.* 6(special issue): 15-25.

Carpenter, J. W. 2010. Diagnosing and treating gastric ileus/stasis in rabbits. *Proceedings:* CVC, Baltimore, USA.

Carter, Christine. 2006. *The Wonderful World of Pet Rabbits.* Pirion Pty Limited: Canberra.

Cheeke, Peter R. 2010. Nutritional Management of Rabbits and Principles of Rabbit Nutrition. Notes, 2010 ARBA National Convention.

Cheeke, Peter R. 1987. *Rabbit Feeding and Nutrition.* Orlando: Academic Press.

Chrenkova, M., L. Chrastinova, M. Polacikova, Z. Formelova, A. Balazi, L'. Ondruska, A. Sirotkin, and P. Chrenek. 2012. The effect of *Yucca schidigera* extract in diet of rabbits on nutrient digestibility and qualitative parameters in caecum. *Slovak. J. Anim. Sci.* 45(3): 83-88.

Clauss, M. 2012. Clinical Technique: Feeding Hay to Rabbits and Rodents. *J. Exo. Pet Med.* 21(1): 80-86.

Coblentz, W. K., J. E. Turner, D. A. Scarborough, K. E. Lesmeister, Z. B. Johnson, D. W. Kellogg, K. P. Coffey, L. J. McBeth, and J. S. Weyers. 2000. Storage Characteristics and Nutritive Value Changes in Bermudagrass Hay as Affected by Moisture Contnet and Density of Rectangular Bales. *Crop Sci.* 40(5): 1375-1383.

Cooke, B. D. 1985. Reduction of Food Intake and Other Physiological

Responses to a Restriction of Drinking Water in Captive Wild Rabbits, *Oryctolagus cuniculus* L.) *Aust. Wldlf. Res.* 9: 247-252.

Denton, D. A., J. F. Nelson, and E. Tarjan. 1985. Water and salt intake of wild rabbits (*Oryctolagus cuniculus* L.) following dipsogenic stimuli. *J. Phys.* 362: 285-301.

Eisermann, K., B. Meier, M. Khaschei, and D. v. Holst. 1993. Ethophysicological responses to overwinter food shortage in wild European rabbits. *Phys. Behav.* 54(5): 973-980.

Ferrets, Rabbits, and Rodents: Clinical Medicine and Surgery. Second edition. 2004. Edited by Katharine E. Quesenberry and James W. Carpenter. St. Louis: Saunders.

Forbes, C. 2002. Mold and Mycotoxins in Rabbit Feed. Accessed 6/17/2010 at http://www.morfz.com/myco.html

Fraser, M. and S. J. Gerling. 2009. *Rabbit Medicine and Surgery for Veterinary Nurses.* Chichester: Wiley-Blackwell.

Gidenne, T., B. Carre, M. Segura, A. Lapanouse, and J. Gomez. 1991. Fibre digestion and rate of passage in the rabbit: effect of particle size and level of lucerne meal. *An. Food Sci. Tech.* 32(1-3): 215-221.

Gidenne, T. and F. Lebas. 2002. Role of dietary fibre in rabbit nutrition and in digestive troubles prevention. *Proceedings:* 2nd Rabbit Congress of the Americas. Habana City, Cuba.

Harcourt-Brown, F. M. 2002. *Textbook of Rabbit Medicine.* Oxford: Butterworth-Heinemann.

Harkness, J. E., P. V. Turner, S. VandeWoude, and C. L. Wheeler. 2010. *Harkness and Wagner's Biology and Medicine of Rabbits and Rodents,* 5th Edition. Ames :Wiley-Blackwell.

Irlbeck, N. A. 2001. How to feed the rabbit (*Oryctolagus cuniculus*) gastrointestinal tract. *J. Anim. Sci.* 79: 343–346.

Jaynes, W. F., R. E. Zartman, and W. H. Hudnall. 2006. Aflatoxin B_1 adsorption by clays from water and corn meal. *Ap. Clay Sci.* 36(1–3): 197–205.

Jin, M, Q. Huang, K. Zhao, and P. Shang. 2013. Biological activities and potential health benefit effects of polysaccharides isolated from *Lycium barbarum. Int. J. Bio. Macromol.* 54:16

Johnson-Delaney, C. A. 2006. Anatomy and Physiology of the Rabbit and Rodent Gastrointestinal System. *Proceedings:* Association of Avian Veterinarians.

Leung, M. C. K., G. Diaz-Llano, and T. K. Smith. 2006. Mycotoxins in Pet Food: A Review on Worldwide Prevalence and Preventative

Strategies. *J. Agric. Food Chem.* 54(26): 9623–9635.

Li, X-M. 2007. Protective effect of *Lyceum barbarum* polysaccharides on streptosotocin-induced oxidative stress in rats. *Int. J. Biol. Macromol.* 40(5): 461-465.

Lowe, J. A. Pet Rabbit Feeding and Nutrition. In: *Nutrition of the Rabbit.* Carlos DeBlas and Julian Wiseman, eds. Wallingford: CABI Publishing.

McWilliams, D. A. 2001. Nutritional Pathology in Rabbits: Current and Future Perspectives. Paper: Ontario Commercial Rabbit Growers Asso. Congress.

The Merck Veterinary Manual. Ninth edition. 2005. Edited by Cynthia M. Kahn. Whitehouse Station: Merck and Co., Inc.

Mezes, M. 2008. Mycotoxins and other contaminants in rabbit feeds. *Proceedings:* 9th World Rabbit Congress, Verona.

Monk, K. A. 1989. Effects of diet composition on intake by adult wild European rabbits. *Appetite.* 13(3): 210-209.

Mugmai, C., A. Dal Bosco, R. Cardinali, R. G. Rebollar, L. Moscati, C. Castellini. 2014. Effect of pasture availability and genotype on welfare, immune function, performanace, and meat characteristics of growing rabbits. *World Rab. Sci.* 22(1): 29-39.

Pearce, M., I. Shahin, and D. Palcu. 2010. Available solutions for mycotoxin binding. Meriden Animal Health Limited. Accessed 7/15/10 at: http://en.engormix.com/MA-mycotoxins/articles/available-solutions-mycotoxin-binding_1500.htm

Richard, J. L. 2007. Some major mycotoxins and their myco-toxicoses—An overview. *Int. J. Food Micro.* 119(1–2):3–10.

Rogers, P. M., C. P. Arthur, and R. C. Soriguer. 1994. The rabbit in continental Europe. In: *The European Rabbit: The history and biology of a successful colonizer.* H. V. Thompson and C. M. King, eds. Oxford: Oxford University Press.

Rompala, Ron. 2002. Molds, Mycotoxins and Feeds: A Brief Summary. Accessed 7/7/2010 at http://www.blueseal.com/techtalks/13/

Saunders, Richard A. and Ron Rees Davies. 2005. *Notes on Rabbit Internal Medicine.* Oxford: Blackwell Publishing.

Somers, N., T. Milotic, and M. Hauffmann. 2012. The impact of sward height, forage quality and competitive conditions on foraging behaviour of free-ranging rabbits *(Oryctolagus cuniculus* L.) *Belg. J. Zool.* 142(1): 74-85.

Sun, Y. et al. 2018. The effects of low levels of aflatoxin B1 on health, growth performance and reproductivity in male rabbits. World Rab. Sci.

26(2): 123-133.

Tschudin, A., M. Clauss, D. Codron, A. Leisengang, and J. M. Hatt. 2011. Water intake in domestic rabbits (*Oryctolagus cuniculus*) from open dishes and nipple drinkers under different water and food regimes. *J. An. Phys. An. Nutr.* 95(4): 499-511.

Uden, P. and P. J. Van Soest. 1981. Comparative digestion of timothy (*Phleum pratense*) fibre by ruminants, equines, and rabbits. *Br. J. Nutr.* 47: 267-272.

Ueno, Y., H. Matsumoto, K. Ishii, and K. Kukita. 1976. Inhibitory effects of mycotoxins on Na+ -dependent transport of glycine in rabbit reticulocytes. *Biochem. Pharm.* 25(18): 2091–2095.

Uhllirova, L., Z. Volek, M. Mareunek, and E. Tumova. 2015. Effect of feed restriction and different crude protein sources on the performance health status and carcass traits of growing rabbits. *World Rab. Sci.* 23(4): 263=272.

Vough, Lester R. Evaluating Hay Quality. Fact Sheet 644, Maryland Cooperative Extension, University of Maryland.

Wang, M-Y, B. J. West, C. J. Jensen, D. Nowicki, C. Su, AfaK. Palu, and G. Anderson. 2002. *Morinda citrifolia* (noni): A literature review and recent advances in Noni research. *Acta Pharmacol. Sin.* 23(12): 1127-1141.

Whitman, Bob D. 2004. *Domestic Rabbits and Their Histories: Breeds of the World*. Leawood: Leathers Publishing.

Yousef, M. I., M. H. Salem, K. I. Kamel, G. A. Hassan, and F. D. El-Nouty. 2003. Influence of Ascorbic Acid Supplementation on the Haematological and Clinical Biochemistry Parameters of Male Rabbits Exposed to Aflatoxin B$_1$. *J. Env. Sci. Health Part B* 38(2): 193-209.

Chapter 7

PHYTOCHEMICALS AND PLANTS

When I began researching this and the following chapter, I quickly realized it would be an impossibility to come up with definitive lists of rabbit-safe and rabbit-toxic plants. Not only do opinions differ as to which plants should be included on which list, the truth is that the safety and/or toxicity of almost any plant depends upon the amount consumed, the form in which it is consumed, individual sensitivities, and many other factors.

Plants contain a huge variety of both simple and complex chemical compounds. Some of these are the macronutrients (proteins, lipids, and carbohydrates, Chapters 3 and 4); others are micronutrients (vitamins and minerals, Chapter 5). Those plant chemicals that are not nutrients are called *phytochemicals* or *phytonutrients*. Most plants contain numerous phytochemicals, some that are potentially beneficial and some that are potentially harmful to those who consume them. For example, there is evidence that the organosulfur compound *allyl isothiocyanate* that gives mustard and horseradish their distinctive "bite" can be carcinogenic in humans, yet it has also been found to *inhibit* the growth of prostate cancer cells. Canavanine, a non-protein amino acid, can cause atherosclerosis in humans but can also inhibit the replication of the influenza virus.

Although I generally dislike making blanket statements, I feel I must make this one: it is impossible for a person or a rabbit to eat enough to live and not consume anything that could potentially be harmful in one way or another. The best one can do is balance the risks and benefits, taking each individuals' health, needs, and sensitivities into account when deciding what foods to give your rabbits.

Quite often, limiting the amount of a potentially harmful substance is all it takes. For example, many rabbit owners have read or heard that rabbits should not consume apple seeds. Apple seeds do contain a chemical that is broken down to cyanide by stomach acid, but the truth is that there is so little of this compound in the seeds that if your rabbit were to consume an entire apple, seeds and all (or even two or three), you would most likely see no negative effect. The same is true of oxalates. While there is no doubt that animals can die of oxalate poisoning, this is most likely to occur only if very large amounts are consumed. A rabbit that ate rhubarb leaves (very high in oxalates) might well suffer serious complications; a rabbit that consumed even a fairly large amount of spinach leaves would be unlikely to be harmed.

As in previous chapters, I have included several tables and charts with information on specific nutrients and phytonutrients found in various rabbit foods. Please remember that data on any nutrient can (and does) vary considerably, depending upon what soil the plant grew in, what part of the plant was analyzed, how old the plant was, what method of analysis was used, and other factors. Values given must be taken as relatives, not absolutes.

SPECIFIC PHYTONUTRIENTS

Plants produce such vast amounts of phytochemicals (over 5,000 are known) that I can only touch upon a very few in this volume. In the years since I wrote the first edition of this book, many new phytochemicals have been described, and new information discovered about those that were already known. Some of these studies have focused on the interactions of phytochemicals with each other and with essential nutrients, for phytochemicals are *bioactive* compounds. That is, they intereact with components of living tissue. Once consumed, the amount of a phytochemical that can be absorbed in the lumen is called its *bioaccessibility*, which in turn affects the amount that will be *bioavailable*.

In simple terms, the above means that when a phytochemical is consumed in food, whether the consuming animal receives any of the potential benefits will depend upon factors such as the food in which it was consumed and what other foods were consumed at the same time. For example, it has been found that lutein uptake by certain cells is inhibited by naringenin but not affected by vitamin C or catechin. Other factors, such as individual genetic differences and the composition of the gut microflora will also affect bioavailability.

THE GARDEN PATCH

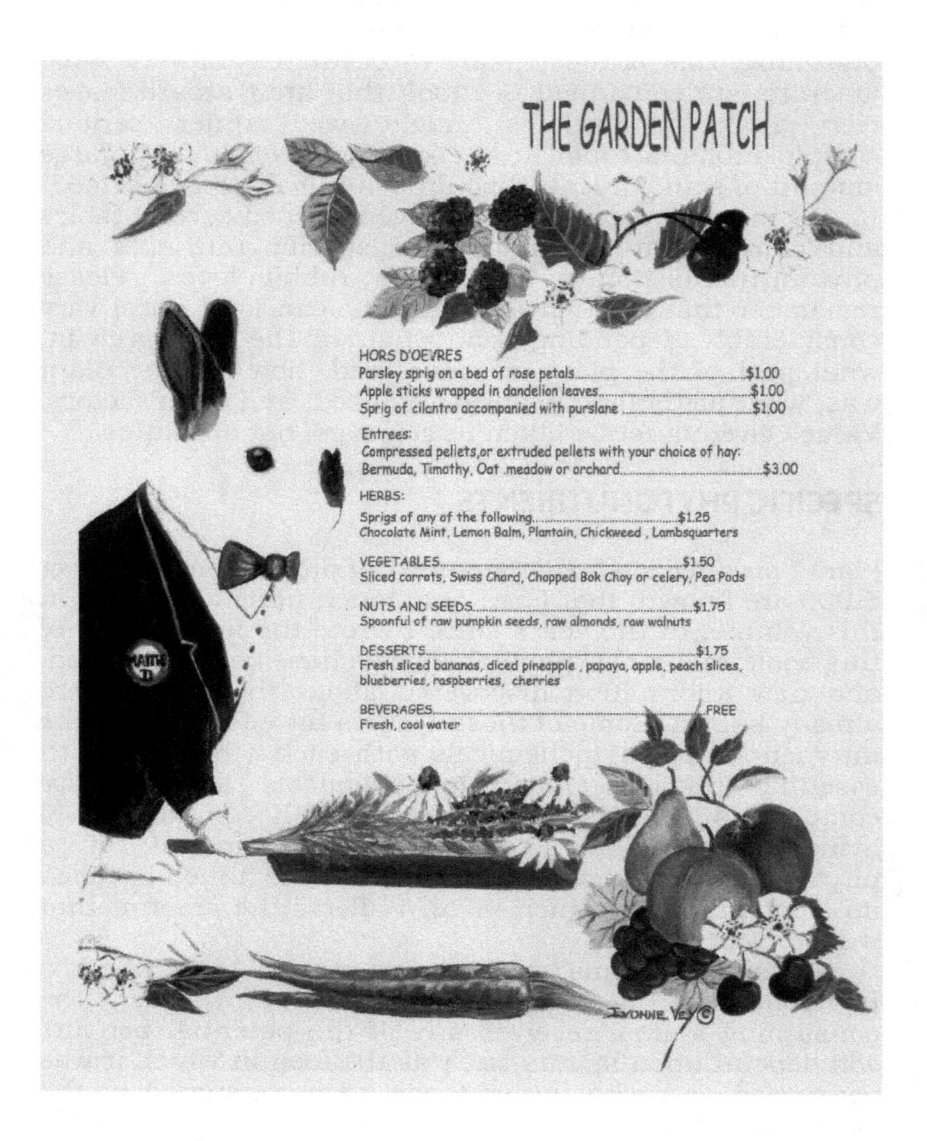

HORS D'OEVRES
Parsley sprig on a bed of rose petals..................................$1.00
Apple sticks wrapped in dandelion leaves..........................$1.00
Sprig of cilantro accompanied with purslane.....................$1.00

Entrees:
Compressed pellets, or extruded pellets with your choice of hay:
Bermuda, Timothy, Oat, meadow or orchard.....................$3.00

HERBS:
Sprigs of any of the following................................$1.25
Chocolate Mint, Lemon Balm, Plantain, Chickweed, Lambsquarters

VEGETABLES..$1.50
Sliced carrots, Swiss Chard, Chopped Bok Choy or celery, Pea Pods

NUTS AND SEEDS..$1.75
Spoonful of raw pumpkin seeds, raw almonds, raw walnuts

DESSERTS..$1.75
Fresh sliced bananas, diced pineapple, papaya, apple, peach slices, blueberries, raspberries, cherries

BEVERAGES..FREE
Fresh, cool water

Yvonne Vey ©

Frankly, most of us have neither the time nor the desire to keep up with the latest developments in nutrition and plant chemistry. Nor is it necessary, for we can safely assume that if we include foods that contain some of the phytochemicals described in this chapter in our rabbits diet, the potential for some benefit will exist. The one aspect of availability that it is worthwhile remembering is that the method of processing fruits and vegetables will affect whatever phytochemicals present. If fresh produce is boiled, most flavonoids will end up in the water, while carotenoids will tend to remain in the plant tissue, although they become more accessible due to the softening of tissues.

In this volume, for the most part I will focus on those phytochemicals that may appear in literature about rabbits or which I think might be of particular interest to those owning rabbits. Much of the information on phytochemicals necessarily contains the names of chemicals. Unless you have an interest in biology, you can ignore the more technical information and focus on the effects of particular phytochemicals and the plants in which they are found.

The words "phenol" and "terpene" will appear with relative frequency. It is not necessary to understand the chemistry of these compounds for the purposes of this book; only to realize they are two major classes of chemical compounds found in plants. But for those who are interested here are brief definitions:

Phenols, or phenolic compounds, are composed of one or more "aromatic rings" and one or more hydroxyl (C-OH) groups and are often attached to sugars. Many essential oils (e.g., clove oil) are phenolic compounds.

Terpenes are chemical compounds of 5-carbon units called isoprene units. There are many classes of terpenes depending upon the number of units (e.g., monoterpene, sesquiterpene). Many plants with terpenes also have noticeable fragrances, such as dill.

Menthol is a monoterpene, as are *geraniol* and *limonene*. Geraniol, found in blackberries, blueberries, carrots, cilantro, lavender, lemon, lime, nutmeg, oregano, and roses, among other plants, has been demonstrated to have fairly strong anti-tumor properties. Limonene, found in the essential oils of citrus (and in other plants), may also have anti-carcinogenic properties. Vitamin A is a diterpene.

Betalains

Once thought to belong to the proanthocyanins (see entry for flavonoids), it was later discovered that betalains have a different alkaloid-like chemical structure. Betalains are antioxidants and, like many other phytochemicals, may have several positive effects (e.g., anticancer, anti-inflammatory) effects on mammals who consume them.

There are two kinds of betalains; yellow betaxanthins and reddish betacyanins. The pigments are restricted to only a few plant groups, and are reduced with cooking. The pigments in beets, bougainvillea flowers, and prickly-pear cactus fruits are betacyanins. Prickly-pear cactus fruits are available in some areas of the southwestern US. Another cactus fruit with betalains is the red-fleshed red dragon fruit or "purple pitaya," also available in some areas. Cactus fruits also contain several micronutrients.

Swiss chard may contain reddish betacyanins or yellow betaxanthins, depending upon the color.

Caffeic acid

Caffeic acid (not related to caffeine, which is an alkaloid (see section on toxic plants later in this chapter) is a phenolic acid found in many foods, including hawthorn, artichokes, pear, basil, thyme, oranges and apples, and which appears to have several potentially beneficial effects on mammals who consume it.

Rosmarinic acid is an ester (organic equivalent of a salt) of caffeic acid and another acid (3, 4 dihydroxyphenyllactic acid). It is found in many herbs, including rosemary, oregano, lemon balm, mints, and sage. Rosmarinic acid is an antioxidant and in addition has been found to have antimicrobial, antiviral, and anti-inflammatory properties. It may have applications for asthma, arthritis, ulcers, and in treating poisoning from various toxins.

Canavanine

This is a non-protein amino acid found in legumes,

including alfalfa. Consumed in large amounts, it has been shown to cause lupus-like symptoms in humans and to increase the risk of atherosclerosis in rabbits. (A positive effect of this amino acid is that it has been found to inhibit the replication of the influenza virus.) The amounts rabbits might consume in alfalfa-based commercial foods are unlikely to cause serious problems in most rabbits.

Cardiac glycosides

These compounds affect the contractions of heart muscle and are toxic to the kidneys. Cardiac glycosides are found in a variety of plants, including Christmas Rose, foxglove, white water lily, and lily-of-the-valley. In general, even fairly small amounts of these compounds can have negative effects on mammals.

Carotenoids

This is a large class of over 600 fat-soluble yellow-to-red pigment compounds that are tetraterpenes. It includes the vitamin A precursors alpha-carotene, betacarotene, and beta-cryptoxanthin, as well as **lycopene, lutein**, and **zeaxanthin**, which are carotenoid pigments but are not vitamin A precursors. Pink guava is very high in carotenoids, and gac (*Momordica cochinchinensis*), mango, red watermelon, papaya, pumpkin, and seaberries (sea buckthorn fruits) are also good sources.

Lutein and zeaxanthin are xanthophylls, which are yellow carotenoid pigments. Lutein is found in red peppers, mustard, broccoli, zucchini, corn, peas, spinach, leeks, collards, and kale. Lutein is an antioxidant, has been found to protect against eye damage, may improve cardiovascular health, and has anti-inflammatory properties.

Zeaxanthin is a yellow pigment that, like lutein, may help protect eyes from age-related disease. It is found in abundance in broccoli, carrots, corn, collards, lettuce, peas, pumpkin, spinach, and wolfberry. Lycopene is the pink-to-red pigment found in gac, guava, pink grapefruit, blood oranges, tomatoes, and watermelon. It has been found to have antioxidant, antifungal, anti-cancer, and antibiotic properties. Lycopene may also help prevent the growth of cataracts.

Although the bioavailability of many phytochemicals is reduced by processing, the bioavailability of carotenoids is increased by chopping, mashing, and cooking.

Chaconine
See entry under solanine.

Coumarin
The polyphenol coumarin, a compound that tastes like vanilla, gives flavor to many plants, including apricots, cherries, cinnamon, lavender, licorice, mullein, strawberries, parsley, and sweet clover. Coumarin also gives cut hay its sweet smell. There is some evidence that coumarin has anti-tumor and antifungal effects as well as blood-thinning properties (when altered to dicoumarol by various fungi). Very high doses of coumarin over long periods of time could potentially be toxic, but this is unlikely to occur in the average diet (rabbit or human).

Cyanogenic glycosides
In the presence of water, these substances release hydrocyanic acid, or prussic acid. Heating, particularly by dry heat, may reduce the toxins. Many mammals can tolerate small amounts of these compounds, but larger amounts can be toxic. Cyanogenic glycosides are found in fruit pits, especially those of the rose family (e.g., apple, pear) and in many other plants such as flax and eucalyptus. Many mammals can tolerate small amounts of cyanogenic glycosides, and it would require high consumption of fruit pits or other cyanogenic glycoside-containing plants for negative effects to appear in a rabbit or human. Ruminants are more sensitive to the compounds than monogastric mammals such as rabbits and humans.

Flavonoids
This is a huge class of phenolic compounds (over 5,000 have been described) that have a chemical structure similar to that of vitamin E, and like vitamin E may function as antioxidants. Water-soluble pigments, such as those in grape skin and autumn leaves, are included in the flavonoids. Some flavonoids may inhibit enzyme

systems in mammals, others may help preserve vitamin C, function as antioxidants, have antibacterial, anti-inflammatory, and/or anti-tumor effects. Others, such as citrus flavonoids naringin and naringenin, have been shown to have an antiatherogenic effect on rabbits.

Flavonoids are found in most plants, including fruits, vegetables, nuts, seeds, herbs, spices, and flowers. Apples, blueberries, red/purple grapes, onions and tea are some common plants particularly high in the compounds. Plants with high concentrations of flavonoids have been used in many traditional systems of medicine, and positive applications for these compounds continue to be discovered. However, it should be noted that not all of the positive effects found in research trials will necessarily be reflected in the mammalian body and that in fact some researchers have found that the bioavailability of flavonoids is low. Still, not all positive effects are lost, and there may yet be many potential applications for these compounds.

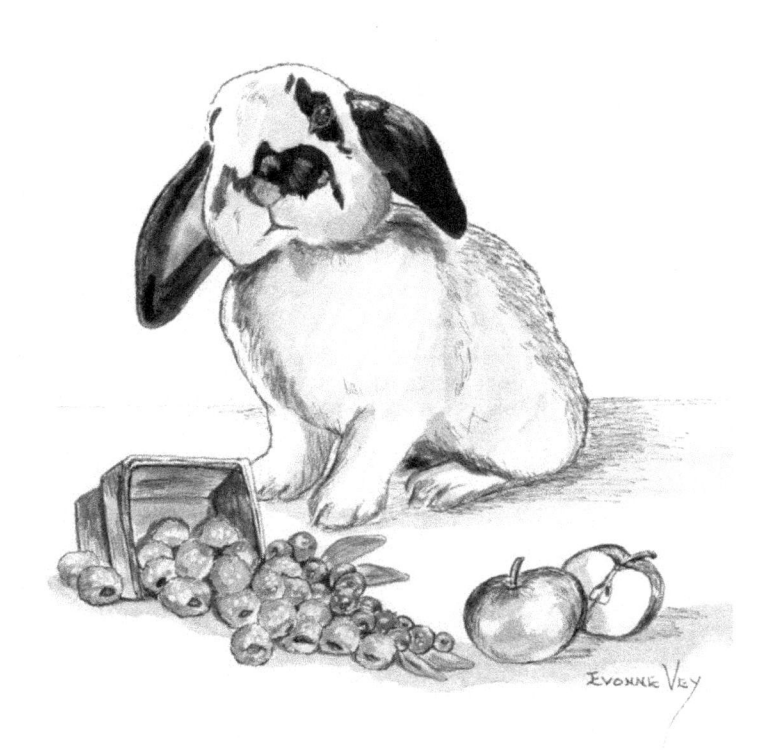

There are seven major subclasses of flavonoids:

- ***Anthocyanidins.*** These are violet and blue plant pigments, which may possibly have some anticarcinogenic effects as well as other beneficial effects to those mammals that consume them. If the anthocyanidin is coupled with sugars, it is called an *anthocyanin.* These compounds are found in many foods but are particularly abundant in avocado, berries (including cranberries), cherries, red cabbage, red onion, mango, plum, purple corn, and rhubarb stalks.
- ***Chalcones.*** A group of yellow pigments that have two aromatic rings. Chalcones are found in apples, ashitaba, bean sprouts, citrus fruits, eucalyptus, licorice, mangosteen, pears, potatoes, strawberries, and tomatoes, among other plants. Chalcones have been found to have antioxidant, antimicrobial, anti-inflammatory and anti-cancer actions, and to positively affect vision and cardiovascular health. Some chalcones also have insulin-like effects.
- ***Flavanols.*** This subclass includes *proanthocyanidins* and *catechins,* among others. Proanthocyanidins are antioxidants and may also have anti-inflammatory and antiatherogenic effects. They are found in foods such as apples, berries, and red grapes. Catechins are also powerful antioxidants. They are found in many plants, including apples, apricots, berries, grapes (seeds and skin) and in green tea leaves. Catechins may help prevent and heal skin damage. Dates and other dried fruits have been found to be extremely high in catechins.
- ***Flavonols*** are colorless or yellow flavonoids found in plant leaves and many flowers. *Quercetin,* the most common flavonoid, may help reduce the risk of cancer, prevent bone loss, and improve lung function and cardiovascular health. Quercetin occurs in apples, blueberries and other berries, broccoli, kale, and tomatoes, among many other foods. *Rutin* is a flavonol that

may have positive effects on the brain. It is found in citrus fruits, parsley, tomatoes, and apricots. *Myricetin*, another flavonol, is found in grapes and walnuts, among other foods, and has anti-inflammatory effects.

- **Flavanones**. *Naringenin*, which may have anti-carcinogenic and anti-inflammatory effects in addition to being an antioxidant, has also been shown to have an anti-atherogenic effect on rabbits. Flavanones are found in citrus fruits and some other plants. *Silybin* is a flavanone in milk thistle.

- **Flavones.** These are yellow pigments found in plant foods such as celery, oranges, palm fruit, parsley, and tangerines. *Luteolin* is a specific flavone that has antioxidant, anticarcinogenic, and anti-inflammatory properties and may help in maintaining healthy blood glucose levels. It is found in celery, green chile, lemons, olives, oregano, parsley, peppermint, rosemary, sage, and thyme, among other plants. *Apigenin*, another flavone, is found in parsley, celery, and chamomile.

- **Isoflavones.** These flavonoids are found in legumes, especially soybeans. Isoflavones have estrogen-like effects and are termed *phytoestrogens*. Although some researchers have found that they may help reduce some cancers, especially breast and prostate cancer, there is no conclusive evidence of this at the time of this writing. Isoflavones have been found to improve semen characteristics in male rabbits.

Glucosinolates (Goitrogenic glycosides, goitrogens)
These are found in plants of the cabbage family (crucifers), and can cause goiter (enlarged thyroid). They are responsible for the bitter, hot taste to mustard and horseradish. There are several different kinds of glucosinates. Some may irritate mucus membranes, others may depress growth, cause liver and kidney lesions, inhibit iodine uptake by the thyroid and inhibit thyroid function. However, it would be necessary for large

amounts to be consumed for the effects to appear. Plants with goitrogens include: Brussels sprouts, broccoli, cabbage, mustard, turnips, bok choy, rutabaga, black mustard, watercress, radish, stinkweed, kale, and kohlrabi. A possible concern with rabbits is that glucosinolates are high in several oil meals used in rabbit feeds, especially in rapeseed meal. Should a feed contain a high percentage of rapeseed meal, it might be helpful to limit the amount given the rabbit.

Isothyocyanates are formed by the hydrolysis of glucosinolates. They have been found to have anticarcinogenic properties. Different isothyocyanates are produced from the different glucosinolates in cruciferous vegetables. *Indole-3-carbinol,* which is produced by the breakdown of a particular glucosinolate (glucobrassicin), may have anticarcinogenic and antiatherogenic effects, in addition to being an antioxidant.

Gossypol

Gossypol is a terpene (dimeric sesquiterpene) found in cottonseeds. It binds to proteins and accumulates in the body. For this reason it may be of concern if the rabbit consumes large amounts of a commercial feed containing cottonseed meal. Its effect on rabbits is primarily on reproduction; bucks may have lowered sperm count. Gossypol is detoxified by heating, and therefore a feed containing cottonseed meal that is heat-treated will most likely be safe for rabbit consumption.

Lectins

Lectins are glycoproteins found in legumes such as raw beans (including soybeans) and peanuts, fungi, lichens, grains, some fruits, and plants of the nightshade family. They are also found in animals; for example, rabbit bone contains lectins. The different lectins are of varying toxicities. Most cause red blood cells (erythrocytes) to clump (agglutinate), although the particularly toxic lectin found in castor beans (ricin) does not. Lectins may be a defense mechanism in plants and may help regulate plant physiological functions. In mammals, consumption of some plant lectins may cause fatty degeneration of the liver, edema, kidney damage, hemorrhages in lymphatic tissue, and digestive problems. In rabbits, the damaging effect of lectins on epithelial cells can cause acute gastrointestinal problems. However, high amounts of the raw foods containing the lectins need to be consumed for signs to appear.

The toxicity of lectins is reduced by steam heating, although dry heat may not reduce toxicity appreciably. It should be realized that any unheated food produced from lectin-containing plants will contains these compounds, including cold-pressed soybean and wheat germ oil.

It has been shown in some studies that rabbits receiving small amounts of foods containing lectins may develop a partial immunity to lectin toxins.

Oxalic acid/oxalates

Oxalic acid is formed from the breakdown of carbohydrates and protein in plants. The oxalic acid may then form water-soluble salts with sodium and potassium or bind with calcium, iron, or magnesium in various insoluble oxalates. The amount and type of these various oxalates in plants will depend upon many factors, including the soil, weather, age of the plant, and plant part. Mammals also synthesize oxalic acid in their bodies, and it may also be produced if excessive vitamin C is consumed.

There is a great deal of sometimes conflicting information on oxalates in the rabbit diet. The effects of oxalates may in fact depend upon a variety of factors, including the form in which they are consumed, the ratio of oxalate to calcium in the plant consumed, amount of ascorbic acid consumed in diet, hydration of the animal consuming the oxalates, amount of magnesium, iron, and calcium in diet, and other factors such as any existing kidney disease. Sometimes apparent toxicity of plants with high levels of oxalates may even be partly from other factors—for example, it is thought that the anthraquinone glycosides in rhubarb leaves are as responsible for their toxicity as are the oxalates. Most oxalates are absorbed in the stomach, sand several factors affect how much oxalate is in soluble form in that organ: pH concentration, calcium, magnesium, and phosphate.

Different forms of oxalate can have different effects upon the rabbits consuming them. That consumed as calcium oxalate crystals may pass through the digestive system mostly undissolved (although the strong acid of the rabbit stomach may dissolve some), and the extremely sharp crystals can irritate the gut as it passes. That consumed in soluble forms and absorbed in the gut then binds to calcium, iron, and magnesium, forming insoluble crystals (these crystals in the bladder may cause urinary urgency in humans) which, under some conditions, may form stones in the kidney. However, calcium oxalate stones are not nearly as common in rabbits as calcium carbonate stones (see entry for calcium in Chapter 5).

Factors that are thought to influence the creation of calcium oxalate stones include insufficient water intake, lack of exercise, high ascorbic acid intake, eating large amounts of plants with high oxalate:calcium ratio (such as sorrel, spinach, beet greens, and purslane) and consistent high consumption of oxalate-rich foods. Factors that may reduce the likelihood of oxalate stone formation in the kidneys include: high fluid consumption, exercise, moderate consumption of plants with high oxalate content and high ascorbic acid content, feeding plants with a low oxalte:calcium ratio (e.g., parsley), choosing plants with most oxalate present in the insoluble forms, consumption of hard water (binds oxalate and decreases its absorption), and giving probiotics, some of which (e.g., *Lactobacillus, Oxalobacter)* "eat" oxalates. It has been found that the amount of *Oxalobacter* in the colon partially controls the amount of free oxalate.

Although some sources claim there is no diet that will help dissolve stones of calcium oxalate, other sources claim that there is some evidence consuming high-acid fruits such as lemon could help dissolve calcium oxalate crystals (although not calcium carbonate crystals) in some cases. In humans, taking potassium-magnesium citrate has been found to help prevent calcium oxalate kidney stones, and some vets recommend giving potassium citrate to rabbits with calcium oxalate stones.

Since oxalates do affect the availability of magnesium, iron, sodium, potassium, and phosphorus, this fact should be considered when feeding high-oxalate foods. If the ratio of oxalate to calcium in foods is high, the oxalate may bind calcium from other foods as well. Interestingly, some vets advise that rabbits with calcium carbonate uroliths be given foods high in oxalate because of this calcium-binding activity.

Overall, controlling potential harm from high-oxalate diets appears to be—as with so many aspects of nutrition—achieved by moderation. Most rabbits consuming reasonable amounts of moderate-oxalate foods along with occasional treats of high-oxalate foods will suffer no adverse effects from oxalates if they are drinking sufficient liquids and getting adequate exercise.

Phloridzin
This is a flavonoid (see earlier entry) found in the roots and bark of certain trees in the rose family (e.g., cherry). This flavonoid can inhibit cellular absorption of glucose in rabbits, possibly interfering with essential cell processes. However, it would take the consumption of high amounts to have this effect. Rabbits consuming moderate amounts of the bark of trees in this family (including apple, pear, and cherry) would be unlikely to suffer any ill effects.

Phthalides (pronounced 'thalides')
Phthalides are members of a group of phytochemicals called *lactones,* cyclic organic esters that give white wines their aroma and taste and are also found in foods as diverse as orange juice and black pepper. The phthalides have the ability to enhance other flavors although they are tasteless themselves. Phthalides can have beneficial effects on mammals because they have been found to cause artery muscles to relax, helping to reduce blood pressure and stress. Some phthalides have also been found to have ani-cancer effects. The phthalides are primarily found in celery, lovage, and species of angelica. The root of European angelica (*Angelica sinensis)*, also known as dong quai or dang gui, has long been used in traditional medicines. The leaves and stems of a Japanese angelica, *Angelica keiskei*, or ashitaba, also contain phthalides (as does parsley) and may be used as a salad herb.

Phytates (phytic acids)
These are found in fairly high amounts in cereal grains such as barley and oats, oil seeds such as sunflower seeds, and legumes such as beans, peas, and lentils. They are found in moderate amounts in roots and tubers, and

leafy greens contain small amounts. Their primary negative effect is that they can form complexes with some vitamins and minerals, preventing the absorption of the micronutrients.

Ruminants such as cows have long been known to utilize these compounds quite well, but since most monogastric mammals do not, foods containing phytates were sometimes listed as unsafe for rabbits. However, it is now known that rabbits utilize phytates quite well, although they may not be able to utilize all the phosphorus since the phytates are not hydrolyzed (broken down) until they reach the cecum, and most phosphorus absorption occurs earlier in the rabbit digestive tract.

Phytosterols
Phytosterols are compounds similar to cholesterol that are produced by plants. They inhibit the absorption of cholesterol in the intestine, and have been found to help lower cholesterol levels. Phytosterols are found in unrefined vegetable oils such as olive oil, sea buckthorn oil, whole grains, legumes, seeds, and nuts.

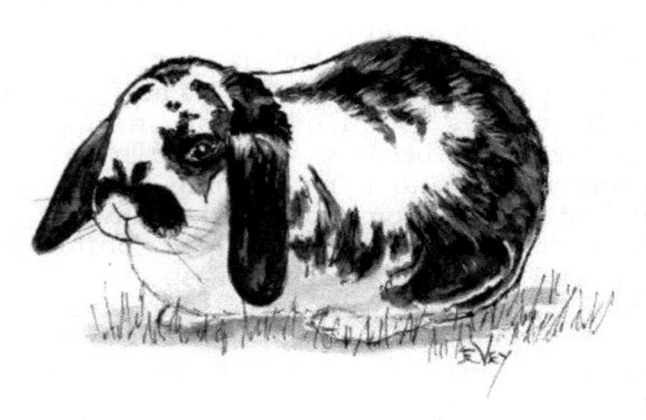

Piperdine/Piperidine
This is the alkaloid that gives black pepper its distinctive taste. It is also the alkaloid found in the extremely toxic poison hemlock (water hemlock has a different toxin, cicutoxin, a terpenoid resin) as well as many other toxic plants, including lupine and tobacco. Piperdine can be fatal if consumed in high amounts, but consumed in smaller amounts piperdine can also increase the

bioavailability of nutrients, and may have antioxidant and antifungal properties. Piperidine has been found to have antidiarrheal effects in rabbits and has been shown to enhance the bioavailability of certain therapeutic drugs in rabbits.

Pyrrolizidine alkaloids
Found in ragwort, comfrey, wooly groundsel, and amaranth, among other plants, these alkaloids can have a very negative effect on many herbivores. However, rabbits have been found to be resistant to their effects.

Quinones
Quinones are phenolic compounds found in many plants. In high concentrations they may have cytotoxic and cardiotoxic effects. They are most toxic in the free state (unbound) and may lose some toxicity when bound to other molecules. Consumption of some flavonoids (see earlier entry) have been found to suppress the cardiotoxic effects of quinones in rabbits. A variety of plants contain quinones, including some legumes, lilies, and verbena. Juglone, found in walnut, is a type of quinone derived from naphthoquinone that can be toxic to rabbits, and walnut bark, shells, and leaves are best not given to rabbits, although the meats are safe in small amounts.

Resveratrol
Resveratrol is a fat-soluble stilbene, which is another polyphenolic compound. It has anticarcinogenic and antiatherogenic effects (including reducing occurrence of thromboses in blood vessels) and may help reduce damage from toxins. It is found in high amounts in berries such as blueberries, cranberries, and mulberries, eucalyptus, red grapes, and peanuts.

Salicylic acid
Salicylic acid is natural aspirin, and has both anti-inflammatory and blood-thinning properties. It is found in high concentration in willow bark, and is also found in many other foods, including almonds, broccoli, chili, cucumbers, spinach, zucchini, tomatoes, dill, thyme, basil, oregano, tarragon, bell peppers, peppermint, berries,

cherries, cantaloupe, guava, oranges, pine nuts, pineapple, plums, and raisins. Salicylic acid has been used to treat skin problems in humans because of its anti-inflammatory effects, and has also been found to reduce the risk of colorectal cancer in humans. However, large amounts of foods containing this phytonutrient should not be given to an animal allergic to NSAIDs or with diabetes or poor circulation.

Saponins

Saponins are glucosides with foaming characteristics. They are found in many plants, including alfalfa, spinach, Christmas rose, daisies, horse chestnut trees, asparagus fern, and oats. Saponins impart a slightly bitter taste to the plant. There are several different kinds of saponins: those found in oats and spinach aid the body's ability to absorb calcium and silica and aid digestion; *sarsaponins* found in yucca may also be beneficial to some animals. Saponins may help lower cholesterol and inhibit the growth of cancer cells.

Some saponins may have negative effects—a few can irritate mucous membranes and destroy red blood cells, high concentrations of other saponins may reduce feed intake and growth rate in some animals. Saponin concentrations found in plants such as English Ivy contain high enough concentrations of saponins with negative effects to be life-threatening to animals that consume large amounts.

Solanine

Solanine and chaconine are glycoalkaloids found in plants of the nightshade family, which includes potatoes and tomatoes. Solanine and chaconine do not accumulate in the body and are not destroyed by heat. They are usually present in highest amounts in green parts of plants, and are also high in potato sprouts. (Potato variety also affects the amounts—in one study mature potatoes of some varieties had higher content than green potatoes of other varieties.) They have been found to destroy rabbit erythrocytes (red blood cells). However, both rabbits and humans would need to consume large amounts for toxic effects to appear. Some glycoalkaloids may also have fungicidal properties.

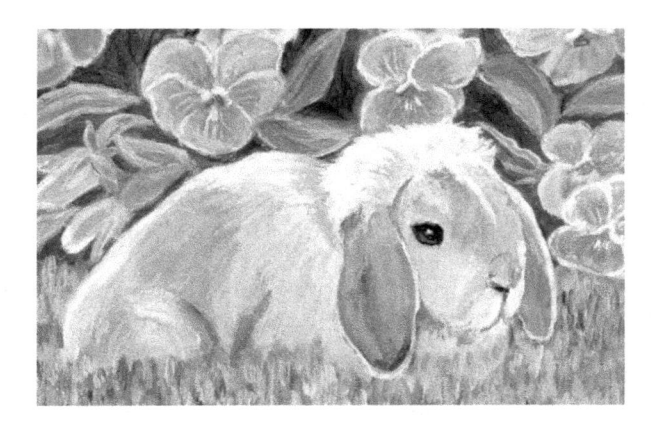

Tannins

Tannins are plant polyphenols that bind and precipitate protein. There are two kinds of tannins, what are called *condensed tannins*, or proanthocyanidins, and *hydrolyzable tannins*. Tannins may occur in leaves, bark, wood, fruit, or roots, and are found in a wide variety of foods, including grapes, persimmons, blueberries, tea, legumes, grasses such as corn and sorghum, and trees such as birch, eucalyptus, maple, oak, pine, and willow. For the plant, they protect against pathogens and discourage possible consumption through their bitter taste. However, if consumed by a mammal in large enough quantities they can reduce feed intake, fiber and organic matter digestibility, and production, depending upon the animal's specific tolerance to tannins. Kidney and gastrointestinal problems can occur. High tannin intake may also increase fecal nitrogen. Drying reduces the solubility of tannins and thereby reduces their ability to complex with proteins.

Condensed tannins, or (technically) oligonetric proanthocyanidins (OPC), are flavonoids (see earlier entry). In some studies they have been found to be more powerful antioxidants than vitamins C and E, although it is possible they lose some of this ability in the process of being digested. They do not interfere with iron absorption as do the hydrolyzable tannins, and have been found to improve cardiovascular health, increase joint flexibility, and have anticarcinogenic effects. Proanthocyanidins are found in particularly high amounts in apples, bilberries, black chokecherries, black currants, brown sorghum, cranberries, grapes, pomegranates and seaberries.

Hydrolyzable tannins (gallotannins, ellagic acid, ellagitannins) are dissolvable in water and are more toxic than condensed tannins. In addition to binding with proteins, they interfere with the absorption of iron. In one study on pikas, another lagomorph, protein and fiber digestibility were lower in pikas consuming a diet high in hydrolyzable tannins.

Many herbivores, including rabbits, can consume low-tannin diets with no ill effects. The age of the tannin-containing plant will affect its toxicity on mammals since the protein-precipitating capacity of the hydrolyzable tannins in plants such as oak decreases as the leaves age and the amount of condensed tannins increases. Therefore, mature oak leaves and ripe acorns can most likely be consumed without ill effect.

Possible positive effects of hydrolyzable tannins are that they are antioxidants, can be toxic to some microorganisms (including *Staphylococcus aureus*) and that some hydrolyzable tannins may prevent toxins from mutating genes, and may therefore have an anti-carcinogenic effect. Ellagic acid is found in raspberries and many nuts.

Xanthones (xanthonoids)

Xanthones are phenolic compounds that are found in many of the members of three plant families. Over 200 xanthones have been identified, but (at this time) they are probably best known for their presence in mangosteen, *Garcinia mangostana,* a white fruit from Southeast Asia. Xanthones, including several of the *mangostins* and *garcinones*, have been found to be powerful antioxidants, to lower cholesterol, suppress tumor growth, and to have anti-inflammatory and antimicrobial effects (including antimicrobial action on MRSA). Mangosteen, mangosteen juice, and other products derived from the fruit are now available in many health food stores.

PHYTONUTRIENTS IN CULTIVATED PLANTS

When considering the pros and cons of feeding rabbits plants with any of the above phytochemicals, it is important to remember that most of the studies that have been done on the various chemicals have been done on the compounds in isolation, and compounds rarely occur in isolation in nature. One very interesting study on the interaction of lectins and tannins found that while both compounds had an inhibitory effect on alpha amylase individually, together they had no significant inhibitory effect on the enzyme. Also, as noted earlier in this chapter, phytochemicals may not have all the effects in a living organism that they have been found to have in isolation.

However, it is also true that many of the studies that have been done on the effect of these compounds on mammals have been done with rabbits. There are multiple studies on many phytochemicals the results of which appear to indicate that some phytochemicals may have positive effects on rabbits when consumed in adequate amounts. Not all phytochemicals have positive effects—some may have negative effects if consumed in high enough amounts or under particular conditions.

Remember that individual rabbit sensitivities vary. One rabbit might be unable to tolerate large amounts of vegetables containing oxalates or tannins, and another might be able to eat high amounts without any ill effects. Introduce new foods into the rabbit's diet one at a time, starting with small amounts. Observe any reactions, and if the rabbit appears able to tolerate the new food, gradually add more.

Another caution I must repeat is that regarding the tables on nutrient content in this volume: listed values are not firm, but are simply averages. Data on any nutrient can (and does) vary considerably, depending upon what soil the plant grew in, what part of the plant was analyzed, how old the plant was, and what method of analysis was used, among other factors. Due to its nature, nutrition is far from an exact science—values given must be taken as relatives, not absolutes.

Greens and Vegetables

Fresh vegetables (both greens and root vegetables) and herbs are not absolutely necessary for a domestic rabbit's diet, but they can be valuable sources of water, protein, vitamins, minerals (including iodine, which is low in most other rabbit foods), and other potentially beneficial phytochemicals such as flavonoids.

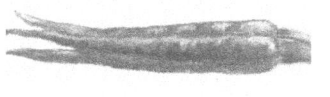

Table 7:1. Nutrient and phytochemical and composition of selected vegetables and herbs. Listings are of those vitamins and minerals present in relatively high amounts; vegetables may contain additional vitamins and minerals. Phytochemicals listed are those discussed in this volume. Oxalate content is given as VL (very low), < 2mg/100g food; L (low), 2–10mg; M (moderate), 11–99mg; H (high), 100–199mg; or VH (very high), > 200mg. *Values compiled from multiple sources.*

Vegetable /herb	fiber (%)	protein (%)	sugar (%)	vitamins	minerals	oxalate	phytochemicals
arugula/ rocket	1.6	2.6	2.1	A, B$_5$, C, folate, choline, K	Ca, K, Mg, Mn	L	betacarotene, glucosinates, indole, lutein, zeaxanthin,
basil	2.7	2.9	0.3	A, C, E, K	Cu, Mg, Zn	H	betacarotene, caffeic acid, limonene, lutein, luteolin, rosmarinic acid, salicylic acid, zeaxanthin
beet greens	3.7	1.8	___	B$_1$, folate, C, K	Ca, Cu, Mo	VH	betacarotene, betacyanins, lutein, oxalate, zeaxanthin
broccoli	3.0	2.98	1.7	A, B$_2$, B$_3$, B$_5$, B$_6$	Cu	VL	alpha and betacarotene, flavonols, glucosinolates, indole, lutein, querctin, salicylic acid, zeaxanthin
cabbage	2.4	1.4	1.2	B$_6$, K	Cu, Si	L	glucosinolates, indole, quercetin
carrot root	4.7	1.0	5.0	biotin B$_6$, folate	Si	M	alfa and betacarotene, betacryptoxanthin, coumarin, geraniol, lycopene, oxalate, zeaxanthin
carrot tops	18.0	13.0	___	A, C, K	K	VH	betacarotene, oxalate
celery (chop before feeding)	1.9	1.46	2.0	A, B$_6$, ribo, fol.ate, choline, K	Fe, K, Mn, Mo, Zn	M	alkaloids, caffeic acid, coumarin, flavones, limonene, luteolin, phthalides, quecetin, zeaxanthin
chard, Swiss	1.6	1.8	1.0	A, B$_3$, C E, K		VH	alpha and betacarotene, betacyanins, betaxanthins, lutein, oxalate, zeaxanthin
cilantro	2.8	2.0	1.0	A, B$_3$, C, E, K, choline	K, Si	M	alpha and betacarotene, geraniol, quercetin
dandelion greens	4.0	1.9	0	A, B$_6$, C, E, K	Fe, Mn	M-H	alpha and betacarotenes, lutein, oxalate, crypto- & zeaxanthin
dill	2.0	3.26	0	A, B$_2$, C, B$_6$, folate	Ca, Fe, K, Mg, Mn, Zn	H	limonene, quercetin, salicylic acid, terpenes

Vegetable/herb	fiber (%)	protein (%)	sugar (%)	vitamins	minerals	oxalate	phytochemicals
kale	2.0	3.1	1.3	A, B_6, C, K	Ca, Co, Cu, K, Mn, Mo	L	alpha and beta-carotene, flavonols, glucosinolates, indole, lutein, quercetin, zeaxanthin
lettuce, leaf	1.3	1.4	0.9	A, B_6, C folate, K	Fe, Ca, Mg. Mn, P	L	alpha betacarotene, quercetin, lutein, anthocyanin (red leaf)
lettuce, Romaine	1.9	1.8	0.7	A, folate, C, K	Cu, K, Mg, Mn	VL	alpha and beta-carotene, lutein, quercetin, zeaxanthin
oregano, fresh	42.8	11.0	0	A, B_6, folate E, K	Fe, Mn	L-M	betacarotene, geraniol, luteolin, rosmarinic acid, salicylic acid
parsley	3.3	2.7	1.0	A, B_3, B_5, folate, C, K	Ca, K, Mn, Se, Zn	VH	betacarotene, coumarin, flavones, lutein, luteolin, oxalate, quercetin, terpenes
peppermint	8.0	4.0	0	A, B_1, B_2, B_3, B_5, folate, C	Ca, Cu, Fe, K, Mn, Se	L-M	luteolin, rosmarinic acid, salicylic acid, tannins
perilla (shisho)	7.0	3.9	0	A, K	Fe, Mo	L-M	anthocyanins, phytosterols, rosmarinic acid, chalcones
pumpkin, canned	3.0	1.0	3.0	A, B_5, E	Co, Cu, Fe, Mn, Si	M	alpha and betacarotene, betacryptoxanthin, lutein, phytic acid
purslane	4.1	2.0	—	A, B_1, B_2, B_3, B_6, C	Fe, K, Mg, Mn	VH	alkaloids, betacarotene, betaxanthins, coumarin, betacyanins, oxalate, saponins, tannins
rosemary, fresh	14.0	3.0	0	A, B_2, B_6, C, folate	Ca, Cu, Fe, K, Mg, Mn	L-M	caffeic acid, limonene, luteolin, rosmarinic acid, tannins, terpenes
spinach	2.7	2.9	0.4	A, B_2, folate, choline C, E, K	Ca, Cu, I, K, Mg Si, Zn	VH	alpha & betacarotene, lutein, oxalate, quercetin, salicylic acid, saponin, zeaxanthin
thyme, fresh	14.0	6.0	0	A, B_2, B_3, B_5, B_6, C.	Ca, Fe, Mg. K	L-M	alpha & betacarotene, caffeic acid, limonene, luteolin, rosmarinic acid, salicylic acid
zucchini	2.0	1.87	0	B_6, folate, C	K, Mn	L	betacarotene, lutein, salicylic acid

Vegetables can also serve to stimulate the appetite of anorexic rabbits and add interest and variety to a healthy rabbit's meals. There have been many studies on the effects of adding various root and/or leaf vegetables to the diets of rabbits, and most show no significant negative effects from such additions, especially if they are made in moderation. However—as with all foods—what may be beneficial in small amounts may not be so in larger amounts. The age, breed, health, and reproductive status of the rabbit need to be taken into consideration. Some rabbits appear to have a sensitivity to greens in particular and will produce very soft cecotrophs if they are given in high amounts (see Chapter 7).

Broccoli is a potent antioxidant and contains phytochemicals that have been found to have anticarcinogenic effects in rabbits. Arugula, a cruciferous vegetable, also contains many cancer-fighting phytochemicals. Tomatoes (technically fruits but mentioned in this section because of their usual inclusion with vegetables) contain flavonols and carotenoids, and are especially high in lycopene, which has been found to have anticancer activity. Broccoli, carrots, collards, lettuce, and spinach all contain zeaxanthin, and lutein is found in spinach, zucchini, collards, mustard, and kale. The lowly vegetable celery is a treasure trove of vitamins, minerals, and phytochemicals, including copper, iron, limonene and quercetins. It is one of the few good sources of phthalides, which have been found to lower blood pressure and reduce stress. (Celery leaves are safe to feed rabbits, and so are the stalks if chopped into small pieces.) The leaves and stems of parsley and the herb ashitaba (*Angelica keiskei*) are another rabbit-safe source of phthalides.

Asian vegetables are available in some areas, and small amounts of many of these can also be given to rabbits with safety. Bok choy (pak choi, *Brassica chinensis*) and Chinese cabbage (Napa cabbage, *Brassica rapa*) are two commonly available Asian vegetables. (Since these are in the cabbage family, extra caution should be observed by giving the rabbit only very small pieces at first until their digestive systems adjust to the new foods.) A lesser-known cabbage is the rosette cabbage, or wu ta cai, a variety of *B. chinensis*. This flat cabbage forms a low rosette of dark-green leaves, and the young leaves in particular are very palatable and rich in nutrition. Ceylon spinach (*Basella alba*), also called Malabar spinach, is another Asian vegetable available in some areas. It is not a true spinach but a perennial vine native to SE Asia, the leaves of which contain large amounts of soluble fiber. Water spinach (*Ipomoea aquatica*), also called kang kong, is another vine, this one related to sweet potato. It is commonly used in SE Asian cuisine and Southern US cuisine.

Herbs

Many herbs have high concentrations of various beneficial phytochemcials and nutrients. Rosemary, oregano, parsley, dill, peppermint, sage, thyme, basil, tarragon, and lemon balm are among the many herbs that contain flavonoids that have antioxidant, anti-inflammatory, and antimicrobial effects. Adding a few herb leaves to a rabbit's diet may help fend off or ameliorate the effects of many diseases. Perilla, or shisho (*Perilla frutescens*), a minty basil-like herb popular in many Asian and SE Asian cuisines, is now available in some grocery markets, as is sawtooth coriander (*Eryngium foetidum*) and ashitaba (*Angelica keiskei*), a type of angelica that is in the celery family. Like the more commonly available herbs, these contain many valuable nutrients and phytonutrients

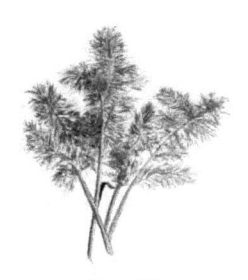

The kind and amount of phytochemicals in herbs and vegetables will vary depending upon the age and part of the plant. Intestinal absorption of phytochemicals is affected by the presence/absence of other phytochemicals and nutrients consumed at the same time, and effects of specific phytochemicals may be reduced or enhanced depending upon those other nutrients. For example, it was found in studies on intestinal absorption in human cells that lutein absorption was impaired by naringenin but was not affected by catechin. But most of us have neither the time nor the inclination to keep up with the latest information on phytochemical bioactivity in rabbits and other mammals. What we can do is add small amounts of vegetables and herbs with potentially beneficial phytochemicals to our rabbits' diets and trust—based on studies on the effects of such phytochemicals in rabbits' diets—that our rabbits will reap some benefits.

Fruits

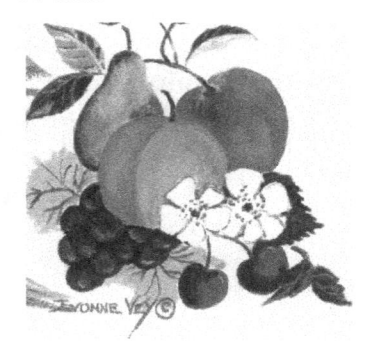

Fruits are often extremely good sources of phytonutrients as well as other nutrients (see chapters 5 and 6). Blueberries and cranberries contain various phytochemicals that have been found to help protect the brain from age-related deterioration, lessen light-induced retinal damage, and prevent bacteria from attaching to the lining of the rabbit urinary tract. Cranberries also have flavanols and proanthocyanidins that help prevent tooth decay and have an anti-inflammatory effect. It has also been suggested by some researchers that cranberries may help protect rabbit kidneys from infection-induced damage. Fresh guava juice has been found to lower the blood sugar of rabbits. The ellagic acid in red raspberries may have anticarcinogenic effects and other phytochemicals may have positive effects on the cardiovascular system. The bromelain in fresh and unpasteurized frozen pineapple helps digest protein and may help reduce inflammation and inhibit the growth of tumors.

Pomegranates and pomegranate juice and extracts have been found to have many potentially beneficial effects. The flavonoids present in pomegranates (feed rabbits juice only) produce anti-inflammatory effects in rabbits and may hold promise in treating diseases such as arthritis. Tannins in the fruit have anti-inflammatory and anti-cancer effects, have been found to inhibit the growth of *Staphylococcus aureus* and may inhibit enterotoxin production; pomegranate peel extracts have been found to have an exterminative effect on rabbit coccidian oocysts; and the juice may help protect from cardiovascular disease.

A variety of fruits from other geographical areas are now available in some groceries and specialty stores, and many of these also have high amounts of various phtochemcials: mangosteen has high levels of xanthones, acai (*Euterpe oleracea*), a dark purple berry from the Amazon, has been found to have cardioprotective effects on rabbits, and seaberry, or sea buckthorn (*Hippophaea rhamnoides*), a plant that is native to northern Asia and

Siberia, contains many carotenoids and flavonoids that have antioxidant, anti-atherogenic and antimicrobial effects. Goji (wolfberry), the fruits of two species of the boxthorn plant in the Solanaceae family, *Lycium chinense and L. barbarum*, have very high levels of beta-carotene and zeaxanthin and are good for eyes and may help prevent heart disease. They also contain compounds (including polysaccharides) that reduce fever, reduce inflammation, have anti-tumor and antimicrobial effects, and protect the liver and kidneys. The xanthones in mangosteen (*Garcinia mangostana*) may have anti-tumor and antimicrobial effects. Starfruit, or carambola, has a very high oxalate content and may be better avoided or given to rabbits in very small amounts. Note: One caution in feeding exotic fruits—feed only pulp or juice, seeds from fruits such as acai, cherimoya, passion fruit, pomegranate, and prickly pear should be removed before giving the fruit pulp to rabbits.

The above are only a few examples; most fruits contain many phytochemicals with potentially beneficial effects. Remember though, that many local fruits such as blueberries and raspberries have high levels of many of the same phytonutrients, so it is not necessary to pay premium prices for you and your rabbits to benefit from the effects of phytonutrients. Nor are the potential benefits of phytochemicals limited to fresh fruits—many dried fruits have been found to have extremely high levels of flavonoids. Dried dates, cranberries, figs, and apricots have been found to have especially high levels of catechins, but these dried fruits should only be fed to **adult** rabbits and in small amounts because of the high sugar content.

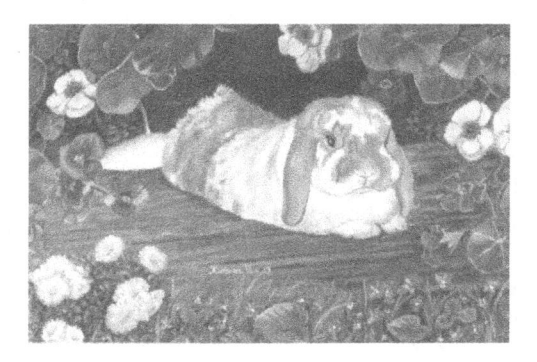

Table 7:2. Nutrient and phytochemical composition of selected fruits. Listings are of those vitamins and minerals present in relatively high amounts; fruits may contain additional vitamins and minerals. Phytochemicals listed are those discussed in this volume. Oxalate content is given as VL (very low), < 2mg/100g food; L (low), 2–10mg; M (moderate), 11–99mg; H (high), 100–199mg; or VH (very high), > 200mg. *Values compiled from multiple sources.*

Fruit	fiber (%)	protein (%)	sugar (%)	vitamins	minerals	oxalate	phytochemicals
acai pulp	29.	8.5	14.	A, E, K	Cu, Fe, K, Zn	M	antho and proanthocyanins, ellagitannin, resveratrol
apple	2.55	0.23	10.4	B$_3$	K, Si	VL	anthocyanidins, caffeic acid, catechins, oxalate, proantho-cyanidins, quercetin
apricot	2.0	1.4	9.24	A, B$_3$, B$_5$, C	Co, K, Mg,	VL	alpha and betacarotene, catechins, coumarin, lycopene, proantho-cyanidins, quercetin
banana	2.5	1.05	12.2	B$_5$, B$_6$, biotin	K, Mg, Mn	L	fructans
blueberry	2.5	0.72	9.96	B$_5$, E	Mn	L	anthocyanidin, catechins, ellagic acid, flavonols, geraniol, oxalate, proanthocyanidins, quercetin, resveratrol, salicylic acid
cherry	1.5	0.92	7.7	C	K, Si	L	anthocyanidins, betacarotene, catechins, coumarin, limonene, lutein, oxalate, proanythocyanidins, quercetin, salicylic acid
cranberries dried	5.8	0.07	65.0	B$_3$, folate K	Mn	L	anythocyanidin, catechins, ellagic acid, lutein, oxalate, proanthocyanidins, quercetin, resveratrol, salicylic acid, terpenes, zeaxanthin
dates, dried	6.7	2.05	68.0	folate	Fe, K, P, Si	VH	catechins (extremely high), tannins
grapes, white	0.9	0.72	17.	B$_1$, B$_2$, B$_6$, C, K	Cu, Fe, Mn	VL	catechins, myricetin, quercetin, rutins, tannins, zeaxanthin
grapes, red/purple	1.0	0.7	15.5	B$_1$, B$_2$, C, E	K	VL	catechins, ellagic acid, oxalate, proanythocyanidins, quercetin, resveratrol, saponins
grapefruit, pink	1.1	0.6	6.98	B$_3$, C	K, Mg	M	coumarin, cryptoxanthin, flavonones, limonene, lycopene, naringen, oxalate
honeydew	0.6	0.5	8.12	B$_3$, C	K, Mg, Zn	VL	lutein, oxalate, zeaxanthin

Fruit	Fiber (%)	protein (%)	sugar (%)	vitamins	minerals	oxalate	phytochemicals
mango	1.8	0.51	14.8	B3, C, E	K	VL	anthocyanidins, alpha and betacarotene, cryptoxanthins, gallic acid, lutein
nectarine	1.6	0.9	7.89	B3	K, Mn	VL	betacarotenes, beta-cryptoxanthin, lutein, lycopene, oxalate
papaya	1.8	0.51	18.0	A, B5, C	K	L	betacarotene, betacryptoxanthin, lutein, oxalate, papain
peach	2.1	0.64	10.6	A, B3, B5, E	Cu, Mg	L	anthocyanidins, betacarotene, cryptoxanthins, lutein, oxalate, proanthocyanidins
pear	2.1	0.4	9.8	B5	Co, K	L	anthocyanidins, caffeic acid, cryptoxanthin, lutein, oxalate
pineapple	1.3	0.45	.26	B3, C	Mn, I, Si	L	bromelain, carotenes, coumarin, salicylic acid
plum	1.5	0.8	9.92	A, E	Cu, K	L	anthocyanidins, alpha and beta-carotene, catechins, coumarin, lutein, oxalate, quercetin, salicylic acid
pomegranate (juice)	0.6	0.98	25.5	B5, folate C, E	Cu, K, P, Zn	M	alkaloids, anthocyanidins, ellagic acid
prickly pear fruit	4.5	0.97	—	A, B3, C, K	Fe, Mg, P, Se, Zn	M	betacyanins, lutein, quercetin
raspberry	6.6	1.0	4.42	B5, C	Mn, Zn	M	anthocyanidins, catechin, ellagic acid, gallotannins, oxalates, phytic acid, quercetin, resveratrol, salicylic acid
strawberry	2.3	0.6	5.0	folate C	K, Mn	L	anthocyanidins, catechins, coumarin, ellagic acid, lutein, oxalate, phytic acid, proanthocyanidins, quercetin, salicylic
tangerine	2.0	1.0	11.0	A, C	K	M	alpha and betacarotene, beta-cryptoxanthin, flavones, geraniol, limonene, lutein, oxalate, zeaxanthin
tomato	1.0	0.9	2.7	A, B3, B5	Co, Cu	M	alpha carotene, chalcones, coumarin, flavonols, lycopene, oxalate, quercetin, rutin, salicylic acid
watermelon	0.45	0.6	6.2	B5	Mg	VL	betacryptoxanthin, lycopene, oxalate

Flowers

Giving a few edible flowers to your rabbit can be an enjoyable way (for both owner and rabbit) to add interest to the rabbit's diet and give a safe treat. Yellow to red flowers such as marigolds, chrysanthemums, and nasturtiums often contain high amounts of carotenoids, and blue to violet flowers often contain proanthocyanidins and other potentially beneficial flavonoids. The following flowers are safe to feed rabbits (feed only petals, not seeds or leaves unless you have specific knowledge they are also rabbit-safe):

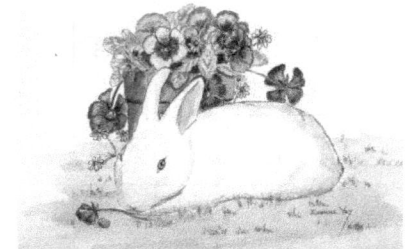

- aster
- carnation
- chrysanthemum
- daisy
- geranium
- geum
- hollyhock
- marguerite
- Michaelmas daisy
- marigold, common (*Tagetes*)[3]
- marigold, pot (*Calendula*)
- nasturtium
- pansies
- roses
- stock
- sunflowers
- violets
- wallflower

Give your rabbit only those flowers you have knowledge were not sprayed or otherwise treated with any pesticides, fungicides, or other toxic compounds. I have purchased special bags of hay with marigold petals added (available at the time of this writing from Kaytee) as a treat for my

---

[3] What is sometimes called "Cape marigold" is not a true marigold, but the weed *Arctotheca calendula,* which is *not* safe to feed rabbits.

rabbits. The rabbits appeared to enjoy the added flavor and it was a simple way to add potentially beneficial phytochemicals to my rabbits' diet.

Nuts, seeds and grains

Nuts and seeds contain many phytonutrients and are also very high in many vitamins and minerals (e.g. magnesium, potassium, vitamin E), providing a good source for some micronutrients that may be lacking in fruits and vegetables. They have other benefits as well. For example, pumpkin seeds have been found to have compounds that help prevent kidney stones and compounds that may have some anti-parasitic action. However, very small seeds (e.g., milo) *can* be a danger to rabbits because of the possibility a rabbit might swallow them whole. Swallowed whole, small seeds could become stuck in the pylorus and cause a serious blockage. Give your rabbit only larger seeds such as sunflower seeds and pumpkin seeds.

Contrary to popular belief, grains do play a role in the diet of many wild populations of *Oryctolagus cuniculus* (see Chapter 1). Small amounts of a grain such as rolled oats can be given to healthy rabbits as a safe low-calcium treat.

Table 7:3. Nutrient and phytochemical composition of selected grains, nuts, and seeds. Listings are of those vitamins and minerals that may be present in relatively high amounts in the listed food and of phytochemicals discussed in this volume. Oxalate content is given as VL (very low), < 2mg/100g food; L (low), 2-10mg; M (moderate), 11-99mg; H (high), 100-199mg; or VH (very high), > 200mg.

Grain/ nut/seed	fi- ber %	pro- tein	vitamins	minerals	oxa- late	phytochemical
barley	17.1	12.24	B_1, B_3, B_6, choline, E	Ca, Fe, Mg, Mo, Se, Zn	VL	fructans, phytic acid
oats, rolled	11.0	22.0	B_1, B_5, folate	Ca, Cu, Fe, K, Mg, Mn, Se, Si, Zn	M	betaglucan, phytic acids, saponins
pumpkin seeds	3.9	24.5	B_1, B_2, B_3, B_5, B_6, choline, E	Cu, Fe, K, Mn, P, Se, Zn	M	betacarotene, phytic acid
sunflower seeds	10.5	22.4	B_1, B_2, B_3, B_5, biotin, folate, choline, E	Ca, Co, Cu, K, Mg, P, Se, Zn	M	phytic acid, oxalate
walnuts	6.8	24.06	B_1, B_3, B_5, B_6, biotin, folate, choline, E	Cu, K, Mg, Mn, P, Se, Si, Zn	H	ellagic acid, oxalate, phytic acid, quer- cetin, resveratrol

Table 7:4. Nutrient and phytochemical composition of selected legumes. Listings are of those vitamins and minerals that may be present in relatively high amounts in the listed food and of phytochemicals discussed in this volume. Oxalate content is given as VL (very low), < 2mg/100g food; L (low), 2-10mg; M (moderate), 11-99mg; H (high), 100-199mg; or VH (very high), > 200mg. *Values compiled from multiple sources.*

Legume	fiber (%)	protein (%)	vitamins	minerals	oxalate	phytochemicals
alfalfa hay	35.0	17.05	A, E, K	Ca, Co, Fe, Mg, Mn, P, Zn	L	isoflavones, saponins
alfalfa sprouts	1.8	3.96	B_1, B_2, B_5, B_6, biotin, folate, B_{12}, K	Co, Fe, K, Mg, Mn, P, Se, Si, Zn	VL	isoflavones, saponins
clover, white	26.9	18.92	A, B_1, B_2, B_3, B_5, B_6, biotin, folate, B_{12}, choline, E, K	Ca, Co, Fe, K, Mg, Mn, P, Se, Si, Zn	H	isoflavones, salicylic acid
peanuts	8.0	24.0	B_1, B_2, B_3, B_5, B_6, biotin, folate, B_{12}, E, K	Co, Fe, K, Mg, Mn, P, Se, Si, Zn	M	isoflavones, lectins, oxalate, proanthocyanins, resveratrol
soybeans	9.3	36.5	B_1, B_2, B_3, B_5, B_6, biotin, folate, B_{12}, choline, E, K	Co, Fe, K, Mg, Mn, P, Se, Si, Zn	M	isoflavones, gallic acid, lectins, oxalate, phytic acid, saponins

Legumes

When I was originally researching this book, particularly as I prepared tables listing the foods that contained various necessary nutrients, I was struck by how often one particular plant came up, even for those nutrients that were harder to find in natural rabbit foods. There really is a rabbit "wonder food," I realized, and it is alfalfa. (My second thought was how many mainstream companion rabbit experts were not going to like that statement!) I finally understood why this plant has been used as the basis for so many commercial rabbit foods.

Alfalfa contains a great many vitamins, minerals, and phytonutrients, along with the macronutrients (carbohydrates, fat, and protein). It can be very difficult to ensure that a rabbit receives adequate amounts of several of these nutrients if it is not given alfalfa in one form or another. Since our domestic rabbits are *not* wild and do not have the opportunity to forage as do their wild relatives, they do not have the opportunity to select foods that would provide nutrients missing in their diet. Instead, they must make do with what we provide. Grass hay is not a particularly nutritious food. Legumes, on the other hand, are nutrient-packed, alfalfa-based pellet or a little alfalfa hay occasionally can help ensure a rabbit receives needed nutrients.

But as with all foods, alfalfa and other legumes should be fed to rabbits according to their needs. While giving a rabbit some of this mineral-and-vitamin-packed, nutrient-dense food can be very beneficial, over-feeding of alfalfa and alfalfa-based foods could potentially lead to obesity or other nutritional ills. Use common sense and observe the health of your rabbits.

GARDENING FOR RABBITS

Although this volume is not intended as an herbal, I have had several requests for more practical information about gardening and the use of various plants for medical conditions. Lisa Hodgson, editor and publisher of *Bunny Mad!* kindly gave me permission to reprint the following article I wrote for her magazine:

Choosing Plants for a Rabbit Garden
by Lucile Moore[4]

Bunnies and gardens just seem to go together—perhaps because they do! Providing garden-fresh produce to one's rabbit helps ensure the bunny's full nutritional needs are met and also makes the rabbit very happy, for most bunnies love to munch on fresh plants.

Because of the emphasis on giving companion rabbits grass hay in much pet rabbit literature, it may come as a surprise that fresh broad-leafed plants are just as critical to a rabbit's diet as grass hay. Due to their small size and high rate of metabolism, rabbits need some succulent nutrient-rich plants for their digestive system to function optimally and to provide necessary energy and nutrients not supplied in grass hay.

Although supermarket produce is certainly beneficial to a companion rabbit, some nutrients are inevitably lost during transport and storage. Growing a few plants for the rabbit's consumption in a small outdoor garden or even in

---

[4] Moore, Lucile. 2016. Choosing Plants for a Rabbit Garden. *Bunny Mad!* Issue 23. Reprinted with permission.

containers on the balcony or windowsill is simple to do, adds variety and nutrients to the rabbit's diet, and can help save time and money.

But what plants are the best choices for a rabbit garden? The answer depends mostly upon one's garden space and personal preferences (and the rabbit's preferences!), for a wide variety of plants are both safe and beneficial for rabbits.

FLOWERS

It is not necessary to grow vegetables to supplement a rabbit's diet with fresh food—flowers do just as well! Giving a few edible flowers to your rabbit can be a fun way to add interest and nutrition to a rabbit's diet while beautifying one's home. Yellow to red flowers contain high amounts of vitamin A precursors and blue to violet flowers such as pansies and violets contain high amounts of potentially beneficial phytochemicals that may have antimicrobial, anti-cancer, anti-inflammatory, and pain-relieving effects. Even white or cream-coloured flowers often have powerful phytochemicals. Because of these potent phytochemicals, flowers are best given to rabbits in small amounts, and should always be added to the diet gradually, starting with only a bite or two.

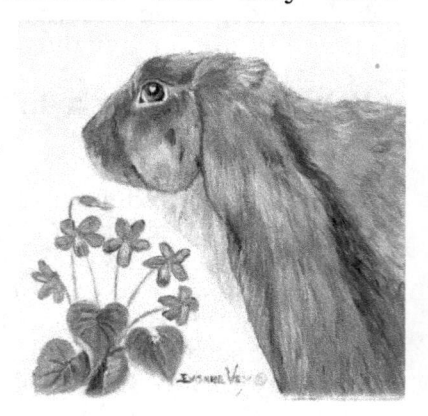

Bunny-safe flowers include:

Aster
Blue cornflower (bachelor's buttons)
Carnation
Chamomile
English Daisy
Geranium (leaves and flowers)
Geum
Goldenrod (leaves and flowers)
Hollyhock (leaves and flowers)
Marguerite

Michaelmas daisy
Marigold (flowers of common and pot marigold, or calendula, but not of cape marigold, which is toxic)
Nasturtium (leaves and flowers)
Pansies (leaves and flowers)
Roses
Stock (gillyflowers)
Sunflowers (leaves and flowers)
Violets (leaves and flowers. Some sources recommend avoiding yellow-flowered violets)
Wallflowers
Yarrow (leaves and flowers)

Note: *Caution should be observed in feeding flowers because many garden flowers are not safe. Give only flower petals and leaves that are known to be safe, and only feed flowers that have not been treated with insecticides or disease-controlling chemicals.*

FRUIT

Many fruits contain high amounts of minerals and phytonutrients that can help reduce inflammation and pain, can have positive effects on the urinary tract, and may help fight cancer and/or tumours. Fruits also contain soluble fibres that can be beneficial to the rabbit digestive tract when given in moderate amounts.

While most fruits are difficult or impossible to grow in limited garden space, some of the smaller fruits such as brambles (blackberries), raspberries, and currants can be grown on small plots, or in the case of strawberries, in containers. Provided no chemicals have been applied to the plants for disease control, the fruits of roses (rose hips) are highly nutritious and may be enjoyed by rabbits.

LEAFY GREENS

"Leafy greens" is a large group that contains a variety of leaf vegetables (and some leafy herbs such as parsley and cilantro) that have high water content and high amounts of many necessary vitamins and minerals as well as potentially helpful phytonutrients that may have antimicrobial, anti-inflammatory, antioxidant, and anticancer effects. In a study I did on health and diet among companion rabbits, greens were the only food the consumption of which had a relationship to the number of episodes of gastrointestinal hypomotility (commonly called stasis): study rabbits given greens in their diet had significantly fewer episodes than those not given greens.

Many greens are readily available in supermarkets and one might wish to grow those that are less commonly available, although even easily purchased greens will have a higher nutrient content if they are consumed shortly after harvesting them from one's own garden. Although greens are both easy to grow and highly beneficial to rabbits, like all foods they should be introduced slowly into a rabbit's diet. Some rabbits are sensitive to particular greens and can only eat very small amounts without producing soft stools.

Lettuces. There is an abundance of lettuce varieties ranging in colour from green to red, spotted, and bronze. Although most are high in nutrients and phytonutrients (the exception being store-bought iceberg lettuce, which it is better not to feed to rabbits), the specific nutrients present will vary with colour, the red, bronze, and spotted lettuces having more vitamin A precursors (carotenes). Lettuces are one of the greens that are easily grown in pots.

Chard. Colourful yellow to purple rainbow Swiss chard contains betalains, a class of phytochemicals that is found in very few plants and which has antioxidant and antifungal effects, and may also help prevent cancer. Chard also contains many minerals and vitamins. Stalks should be chopped before feeding to rabbits

Chicory, endive/escarole and spinach. These greens have received some bad press because of their high calcium and oxalate content, but much of that is bound in an insoluble form and the greens can be safely given to healthy rabbits in moderate amounts. However, they are best given in only very small amounts to rabbits with existing bladder or kidney disease or to those rabbits at high risk of developing such disease (obese, inactive or drinks little water). These greens have high carotene content and also contain many minerals and phytochemicals.

Cruciferous greens. Greens that are members of the cabbage family, such as rocket (arugula), kale, mustard, and the various cabbages contain cancer-fighting chemicals as well as many vitamins and minerals. Because of their gas-producing potential it is important to introduce them slowly into a rabbit's diet, and it is best to give only moderate amounts even to those rabbits accustomed to eating them.

HERBS

In addition to high amounts of vitamins and minerals, herbs contain many potentially beneficial phytochemicals (e.g geraniol, rosmarinic acid, limonene) that give these plants their distinct aroma and flavour and which may have antimicrobial, anti-inflammatory, antioxidant, antiatherogenic, analgesic, and cancer-fighting properties. Because of these potent phytochemicals, herbs are best given to rabbits in small to moderate amounts, always beginning with just a bite or two. Many herbs (such as basil and parsley) adapt well to container gardening and can be grown in pots on the windowsill.

Some of the herbs that are easy to grow include:

Basil
Cilantro
Dill
Fennel
Mint (spearmint and peppermint)
Parsley, curly and flat-leafed
Rosemary
Sage
Thyme

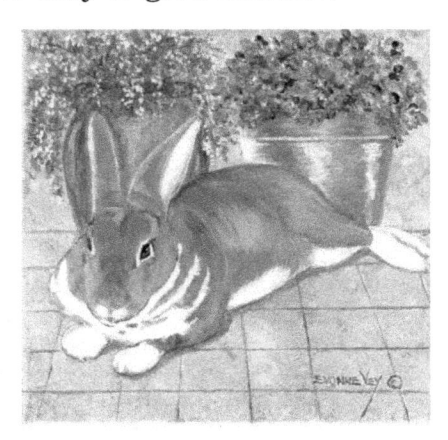

WEEDS

Some of the plants that are intentionally removed from gardens actually make excellent bunny food, although they should only be given if one knows no poisonous chemicals have been applied to their foliage or to the soil in which they grow. In addition to high vitamin and mineral content, many weeds contain high amounts of phytochemicals and can have antimicrobial, pain-relieving, anticancer, antioxidant and other potentially beneficial health effects.

Weeds that are safe to give in small amounts include:

Chickweed (starweed, starwort)
Dandelion: greens and flowers
Lamb's quarter (fat hen, goosefoot)
Loveage. Occurs as a weed in some areas of the UK. Stems should be chopped.
Ribwort plantain
Purslane (pursley, hogweed, pigweed)
Shepherd's purse

Dandelion greens, ribwort plantain, and lamb's quarter have high vitamin and mineral content and the leaves have a diuretic effect. Loveage contains phytochemicals that can reduce stress, as well as many other nutrients. Purslane has very high vitamin E content, as well as high amounts of many minerals. Dandelion leaves have some oxalate and should be given in moderate amounts; purslane and lamb's quarter have very high oxalate content and should only be given in very small amounts.

RABBIT MANURE
Not only can a garden benefit your rabbit, but your rabbit can benefit the garden! Rabbit manure is a wonderful manure. It contains much higher levels of nitrogen and phosphorous than do steer, sheep, horse and chicken manures and has the added benefit that it does not have to be aged or composted. Unlike most other manures, rabbit droppings can be added directly to the soil around the plants without danger of burning. So the next time you clean your rabbit's area, take the rabbit poop and sprinkle it on top of the garden soil or scratch it into the dirt. Or make manure tea for garden plants by adding a quart of water to a cup or so of droppings in a bucket and letting it steep for a day or two.

DISEASES AND PLANTS THAT MAY HELP ALLEVIATE THEIR SYMPTOMS
Fresh plants contain many nutrients that may help prevent and/of alleviate symptoms of common rabbit ailments. Only plants that have been discussed in the article are listed.

Arthritis *(pain and inflammation):* Leafy greens, dandelion greens, ribwort plantain, mint, parsley, basil, rosemary, chickweed, loveage, black currants, pot marigold flowers, Michaelmas daisy, goldenrod, chamomile, carnation petals, and yarrow.

Cancer/tumours*:* Leafy greens (especially cruciferous greens), rosemary, chamomile flowers, Michaelmas daisy, yarrow, violet leaves and flowers, fruits and leaves of bramble, raspberry, and strawberry.

Cardiovascular disease: Dark leafy greens, dill, parsley, rosemary, thyme, loveage, chickweed, dandelion greens, purslane, bramble, raspberry, and strawberry leaves and fruits, hollyhock, pot marigold (calendula) flowers, violets.

Digestive disorders: Rose hips, parsley, sage, rosemary, cilantro, chickweed, chamomile, spearmint, pot marigold flowers, daisy, hollyhock, yarrow. Carminatives (help prevent or reduce gas) include dill, fennel, chamomile, peppermint, thyme, carnation flower petals.

Fever*:* Chamomile, thyme, sage, peppermint, spearmint, hollyhock.

Frequent infections*:* Dark leafy greens, lamb's quarter, ribwort plantain, basil, sage, thyme, cilantro, parsley, mint, bramble leaves, goldenrod, yarrow, dandelion greens, nasturtium leaves and flowers, rose petals.

Respiratory: Fennel, thyme, rose petals, flowers and leaves of English daisy, hollyhock, Marguerite daisy, nasturtiums, violets, and sunflowers.

Disease affecting ***skin and fur:*** Dark leafy greens, mint, parsley, basil, chickweed, lamb's quarter, dandelion greens, bramble and raspberry leaves, purslane, marigold flowers, violet and pansy leaves and flowers.

Stress: Loveage, celery, chamomile, leafy greens, parsley, cilantro, carnation and rose petals.

Urinary tract disease*:* Dandelion leaves, dark leafy greens, cilantro, parsley, ribwort plantain, lamb's quarter, shepherd's purse, strawberry leaves, peppermint, Marguerite, nasturtium leaves, marigold flowers. Diuretics (promote production and excretion of urine) include loveage, parsley, dandelion greens, ribwort plantain, spearmint, goldenrod, geum flowers, wallflowers.

SAFETY

This is only a sampling of bunny-safe plants and there are many other plants, both wild and cultivated, that are safe to give rabbits. The rabbits' well-being should always be the first priority, so only give a rabbit plants that one can positively identify and which one is certain are safe and which have not been treated with disease or insect-controlling chemicals.

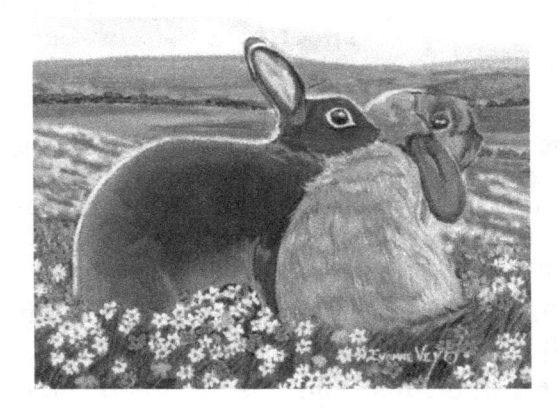

References

Akiyama, H., K. Fujii, O. Yamasaki, T. Oono, and K. Iwatsuki. 2001. Antibacterial action of several tannins against *Staphylococcus aurues*. *J. Antimicrob. Chemother.* 48: 487–491.

Al-Mamary, M., A-H Molham, A. Abdulwali, and A. Al-Obedi. 2001. *In nino* effects of dietary sorghum tannins on rabbit digestive enzymes and mineral absorption. *Nutr. Res.* 21(10): 1393–1401.

Amr, A. R. and E. E-K Abeer. 2011. Hypolipidemic and hypocholestermic effect of pine nuts in rats fed high fat cholesterol diet. *World App. Sci. J* 15(12): 1667-1677.

Aviram, M. and L. Dornfield. 2001. Pomegranate juice consumption inhibits serum angiotension convertin enzyme activity and reduces systolic blood pressure. *Athero.* 158(1): 195-198.

Bakirel, T., U. Bakirel, O. U. Keles, S. G. Ulgen, amd H. Yardibi. 2008. *In vivo* assessment of antidiabetic and antioxidant activites of rosemary (*Rosmarinis officinalis*) in alloxan diabetic rabbits. *J. Ethnopharm.* 116(1): 64-73.

Balch, Phyllis A. and James F. Balch. 2000. *Prescription for Nutritional Healing.* New York: Avery.

Basu, M., R. Prasad, P. Jayamurthy, K. Pal, C. Arumughan, and R. C. Sawhney. 2007. Anit-atherogenci effects of sea buckthorn (*Hippophaea rhamnoides*) seed oil. *Phytomed.* 14(11): 770-777.

Bayo, N. O., O. D. Eyarefe, and R. O. A. Arowolo. 2010. Effects of Tahitian Noni Juice on Ketamine Anaesthesia in Some Local Rabbits. *Br. J. Pharmacol. Toxicol.* 1(2): 81-84.

Bialecka, M. 1997. The effect of bioflavonoids and lecithin in the course of experimental atherosclerosis in rabbits. *Ann. Acad. Med. Stetin.* 43: 41–56.

Braga, L. C., J. W. Shupp, C. Cummings, M. Jett, J. A. Takahashi, I. S. Carmo, E. Chartone-Souza, and A. M. A. Nascimento. 2005. *J. Ethnophar.* 96(1-2): 335-339.

Briske, D. D. and B. J. Camp. 1982. Water Stress Increases Alkaloid Concentration in Threadleaf Groundsel (*Senecio longilobus*) *Weed Sci.* 30:106–108.

Buhler, D. R. and C. Miranda. 2000. Antioxidant Activities of Flavonoids. Accessed 7/21/10 at http://lpi.oregonstate.edu/f-w))/flavonoid.html

Butkute, B., A. Dagilyte, R. Benetis, A. Padarauskas, J. Ceviciene, V. Olsauskaite and N. Lemeziene. 2018. Mineral and Phytochemical Profiles and Antioxidant Activity of Herbal Material from Two Temperate *Astragalus* Species. *BioMed Res, Int.* Vol. 2018, article ID 6318630, 11 pp.

Burke, D. S., C. R. Smidt, and L. T. Vuong. 2005. *Momordica cochinchinensis, Rosa roxburghii,* wolfberry, and sea buckthorn- highly nutritional fruits supported by tradition and science. *Current Topics Nutraceut. Res.* 3(4): 259-266.

Cannas, A. 2008. Tannins: fascinating but sometimes dangerous molecules. Accessed 7/22/10 at http://www.ansci.cornell.edu/plants/toxicagents/tannin.html

Challen, J. 1998. The Power of Flavonoids' Antioxidant Nutrients in Fruits, Vegetables, and Herbs. Accessed 7/21/10 at http://www.thenutritionreporter.com/power_of_flavonoids.html

Cheeke, P. R. Feeding systems for tropical rabbit production emphasizing roots, tubers and bananas. Accessed 7/24/10 at http://www.fao.org/docrep/003/t0554e/T0554E16.htm

Chen, C-Y O. and J. B. Blumberg. 2008. Phytochemical composition of nuts. *Asia Pac. J. Clin. Nutr.* 17(S1): 329-332.

Dearing, M. D. 1996. Effects of *Acomastylis rossii* tannins on a mammalian herbivore, the North American pika, *Ochotona princes*. *Oeco.* 109(1) 122–131.

Deineka, V. I., V. N. Serokopudov, L. A. Deinka, and M. Y. Tret'yakov. 2007. Flowers of marigold (Tagetes) species as a source of xanthophylls. *Pharm. Chem. J.* 41(10):540–542.

De Souza, M. O., M. Silva, M. F. Silva, R. d-P. Oliveira, and M. L. Pedrosa. 2010. Diet supplementation with acai (*Euterpe oleracea* Mart.) pulp improves biomarkers of oxidative stress and the serum lipid profile in rats. *Nutr.* 26(7-8): 804-810.

Diab, S. M. 2004. The Chemistry of Juglone: A detective story of unsolved mystery. Accessed 7/22/10 at http?/www.stfrancis.edu/ns/diab/CRT/Juglone.ppt

Dr. Duke's phytochemical and Ethnobotanical Databases. Http://www.ars-grin.gov/duke/

Drewnowski, A. and C. Gomez-Carneros. 2000. Bitter taste, phytonutrients and the consumer: A review. Accessed 4/7/16/www.m.ajen.nutrition.org/content/72/6/143.

Feio, C. A., M. C. Izar, S. S. Ihara, S. H. Kasmas, C. M. Martins, M. N. Feio, L. A. Maues, N. C. Borges, R. A. Moreno, R. M. Povoa, and F. A. Fonseca. 2012. *Euterpe oleracea* (acai) modifies sterol metabolism and attenuates experimentally-induced atherosclerosis. *J. Athero. Throm.* 19(3): 237-245.

Fenwick, D. E. and D. Oakenfell. 1983. Saponin content of food plants and some prepared foods. *J. Sci. Food Agric.* 34(2): 186–191.

Fish, B. C. and L. U. Thompson. 1991. Lectin-Tannin Interactions and Their Influence on Pancreatic Activity and Starch Digestibility. *J. Agric. Food Chem.* 39: 727–731.

Gasmi-Boubaker, A., R. M. Losada, H. Abdouli, and A. Riguerio. 2012. Importance of Mediterranean forest products as food resources of domestic herbivores:the case of oak acorn. *Eur. Fed. An. Sci.* 129: 123-6.

Gohara, A. A. and M. M. A. Elmazar. 1997. Isolation of hypotensive flavonoids from *Chenopodium* species growing in Egypt. *Phytother. Res.* 11(8): 564–567.

Gross, P. Acai, a Potent Antioxidant Superfruit. Accessed 3/22/13 at: http://chetday.com/acaisuperfruit.htm

Harcourt Brown, Frances. 2002. *Textbook of Rabbit Medicine.* Oxford:Butterworth Heinemann.

Imamura, Y., T. Migita, Y. Uriu, M. Otagiri, and T. Okawara. 2000. Inhibitory Effects of Flavonoids on Rabbit Heart Carbonyl Reductase. *J. Biochem.* 127(4): 653–658.

Jaeger, P. and W. G. Robertson. 2004. Role of Dietary Intake and Intestinal absorption of Oxalate in Calcium Stone Formation. *Nephron. Phys.* 98: 64-71.

Janakiraman, K. and R. Manavalan. 2008. Studies on effect of Piperine on Oral Bioavailability of Ampicillin and Norfloxacin. *Afr. J. Tradt. Compl. Altern. Med.* 5(3): 257–262.

Jin, Mingliang, Q. Huang, K. Zhao, and P. Sheng. 2013. Biological activities and potential health benefits of polysaccharides isolated from *Lycium barbarum* L. *Int. J. Bio. Macromol.* 54: 16-23.

Joythi, B. A., K. Venkatesh, P. Chakrapani, and A. R. Rani. 2011. Phytochemical and Pharmacological Potential of *Annona cherimola*—A Review. *Int. J. Phytomed.* 3: 439-447.

Kan, W. L., C. H. Cho, J. A. Rudd and G. Lin. 2008. Study of the antiproliferative effects and synergy of phthalides from *Angelica sinensis* on colon cancer cells. *J. Ethnopharmacol.* 120: 36-43.

Kim, D-J, H-K Kim, M-H Kim and J-S Lee. 2007. Analysis of Oxalic Acid of Various Vegetables Consumed in Korea. *Food Sci. and Biotech.* 16(4): 650–654.

Kim, J-S, Y-S Kwon, Y-J Sa, and M-J Kim. 2010. Isolation and Identification of Sea Buckthorn (*Hippophae rhamnoides*) Phenolics with Antioxidant Activity and α-Glucosidase Inhibitory Effect. *J. Agri. Food Chem.* 59(1): 138-144.

Kubola, J. and S. Siriamornpun. 2011. Phytochemicals and antioxidant activity of different fruit factions (peel, pulp, aril and seed) of thai gac (*Momordica cochinchinensis* Spreng.). *Food Chem.* 127: 1138-1145.

Lako, J., V. C. Trenerry, M. Wahlqvist, N. Wattanapenp- aiboon, S. Sotheeswaran, and R. Premier. Phytochemical flavonols, carotenoids and the antioxidant properties of a wide selection of Fiijian fruit, vegetables and other readily available foods. *Food Chem.* 101(4): 1727-1741.

Lansky, E. P. and R. A. Newman. 2007. *Punica granatum* (pomegranate) and its potential for prevention and treatment of inflammation and cancer. *J. Ethnophar.* 109(2): 177-206.

Lebas, F. 2004. Reflections on Rabbit Nutrition with a Special Emphasis on Feed Ingredients Utilization. Proc. 8th World Rabbit Congress. Puebla.

Lee, C-H, T-S Jeong, Y-K Choi, B-H Hyun, G-T Oh, E-H Kim, J-R Kim, J-I Han and S-H Bok. 2001. Anti-Atherogenic Effect of Citrus Flavonoids, Maringin and Naringenin, Associated with Hepatic ACAT and Aortic VCAM-1 and MCP-1 in High Cholesterol-Fed Rabbits. *Biochem. Biophys. Res. Comm.* 284(3): 681–688.

Li, X-M. 2007. Protective effect of *Lycium barbarum* polysaccharides on streptozotocin-induced oxidative stress in rats. *Int. J. Biol. Macromol.* 40(5): 461-465.

Libert, B. and V.R. Franceschi. 1987. Oxalate in crop plants. *J. Agri. Food Chem.* 35(6): 926–938.

Linus Pauling Institute at Oregon State University. Website: http://lpi.oregonstate.edu/

Liu, S-H, L-T Lee, N-Y Hu, K-K Huange, M-C Shih, I. Munekazu, J-M li, T-Y Chou, W-H Wang, and T-S Chen. 2012. Effects of alpha-mangostin on the expression of anti-inflammatory genes in U937 cells. *Chin. Med.* 7(1): 19.

Liu, Y., X. Song, Y. Han, F. Zhou, D. Zhang, B. Ji, J. Hu, Y. Lv., S. Cai, F. Gao, and X. Jia. 2011. Identification of Anthocyanin Components of Wild Chinese Blueberries and Amelioration of Light-Induced Retinal Damage in Pigmented Rabbit Using Whole Berries. *J. Agri. Food Chem.* 59(1): 356-363.

Livingston, A. L., D. Smith, H. L. Carnahan, R. E. Knowles, J. W. Nelson, and G. O. Kohler. Variation in the xanthophylls and carotenen content of Lucerne, clovers, and grasses. *J. Sci. Food Agric.*19(11):632-6.

Maiyoh, G. K., J. E. Kuh, A. Casaschi, and A. G. Theriault. 2007. Cruciferous Indole-3-Carbinol Inhibits Apolipoprotein B secretion in HepG2 Cells. *J Nutr.* 137: 2185–2189.

Marounek, M., D. Duskova, and V. Skrivanova. 2003. Hydrolysis of phytic acid and its availability in rabbits. *Br. J. Nutr.* 89: 287–294.

Martin, R. J., D. R. Lauren, W. A. Smith, D.J. Jensen, B. Deo, and J. A. Douglas. 2006. Factors influencing silymarin content and composition in variegated thistle (*Silybum marianum*) *New Zea. J. Crop Hort. Sci.*34: 239–245.

Mazzio, E. A. and K. F. A. Soliman. 2009. *In Vitro* Screening for the Tumoricidal Properties of International Medicinal Herbs. *Phytother. Res.* 23(3): 385-398.

Menser, H. A., W. M. Winant, and O. L. Bennett. 1970. Elemental composition of common ragweed and Pennslyvania smartweed spray-irrigated with municipal sanitary landfill leachate. *Env. Poll.*18(2):87–95.

The Merck Veterinary Manual. Ninth edition. 2005. Edited by Cynthia M. Kahn. Whitehouse Station: Merck and Co., Inc.

Mohandes, J., A. F. Chennel, G. G. Duggan, J. S. Horvath, and D. J. Tiller. 1986. Sex-dependent activities of quinine reductases in rabbits indicate higher risk of bladder cancer in the male. *Carcinog.* 7(3): 353–6.

Movahedian, A., A. Ghannadi, and M. Vashirnia. 2007. Hypocholesterolemic Effects of Purslane Extract on Serum Lipids in

Rabbits Fed with High Cholesterol Levels. *Int. J. Pharmacol.* 3: 285–289.

Mullen, W., J. McGinn, M. E. J. MacLean, M. R. MacLean, P. Gardner, G. G. Duthie, T. Yokota, and A. Crozier. 2002. Ellagitannins, Flavonoids, and Other Phenolics in Red Raspberries and Their Contribution to Antioxidant Capacity and Vasorelaxation Properties. *J. Agri. Food Chem.* 50(18): 5191-5196.

Noonan, S. C. and G. P. Savage. 1999. Oxalate content of foods and its effect on humans. *Asia Pac J Clin Nutr* 8(1): 64–74.

Norazmir, M. N. and M. Y. Ayub. 2010. Benficial Lipid-Lowering effects of Pink Guava Puree in High Fat Diet Induced-Obese Rats. *Mal. L. Nutr.* 16(1): 171–185.

Orlikova, B., D. Tasdemir, F. Golais, M. Dicato, and M. Diederich. 2011. Dietary chalcones with chemopreventative and chemotherapeutic potential. *Genes Nutr.* 6(2): 125-147.

Padhye, S., A. Ahmad, N. Oswal, and F. H. Sarkar. 2009. Emerging role of Garcinol, the antioxidant chalcone from *Garcinia indica* Chois, and its synthetic analogs. *J. Hematol. Oncol.* 2: 38.

Paterson, R.T. 1993. Use of Trees by Livestock: Quercus. Accessed 7/24/10 at http://www.smallstock.info/research/reports/R5732/NR08UE/ B1701_5.HTM

Pedraza-Chaverri, J., N. Cardenas-Rodriguez, M. Orozco-Ibarra, and J. M. Perez-Rojas. 2008. Medicinal properties of mangosteen (*Garcinia mangostana*). *Food Chem. Tox.* 46(10): 3227-3239.

Pepsi, A., C. P. Ben and S. Jeeva. 2012. Phytochemical Analysis of Four Traditionally Important Aquatic species. *Int. Res. J. Biol. Sci.* 1(5): 66-69.

Perry, A., H. Rasmussen, and E. J. Johnson. 2009. Xanthophyll (lutein, zeaxanthin) content in fruits, vegetables and corn and egg products. *J. Food Comp. Anal.* 22: 9–15.

Phan, M., M. Bucknall, and J. Arcot. 2018. Effect of Different Anthocyanidin Glucosides on Lutein Uptake by Caco-2 Cells, and their Combined Activities on Anti-oxidation and Anti-inflammation In Vitro and Ex Vivo. *Molecules* 23(8):2035.

Powell, J. J., S. A. McNaughton, R. Jugdaohsingh, S. H. C. Anderson, J. Dear, F. Khor, L. Mowatt, K. L. Gleason, M. Sykes, R .P. H. Thompson, C. Bolton-Smith, and M. J. Hodson. 2005. A provisional database for the silicon content of foods in the United Kingdom. *Br. J. Nutr.* 94: 804–812.

Puotinen, C.J. 2000. *The Encyclopedia of Natural Pet Care.* New York: McGraw-Hill.

Ravindran, V., G. Ravindran, and S. Sivalogan. 1993. Total and phytate phosphorus contents of various foods and feedstuffs of plant origin. *Food Chem.* 50(2): 133–136.

Rebecca, O. P. S., A. N. Boyce, and S. Chandran. 2010. Pigment identification and antioxidant properties of red dragon fruit (*Hylocereus polyrhizus*). *Af. J. Biotec.*9(10): 1450-54.

Rogosic, J., T. Saric, J. A. Pfister, and M. Borina. 2012. Importance of plants with medicinal properties in herbivore diets. *Eur. Fed. An. Sci.* 131: 45-56.

Romanova, A. S., A. V. Patudin, and A .I. Ban'kovskii. 1977. Quinones of higher plants as possible therapeutic agents. *Khimiko-Farmats. Z.* 11(7): 53–65.

Sajjadi, S. E., Y. Shokoohinia, and P. Mehramiri. 2003. Isolation and characterization of steroids, phthalide and essential oil of the fruits of *Kelussia odoratissima* Mozaff., an endemic mountain celery. *Br. J. Pharma.* 140(5): 948-954.

Samkol, P. and S.D. Lukefahr. 2008. Feed Resources for Rabbits. WRSA Proc. 1479–1497. Verona.

Shabaan, W. F., T. A. Taha, F. D. El-Nouty, A. R. El-Mahdy, and M. H. Salem. 2008. Reproductive toxicological effects of gossypol on male rabbits: biochemical, enzymatic, and electrolytic properties of seminal plasma. *Fert. Steril.* 89(5 Suppl.): 1585–1593.

Subramanian, S., D. S. Kumar, and P. Arulselvan. 2006. Wound Healing Potential of *Aloe vera* Leaf Gel Studied in Experimental Rsabbits. *Asian J. Biochem.* 1(2): 178-185.

Taqui, S H., A .J. Shah, and A. H. Gilani. 2009. Insight into the possible mechanism of antidiarrheal and anitispasmodic activities of piperine. *Pharmacom. Biol.* 47(8):660–664.

Terao, J., Y. Kawai, and K Murota. 2008. Vegetable flavonoids and cardiovascular disease. *Asia Pac. J. Clin. Nutr.* 17(S1): 291–293.

Thakur, M., M. Kumari, and C. S. Pundir. 2001. Determination of oxalate in foodstuffs with arylamine glass-bound oxalate oxidase and peroxidase. *Current Sci.* 81(3): 248–251.

Turroni, S., B. Vitali, C. Bendazzoli, M. Candela, R. Gotti, F. Federici, F. Pirovano, and P. Brigidi. 2007. Oxalate consumption by lactobacilli: evaluation of oxalyl-CoA decarboxylase and formyl-CoA transferase activity in Lactobacillus acidolphilus. *J. Appl. Microbiol.* 103(5):1600–1609.

Tsai, J-Y, J-K Huang, T. T. Wu, and Y. H. Lee. 2005. Comparison of Oxalate Content in Foods and Beverages in Taiwan. *JTUA* 16: 93–98.

Tyystjarvi, P. S. E. 1993. Stearidonic and y-linolenic acid contents of common borage leaves. *Phytochem.* 33(5): 1029–1032.

Umar, K. J., L. G. Hassan, S. M. Dangoggo, and M. J. Ladan. 2007. Nutritional Composition of Water Spinach Leaves. *J. Appl. Sci.* 7:803-9.

Verhoeven, D. T., H. Verhagen, R. A. Goldbohm, P. A. van den Brandt, and G. Poppel. 1997. A review of mechanisms underlying anticarcinogenicity by brassica vegetables. *Chem. Bio. Interact.* 103(2): 79–129.

Vinh, L.T. and E. Dworschak. 1983. Phytate Content of some Foods from Plant Origin from Vietnam and Hungary. *Food* 29(2): 161–166.

Vinson, J. A., L. Zubik, P. Bose, N. Samman, and J. Proch. 2005. Dried Fruits: Excellent *in Vitro* and *in Vivo* Antioxidants. *J. Am. Coll. Nutr.* 24(1): 44–50.

Vreman, H. J., D. Thorning, and M.W. Weiner. 1980. Effects of dietary acetate and bicarbonate on experimental atherosclerosis in rabbits. *Atheroscl.* 35(2): 145–53.

Vuong, L. T., A. A. Franke, L. J. Custer and S. P. Murphy. 2006. *Momordica cochinchinensis* Spreng. (gac) fruit caro-tenoids reevaluated. *J. Food Comp. Anal.* 19(6-7): 664-668.

Wang, M-Y, B. J. West, C. J. Jensen, D. Nowicki, C. Su, AfaK. Palu, and G. Anderson. 2002. *Morinda citrifolia* (noni): A literature review and recent advances in Noni research. *Acta Pharmacol. Sin.* 23(12): 1127-1141.

Wang, X-D., S-J Sheng, J-P Zhu, J-P Cui, and X-Y Xie. The Extermination Effect of Pomegranate Peel Extracts on Rabbit Coccidian Oocysts Cultured *in Vitro*. *China An. Husb. Vet. Med.*

Webb, M. A. 1999. Cell-Mediated Crystallisation of Calcium Oxalate in Plants. *Plant Cell.* 11: 751–761.

Woo, K. K., F. H/ Ngou, L. S. Ngo, W. K. Soong, and P. Y. Tang. 2010. Stability of betalain pigments from red dragon fruit (*Hylocereus polyrhizus*). *Am. J. Food Technol.* 6: 140–148.

Yousef, M. I., A. M. Esmail, and H. H. Baghdadi. 2004. Effect of Isoflavones on Reproductive Performance, Testosterone Levels, Lipid Peroxidation, and Seminal Plasma Biochemistry of Male Rabbits. *J. Env. Sci. Health Part B* 39(5-6): 819-833.

Yu, Y-M, W-C Chang, C-H Wu, and S-Y Chiang. 2005. Reduction of oxidative stress and apoptosis in hyperlipidemic rabbits by ellagic acid. *J. Nutri. Biochem.* 16(11): 675-681.

Zeweil, H. S. and Y. M. El-Gindy. 2017. Effects of parsley supplementation on the seminal quality, blood lipid profile, and antioxidant status of young and old male rabbits. *World Rab. Sci.* 25 (3): 215-223.

Chapter 8

WILD PLANTS AND TOXIC PLANTS

Many people who have rabbits feed their pets wild plants. They enjoy collecting the plants for their rabbits (or enjoy allowing the rabbits to graze on the plants outdoors) and feel they are providing a nutritious and safe treat for their pets. In most cases this is true—many wild plants have high micronutrient content and the rabbits usually enjoy eating them as much as the owners enjoy feeding them to their rabbits. However, there are two cautions to keep in mind:

- Wild plants are not always easy to identify correctly.
- Even if correctly identified, a plant may not always be safe to feed rabbits due to chemical sprays or other contaminants.

Identifying wild plants is not simple. I have known both extension service range workers and professors of botany to make mistakes on plant IDs in the field, and I have found misidentified plants in university herbarium collections. During my semesters of studying agrostology and plant taxonomy I spent many hours dissecting plants under microscopes, making identifications based on millimeter measurements of plant parts. Caution is much safer than over-confidence in identifying plants. I strongly recommend that anyone considering giving their rabbits wild plants first purchase a good book on the local flora. Please, *if you are not 100% certain of a plant's identity, do not feed it to your rabbits.* Although in most cases a misidentification would probably lead to no lasting harm, in others it could. For example, the deadly poison hemlock could be mistaken by a novice for a harmless member of the carrot family.

Another problem that may arise in plant identification is the use of multiple common names. For example, there are at least three different plants that have the common name "pigweed," and each one also has several other common names. The same species of plant may have a different appearance depending on where it is growing—a plant growing in a high-moisture area of the eastern US — may look very unlike the same species growing in the arid southwest.

Even correctly-identified wild plants may not be safe if they have been sprayed with pesticides or other chemicals. Do not collect plants anywhere unless you know for certain no chemicals have been applied. And always wash the wild plants before feeding them to rabbits in order to remove dust, bacteria, fungal spores, feces, urine, and parasite eggs. Also be sure to remove any discolored or moldy-looking areas to prevent possible mycotoxin poisoning.

FIFTEEN GENERALLY RABBIT-SAFE WILD PLANTS

There are many plants besides the fifteen I am listing that may be safe to feed your rabbits. Rather than attempt to list all possible bunny-safe wild plants, I have chosen to list a few that have broad distributions and are fairly easy to identify. But unless you are sure of your identification, do not risk feeding the plant to your rabbit.

Remember, any rabbit can have a sensitivity to any plant. If you have not given a particular plant to your rabbit before, start with just a leaf or two the first day. If no negative symptoms appear, you can try giving a few more leaves the next day, and so on. It is best to introduce only one new plant to your rabbit's diet at a time so you can be fairly certain that any symptoms that might appear would be from that plant's consumption.

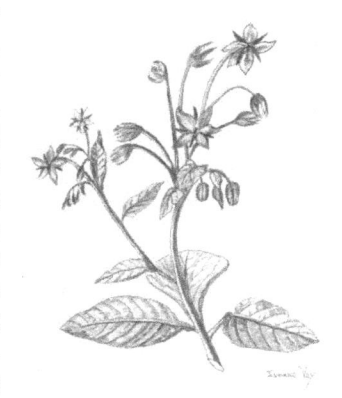

1. Borage. *Borago officinales*, or common borage, is a coarse, rough, hairy plant with bright blue 5-petalled flowers. Borage is high in beta carotene, vitamins B_1, B_2, and B_3, choline, vitamin C; the minerals Ca, Fe, K, Mg, Zn, and P. Gamma linoleic acid and stearidonic acids are two fatty acids found in borage leaves. In some mammals, borage acts as a diuretic, increases milk production, and can lower fever. Comfrey, *Symphytum officianle,* is also in the borage family. Although it has some pyrrhidozole alkaloids, rabbits are resistant to these compounds and small amounts of comfrey can be fed safely. Comfrey contains, among other compounds, allantoin, beta-carotene, vitamins B_1, B_2, and B_3, vitamin C, Ca, Fe, K, Mg, Mn, P, Se, and Zn. Allantoin stimulates cell growth, and comfrey has been used medicinally for many years, especially as a healing poultice for wounds. It is not recommended to feed the seeds to rabbits.

   2. **Raspberries and blackberries** (*Rubus* spp.), members of the rose family, are found in many parts of the world and have been used medicinally in many cultures. All the above-ground parts are safe to feed rabbits, including the leaves, stems, and fruits, although one should make certain no chemicals have been applied to the plants. Bramble leaves are astringent and infusions made with them have been used to lower fever and increase milk production in humans. The leaves contain alpha-carotene, beta-carotene, caffeic acid, lutein, vitamins B_1, B_2, and B_3, vitamin C, the minerals Ca, Fe, Mg, Mn, P, K, Se, Si, Zn, and hydrolyzable tannins.

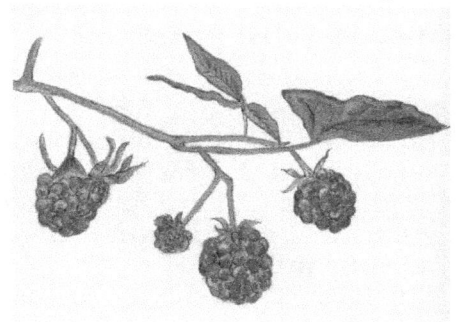

   3. **Chickweeds**, also called starweeds and starworts, are members of the pink family. *Stellaria media* grows along the ground and has light green oval leaves and small white star-like flowers. The plants contain beta-carotene, vitamins B_1, B_2, B_3, B_6, vitamins C and E; fatty acids, and the minerals Ca, Fe, K, Mg, Mn, P, S, Se, Si, and Zn. Chickweed may lower blood lipids, may have anti-inflammatory properties, and is good for the skin when applied topically.

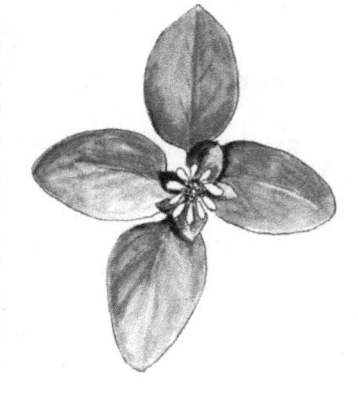

4. **Clover**, also called trefoil. Clover belongs to the legume, or pea family. Both white clover (*Trifolium repens*) and red clover (*Trifolium pratense*) are safe for rabbits to eat in small amounts. Red clover, also called bee-bread, meadow trefoil, and cow flower, contains isoflavones (phytoestrogens). The flowers contain beta-carotene, caffeic acid, coumarin, salicylic acid, Ca, Fe, Mg, Mn, P, K, Se, Zn, vitamin B_3, C, and E. They have a calming effect on the digestive system. Sweet clover is another legume. It has light green lance-shaped leaflets and flowers in spikelike clusters. White sweet clover (*Melilotus alba*) and yellow sweet clover (*Melilotus officinalis*) are bunny safe if untreated and given in small amounts. These common plants are very sweet-smelling because of melilotin and other vanilla-like phytochemicals called coumarins, used in making perfumes (and which, if clover is spoiled, can cause serious illness). Other phytochemicals found in sweet clover include caffeic acid, flavonoids, and monoterpenes. All the clovers have fairly high oxalate content.

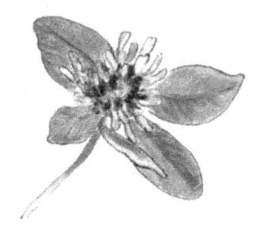

Giving large amounts of any clover is not recommended, both because of its richness and its potential to be contaminated with life-threatening molds if it is the least bit spoiled. Also, when sweet clover is not dried properly, molds may break coumarin down to dicoumerol, which is an anticoagulant. Great caution should be taken in giving any clover, fresh or dried, to bunnies less than three months old; give a leaf or two only if it is desired to accustom the rabbit's gut to the plant.

5. **Dandelion**. *Taraxacum officinale.* This common weed needs no description. Both leaves and flowers are safe for rabbits to eat, but as this plant is considered a pesky weed by most, the utmost care must be taken to be sure any plants given to rabbits have not been treated chemically. Dandelion has long been used for many medicinal purposes, and has been found to

strengthen blood vessels and relieve arthritis symptoms. The leaves contain protein, saponins, betacarotene, caffeic acid, lutein, coumarin, lactones, terpenes, vitamins B_1, B_2, and B_3, vitamin C, Ca, Fe, Mg, Mn, P, K, S, Se, Si, and Zn. The leaves may act as a diuretic, improve kidney and liver function, reduce serum cholesterol, and have laxative action. The blossoms are also a good source of vitamin A. Helenin, a phytochemical found in the flowers, has been found to help with night blindness in humans.

6. Knotweed, *Polygonum aviculare,* also called smartweed, hogweed, wireweed, and lady's thumb, belongs to the buckwheat family. It grows low along the ground, has dark-green lance-shaped leaves and dense spikes of pinkish flowers. Knotweed has fairly high amounts of Ca, Mg, Mn, and Zn, and also has diuretic qualities. Under certain conditions it is possible knotweed may accumulate high amounts of Mn, and only small amounts should be given rabbits.

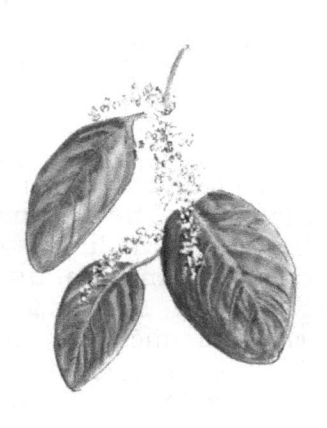

Two other members of the buckwheat family that are safe to feed rabbits are sorrel, *Rumex acetosella,* and dock, *Rumex crispus*. Both these are fairly high in oxalic acid and soluble oxalates and should be fed to rabbits in amounts similar to spinach. Sorrel and dock are fairly high in vitamins A and C, have moderate amounts of vitamin K, and moderate amounts of Ca and Mg. The seeds of these plants should not be fed to rabbits.

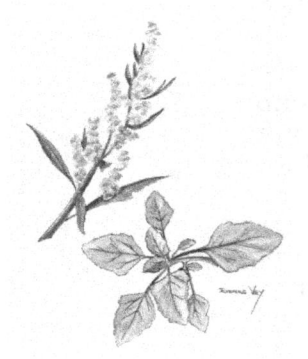

7. Lamb's quarter, *Chenopodium album,* is also called fat hen and goosefoot. This plant has long been used as a vegetable by humans, and is also bunny-safe. The leaves have an irregular wedge shape and are medium-green with whitish undersides. Lamb's quarter is high in vitamin A and the minerals Ca, K, and P. It is also a good source of protein and fiber, and contains several trace minerals. Lamb's quarter is extremely high in oxalates, however, and should not be given too frequently for this reason. Compounds in the seeds have been found to kill rabbit sperm, but it is not recommended that the seeds be given to rabbits.

8. Lovage, *Levisticum officianle.* This bunny-safe herb that can be used as a celery substitute was once widely-cultivated as a green in Britain, but today is usually considered a weed. It grows up to 5 feet tall, has leaves rather like coarse celery leaves, and yellow carrot-like flowers. It contains many of the same phytochemicals as celery (e.g., phthalides) and is extremely high in the flavonoid quercetin. Other phytochemicals lovage contains includes resins, ligulin, and an unsaturated organic acid called *angelic acid* that is used in the perfume industry. It has diuretic qualities, has been used for bladder and kidney problems, rheumatism, and to relieve indigestion and gas.

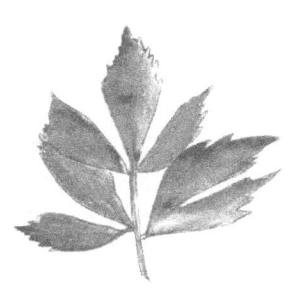

9. Mallow. The common mallow, *Malva sylvestris,* may grow to three feet high, has lobed round broad leaves similar to hollyhocks or geraniums, and has pinkish-lavender flowers which are also safe for rabbits to eat. Mallow is high in thiamine, protein, carbohydrate, iron, and calcium. It also contains several flavonoids, including anthocyanidins, pro-anthocyanidins, rosmarinic acid, and tannins. The mucilage present in the stems and leaves soothes mucous membranes, and has been used for digestive disorders. The leaves also soothe mucous membranes and are often used topically to make poultices for insect bites and skin ailments.

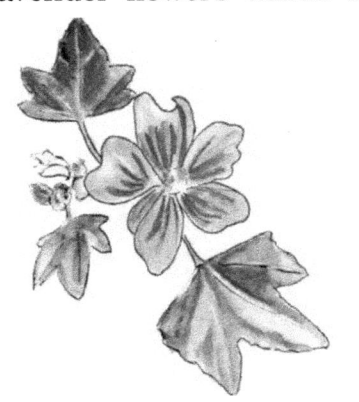

10. Milk thistle. There are two different plants known by the common name milk thistle, depending upon where you live. True milk thistle, or *Sylibum marianum (Caduus marianus* L.), is also known as lady's thistle, holy thistle, and St. Mary's thistle. It has distinctive light-green leaves with blotchy white areas and purple flowers. Milk thistle fruit seeds contain beta-carotene, fatty acids, Ca, Fe, Mg, Mn, P, K, Se, Zn, and compounds known as silymarins. These compounds have been found to protect the liver from toxins, boost liver regeneration, and to be one of the only antidotes to poisoning from *Amanita* mushrooms. Silymarins have been shown to have antiatherogenic effects on rabbits and may also have antimicrobial and anti-tumor properties. However, the compounds are *not* found in the leaves, which have no special therapeutic effects other than possible soothing effects from the mucilage. Their nutritive content is similar to that of alfalfa, and they can be a good source of fiber and protein. It is not recommended the fruits or seeds be fed to rabbits. If the benefits of milk thistle seeds are desired, it is best to purchase a milk thistle seed extract.

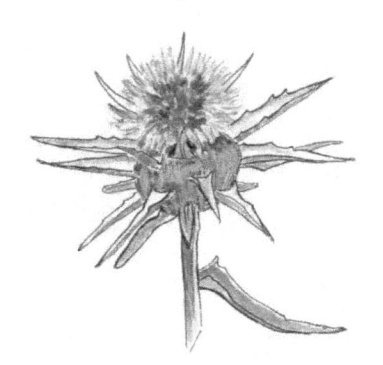

Sow thistle, *Sonchus oleraceus,* is also known as milk thistle in some areas. Sow thistle has broad light-green leaves and small yellow flowers. Sow thistle is safe to feed rabbits and contains vitamins A, B-complex, C, and some minerals.

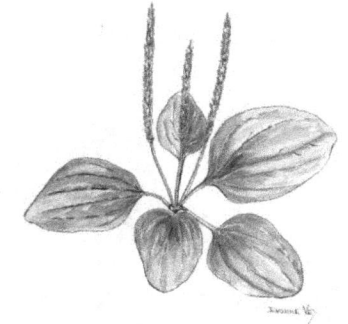

11. Plantain, also called ribwort. Several members of the genus *Plantago* are safe for rabbits to eat, including *P. major* (broad-leafed plantain) and *P. lanceolata* (narrow-leafed plantain). Leaves of both plants form a rosette at the base, and the flower stems arise from the center. Leaves have obvious "ribs," and generally this is an easy plant to identify. Ribwort leaves have many phytochemicals, including allantoin, coumarin, tannin, caffeic acid, cinnamic acid, salicylic acid, and vanillic acid. They are also a source of vitamins A and potassium. The leaves have astringent and diuretic qualities, lower fever, soothe mucous membranes, and are good for indigestion. Applied topically, the leaves have healing and antibiotic effect on wounds and insect bites.

12. Purslane, *Portulaca oleracea,* is also called pursley, hogweed and pigweed. Common purslane is a low-growing succulent with thick reddish-pink stems, fat small bronze-green leaves and small yellow flowers. It is related to the moss rose and has a peppery flavor. Although it is included on some lists of potentially toxic greens because of its high oxalate content, it is safe in small amounts for healthy adult rabbits, as are other greens with high oxalates such as spinach.

Common purslane is a weed of interest at this time because of the high amounts of vitamins C and E and alpha linoleic acid (one of the omega-3 fatty acids) it contains, and is even being served at some upscale restaurants. It is high in protein, is a powerful antioxidant, and contains flavonoids, coumarin, dopamine, and vitamins A, C, and E. In one study it was found to be useful in lowering cholesterol in rabbits. It may also have analgesic, anti-inflammatory, anti-convulsant, anti-ulcerogenic, antifungal, and wound-healing properties.

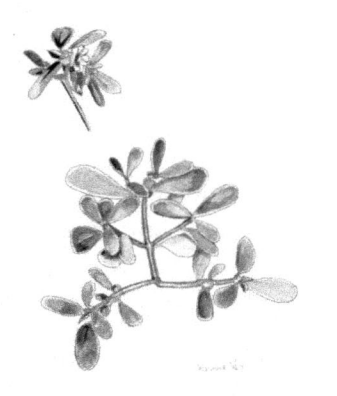

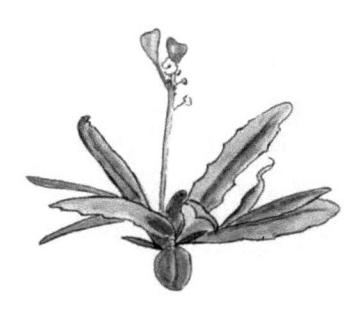

13. Shepherd's purse, *Capsella bursa-pastoris,* also called caseweed and shovelweed, has a rosette of deeply-toothed or heart-shaped leaves at the base and erect flower stalks with tiny white flowers. Seed pods are thought to be purse-shaped. This plant is high in protein and vitamin K, and also contains vitamins A, B$_1$, and C, choline, the minerals Fe, S, and K, and many flavonoids, including saponins. It is a low-oxalate green. Although extracts have been used to increase the rate of blood clotting in humans, not all studies have shown similar effects on rabbit blood. However, it may help reduce urinary tract irritation.

14. Wild strawberries, *Fragaria spp.,* are members of the rose family. Both leaves and fruits are safe for rabbits to consume. The leaves contain Ca, Cu, Fe, K, Mg, Mn, and Zn, as well as many phytochemicals such as tannins, proanthocyanins, flavonoids, salicylic acid, and caffeic acid. The leaves may have antidiarrheal and diuretic effects. The fruits contain anthocyanidins, coumarin, ellagic acid, and quercetin, among other flavonoids. Both fruits and leaves have been found to have anticarcinogenic effects and have been used to treat urinary tract infections in humans.

15. Sunflower, *Helianthus annuus*. Like dandelions, sunflowers need no description. All parts of the plant are safe for rabbits to eat. Sunflower seeds are high in unsaturated fats and B-vitamins. The broad triangular leaves have a protein and carbohydrate content similar to that of grass. They also contain fatty acids and are fairly high in lignin content.

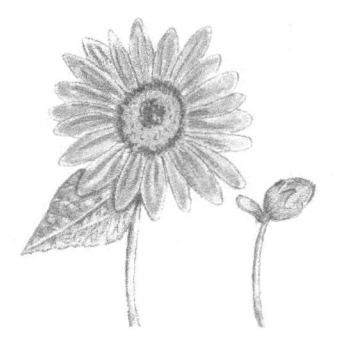

If you choose to collect any of the above plants for your rabbit, be certain you are doing so in an area that has not been treated with any pesticides or herbicides. Wash the plants thoroughly, pat dry in a towel or between paper towels, and store in the refrigerator.

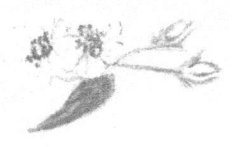

Other rabbit-safe wild plants

Rabbit expert Christine Carter resides in Australia and recommends several other wild plants for rabbit consumption in addition to those I have already listed. Following is an excerpt on feeding rabbits wild plants from her book, *The Wonderful World of Pet Rabbits* (used with her permission).

THE WONDERFUL WORLD OF WEEDS
by Christine Carter

There is a wise saying that goes 'nature knows no weeds' but unfortunately few people appreciate the true value of these plants. Rather than go out and harvest a collection of weeds for their bunnies, many owners find it easier just to feed them pellets along with some purchased vegetables.

The Collins English Dictionary describes a weed as 'a plant growing where undesired' or 'any plant that grows wild and profusely, especially among cultivated plants.' Even plants that were once popular for aesthetic or consumption purposes are now looked upon as noxious weeds because they are no longer useful. For rabbit owners however, weeds need not be worthless or a nuisance—many varieties make up part of a nutritious, fibrous diet for our pets. I believe that by providing our rabbits with a variety of herbs and weeds we are giving them the choice to select a more natural diet. In fact, many edible weeds contain more nutrients than some commercial vegetables.

Before the wonders of modern medicine, we were able to find cures for many ailments in plants, and even to this day many commercial drugs and medicines contain various plant extractions. Animals feeling poorly will instinctively seek out and eat whatever therapeutic plants are needed at the time.

Weeds have valuable medicinal and nutritional value for animals and humans—yes, we can benefit by eating weeds too!

Numerous herb plants contain either one or both astringent (prevents/remedy for diarrhoea) and laxative properties and are useful in symptomatic cases of constipation (gastrointestinal statis). Many also have a reputation for acting as a diuretic and therefore may be helpful in preventing or in part, remedying bladder sludge/stones. In the information about weeds, I have included a few snippets about the renowned correlation between herbal weeds and their beneficial medicinal properties to humans and animals. I hope the information provides reassurance to those reluctant to feed weeds to their bunnies. However, the noted (possible) health benefits do not necessarily endorse my personal recommendation to use them as home remedies to prevent or cure illness or disease.

A wonderful array of rabbit food is probably sitting in your garden just waiting for harvesting. I enjoy weeding (it is true) and derive satisfaction in the knowledge that every weed I feed to my bunnies is wholesome and thoroughly enjoyed. I am also one of the rare individuals who deliberately allows selected weeds to go to seed—by encouraging reproduction I can guarantee an ongoing supply.

My favourite weeds are regularly fed to my rabbits for many years, and I can wholeheartedly vouch for their merits. Some weeds are only available seasonally while others are present all year round, in my garden and locally. Please note the list is not restricted to my surrounding district, these weeds are generally available throughout many countries.

When harvesting weeds be sure to shake off most of the soil that is attached to the roots. Bunnies do not need wads of dirt accumulating in their hutch and if they wish to nibble at the plant's roots, the less dirt on them the better. Instead of uprooting entire plants you could just pick the foliage – due to their hardiness, weeds will regrow to yield a succession of crops.

Generally, you should feed most weeds (unless otherwise indicated) as side dishes, not in bulk as you would feed grass or hay.[5]

- Cat's Ear (*Hypochoeris glabra*) and Flatweed (*Hypochoeris radicata*) are related to dandelion and look similar.
- Curled dock (*Rumex cripus*) and broad-leaved dock (*Rumex obtusifolius*): Dock contains generous amounts of iron, four times the vitamin A content of carrots and twice the vitamin C content of oranges. The dock weed could be useful as a diuretic or help treat diarrhoea. Because they accumulate oxalates—especially at the flowering stage—only feed dock to your rabbits in limited amounts.
- Fennel (*Foeniculum vulgare*): therapeutically recommended for rabbits for increasing a nursing does' milk supply as well as aiding digestion and stomach upsets.
- Groundsel (*Senecio vulgaris*): groundsel is quite similar in appearance, and is in the same 'sunflower' family group, as the common sow thistle. Groundsel is a good source of minerals and is beneficial to rabbits.
- Prickly lettuce (*Lactuca serriola*) can safely be fed to our bunnies in generous quantities. Prickly lettuce and the non-prickly variety wild lettuce (*Lactuca satigna*) are ancestors to cultivated lettuce and their tender

---

[5] The list of Christine Carter's favorite wild plants has been edited to remove duplications from my list. I recommend that those interested in rabbit-safe wild plants occurring in Australia refer to her book, *The Wonderful World of Pet Rabbits,* published by Pirion Pty. Ltd.

young leaves have been collected as a salad vegetable for centuries.

- Turnip weed (*Rapistrum rugosum*); wild turnip (*Brassica tournefortii*); buchan weed (*Hirschfeldia incana*); sand rocket or Lincoln weed (*Diplotaxis tenuifolia*): these weeds are related to the Brassica family and have been grouped together because they are very similar in appearance. Sand Rocket has high crude protein in the early stages of growth but once mature (as with the majority of plants) this will decline. I recommend feeding these weeds in moderate amounts.

- Burdock (*Articum minus*) is grown commercially and consumed by humans. It tastes similar to celery and is claimed to prevent cancer.

- Nettles, known as small nettles (*Urtica urens*): these tend to be regarded as noxious weeds due to their stinging hairy leaves. Nettles contain significant amounts of calcium, iron, phosphorus and protein and are also high in vitamin D. Feed the entire plant to your rabbits, but let it wilt a little first. Nettles can also be dried and used as nutritious rabbit fodder during winter. To treat stinging or nettle rash, apply some juice from a nettle stem or some crushed dock or bracken leaves to the affected area.

Only pick healthy, appetising looking weeds —for example reject any that appear fungus or frost affected. Do not feed your rabbits sprayed or poisoned weeds and notify immediate neighbours that you have sensitive pet rabbits so they might take care not to spray near boundary fences.

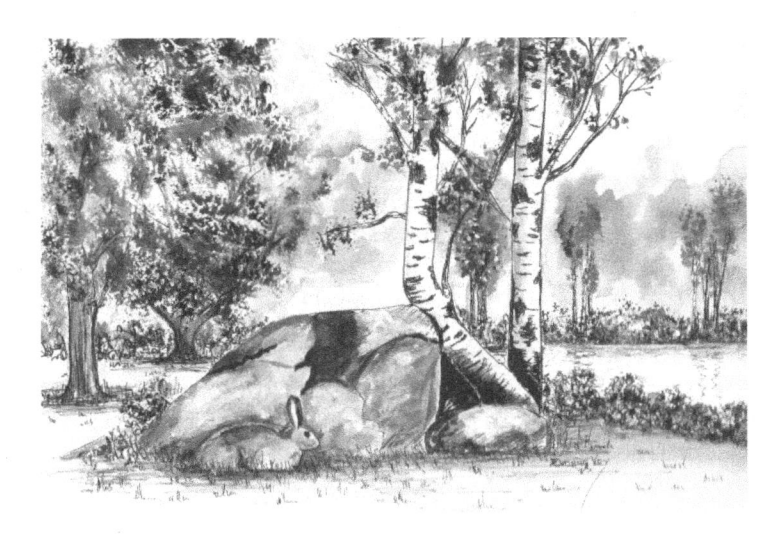

TOXIC PLANTS

As we saw in the chapter on cultivated plants, the issue of the toxicity or safety of any plant is not always black-and-white. Plant toxicity to a mammal can depend upon what age the plant is when it is eaten, where it is growing, what time of year it is, the part of the plant that is consumed, and/or in what quantity it is eaten. Plants growing under drought conditions may accumulate higher concentrations of some toxins in their tissues, as may plants experiencing a growth surge after receiving high nutrient fertilizer or treated water. Factors such as the age, health, and sensitivities of the animal consuming the plant will also come into play. Perhaps the best solution to the question of the toxicity of a plant is this: *unless you have absolute knowledge that a particular plant is safe for your rabbit to consume, assume it is not until you find out otherwise.* Don't take chances.

The following table of plants potentially toxic to rabbits (Table 8:1) is not an exhaustive list of all plants that could potentially be toxic. I have chosen to include some of the plants most likely to be encountered and/or those that are exceptionally toxic, even in small quantities, such as poison hemlock. I have not listed all plants with bulbs containing toxic compounds because there are so many. Assume any bulb, corm, rhizome, or other fleshy underground part is toxic unless you have specific knowledge it is not.

Some of the toxins found in these plants (e.g., saponins) were discussed in the previous chapter. Here are brief definitions of a few others: **Alkaloids**—organic compounds that usually contain at least one nitrogen atom, formed from the breakdown of proteins and thought to play a role in discouraging predation by herbivores. They have a bitter taste. Caffeine (not related to caffeic acid) is an alkaloid. **Phenols**—weakly acidic organic compounds with one or more OH (hydroxyl) groups bound to an aromatic ring. Phenols have both antiseptic and antibacterial qualities, but can damage the liver. Rabbits appear to be sensitive to phenols, and can develop respiratory problems from breathing phenols such as those in some fresh wood shavings. *Resinoids*—resin-like substances. (Resins are plant exudates that are not soluble in water—semi-solid to solid organic substances such as copal and amber.) **Terpenes**—chemical compounds of 5-carbon units called isoprene units. There are many classes of terpenes depending upon the number of units (e.g., monoterpene, sesquiterpene). Menthol is a monoterpene. Vitamin A is a diterpene.

There can be overlap among the various classes of compounds. For example, saponins are glycosides linked to steroids or triterpenes. Not all alkaloids, phenols, resinoids, and terpenes are necessarily toxic, and almost all plants contain potentially toxic substances. It is usually the amount of a particular compound that is present which determines toxicity. Because so little has been researched regarding what plants are actually toxic to rabbits, many of the plants in the following chart will be plants that are known toxins to other animals, especially other herbivores. Sometimes—as with pyrrolizidine and atropine—rabbits are not as sensitive to specific toxins as are other herbivores, and I have not listed several plants containing those compounds for that reason. Rabbits may be *more* sensitive to yet other toxins (e.g., aflatoxin, discussed in Chapter 6). Until the actual toxicities of the various chemical compounds to rabbits are known, caution is best.

I have chosen to list plants by common name only because in many cases there are multiple species (and sometimes multiple genera) that contain the same compounds.

Table 8:1. Selected plants potentially toxic to rabbits. *Values compiled from multiple sources.*

Plant common name	Where found	Toxic compounds	Comments
Autumn crocus	Native to Europe and N. Africa; cultivated; naturalized many areas	Alkaloid colchicines found in every part of plant; esp. high in bulb.	
Avacado	Cultivated tree.	Monoglyceride in all above-ground parts.	May cause severe respiratory distress. Toxic to rabbits.
Black locust	Native to N. and Central America; cultivated.	High oxalate content in seeds, leaves, young shoots, and inner bark.	
Black walnut	Native to N. America; cultivated	Juglone. Hulls and bark unsafe for rabbit to eat; bedding from walnut shavings may be unsafe.	Hulls tend to become moldy rapidly and may have mycotoxins.
Bleeding heart	Native to Japan and N. America; widely cultivated in gardens.	Alkaloids in all parts of plants.	
Bracken fern	Found in N. and S. America, Australia, Asia, and Europe	Thiaminases destroy vit. B_1. May contain carcin-ogens and bone marrow toxins.	Can be very toxic to cattle, sheep, and horses.
Caladium	Ornamental and houseplant, native to tropic Americas	High concentrations of calcium oxalate crystals	Crystals present throughout plant
Capeweed	Native to S. Africa; weed in Australila and N. America	Can have toxic levels of nitrates under some growing conditions.	Some purchased hay may contain this weed.
Castor bean	Native to tropical Africa; ornamental & crop plant; naturalized some areas.	Ricin (a lectin) in all plant parts, but especially in seeds.	Seeds highly toxic.
Daphne/ spurge laurel	Woody shrub native to Eurasia, cultivated in US, naturalized some areas	Diterpenes (mezerein) which are strong skin irritants	Toxins present in bark, leaves, fruit; can be fatal
Death camus	Native to Canada and US; also cultivated in gardens.	Steroidal alkaloids, glycoalkaloids, ester alkaloids. Toxins in all plant parts, esp. bulb and leaves.	One of the most poisonous plants found in N. America.
Delphinium /larkspur	Widely cultivated in gardens; native species in many areas.	Delphinine and other alkaloids in all plant parts.	Young plants and seeds are most toxic.
Dieffen-bachia/ dumbcane	Common ornamental & house plant; native to tropic Americas	High oxalate content; toxic proteins in all plant parts.	
Dogbanes	Native to N. America; naturalized elsewhere	Resinoid glucoside	.

Plant common name	Where found	Toxic compounds	Comments
Dragon tree	Palm-like houseplant and ornamental	Alkaloids, saponins.	
English ivy	Native to Europe; naturalized grown elsewhere	Saponins in berries and leaves.	
Eucalyptus	Australia native; ornamental; naturalized.	Cyanogenic glycosides.	
Flax	Widely cultivated and native in many areas	Nitrates, cyanogenic glycosides all plant parts	Reported dry heat reduces cyanides
Foxglove	Native Europe; widely cultivated gardens.	Alkaloids, cardiac glycol-sides, saponins.	Toxins in leaves, seeds, and flowers.
Georgina gidyea	Australia	Fluoroacetic acid (cardiac toxin) in pods & young foliage	
Horse chestnut/ buckeye	Ative to Eurasia and North America	Glycosidic saponin (aesculin), alkaloid	In leaves, flowers, sprouts and seeds; affects nervous system
Hydrangea	Native to Japan, planted as orna-mental.	Cyanogenic glycoside	Toxin present in leaves, branches and buds
Jimson weed/ thornapple dautra/ angel's trumpet	Native to Americas and Asia; ornamental, naturalized some areas	Tropane alkaloids in leaves, juice, and seeds	
Jute	Native to Asia; cultivated.	Cardiac glycosides	
Lantana	Native tropical Americas, houseplant, naturalized	Triterpenes in all plant parts	
Lily-of-the-valley	Native Euasia; cultivated, wild spp. southern US.	Cardiac glycosides in all plant parts	
Lupine/ bluebonnet	Native Europe and N. America; also cultivated	All parts contain alkaloids piperidine, quinolizidine	

Milkweeds	Native to N. Amer; common weed elsewhere	Steroid glycosides, resinoids	Toxins in all plant parts, green or dry
Oak	Native to temperate zones; clutivated	Gallotannins high in young leaves, unripe acorns	Rabbits eat mature lvs and acorns w/ no apparent harm
Oleander	Native to Asia and Africa; ornamental	Cardiac glycosides	Entire plant very toxic
Philoden-dron	Native S. & Central America; house plant	All parts high oxalate	Mildly toxic
Poison hemlock	Native Europe; naturalized many areas	Piperidine alkaloids in all parts	Stems hollow, may be purple-spotted
Privet	Native Europe and N. Africa; ornamental	Resinoid (andromedo-toxin) and other toxins in all plant parts	Some of toxins are GI irritants; most livestock affected.
Rhododen-dron/ azalea	Native N. America and Asia; ornamental.	Resinoid (andromeda-toxin) in all parts.	Honey from flowers also toxic.
Sanseviera	Houseplant	Hemolytic saponin	
Sneeze-weeds	Native N. Amer.; some cultivated	Many contain sesquiter-penes in all parts	Toxic to sheep, cattle, horses
Sorghum/ Johnson grass	Cultivated	Hydrocyanic acid and nitrates. New shoots contain highest toxins	Dried grasses may be safe for cyanides but not nitrates
Spotted emu bush	Australia	Cyanogenic glycosides	Young leaves are esp. toxic
Yew, trees and shrubs	Native Europe, Japan, N. America; cultivated	Alkaloids (inc. taxine & ephedrine), cyanide, volatile oils in foliage, seeds, and bark.	Highly toxic.

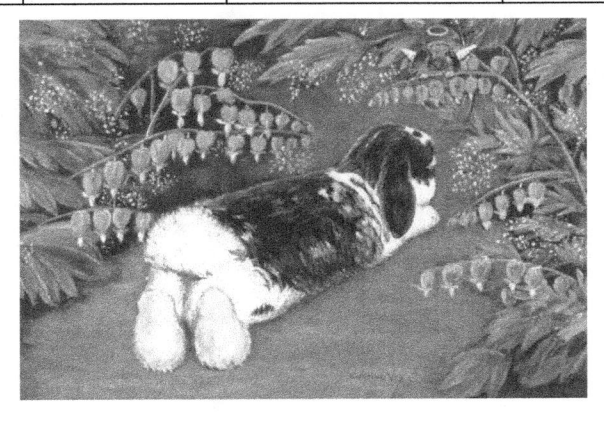

References

Al-Mamary, M., A-H Molham, A. Abdulwali, and A. Al-Obedi. 2001. *In vivo* effects of dietary sorghum tannins on rabbit digestive enzymes and mineral absorption. *Nutr. Res.* 21(10): 1393–1401.

Balch, Phyllis A. and James F. Balch. 2000. *Prescription for Nutritional Healing.* New York: Avery.

Bialecka, M. 1997. The effect of bioflavonoids and lecithin in the course of experimental atherosclerosis in rabbits. *Ann. Acad. Med. Stetin.* 43: 41–56.

Briske, D. D. and B. J. Camp. 1982. Water Stress Increases Alkaloid Concentration in Threadleaf Groundsel (*Senecio longilobus*) *Weed Sci.* 30:106–108.

Cannas, A. 2008. Tannins: fascinating but sometimes dangerous molecules. Accessed 7/22/10 at http://www.ansci.cornell.edu/plants/toxicagents/tannin.html

Carter, Christine. 2006. *The Wonderful World of Pet Rabbits.* Canberra: Pirion Pty. Ltd.

Diab, S. M. 2004. The Chemistry of Juglone: A detective story of unsolved mystery. Accessed 7/22/10 at http://www.stfrancis.edu/ns/diab/CRT/Juglone.ppt

Gohara, A. A. and M. M. A. Elmazar. 1997. Isolation of hypotensive flavonoids from *Chenopodium* species growing in Egypt. *Phytother. Res.* 11(8): 564–567.

Harcourt Brown, Frances. 2002. *Textbook of Rabbit Medicine.* Oxford: Butterworth Heinemann.

James, Wilma Roberts. 1973. *Know Your Poisonous Plants.* Happy Camp: Naturegraph Pub.

Martin, R. J., D. R. Lauren, W. A. Smith, D.J. Jensen, B. Deo, and J. A. Douglas. 2006. Factors influencing silymarin content and composition in variegated thistle (*Silybum marianum*) *New Zea. J. Crop Hort. Sci.*34: 239–245.

Menser, H. A., W. M. Winant, and O. L. Bennett. 1970. Elemental composition of common ragweed and Pennslyvania smartweed spray-irrigated with municipal sanitary landfill leachate. *Env. Poll.* 18(2): 87–95.

The Merck Veterinary Manual. Ninth edition. 2005. Edited by Cynthia M. Kahn. Whitehouse Station: Merck and Co., Inc.

231

Movahedian, A., A. Ghannadi, and M. Vashirnia. 2007. Hypocholesterolemic Effects of Purslane Extract on Serum Lipids in Rabbits Fed with High Cholesterol Levels. *Int. J. Pharmacol.* 3: 285–289.

Oglesbee, Barbara. 2006. *The 5-Minute Veterinary Consult: Ferret and Rabbit.* Oxford: Wiley Blackwell.

Paterson, R.T. 1993. Use of Trees by Livestock: Quercus. Accessed 7/24/10 at http://www.smallstock.info/research/reports/R5732/NR08UE/B1701_5.HTM

Tyystjarvi, P. S. E. 1993. Stearidonic and y-linolenic acid contents of common borage leaves. *Phytochem.* 33(5): 1029–1032.

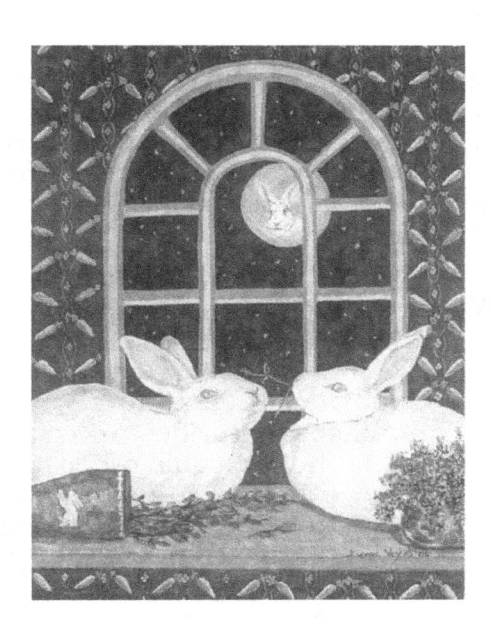

Chapter 9

PREBIOTICS, PROBIOTICS, AND OTHER FEEDING ISSUES

Often when writing a non-fiction book such as this one there are a few topics the author feels should be addressed within the compass of the book that do not fit neatly into any of the other chapters. The subjects addressed in this chapter are such topics. Prebiotics and probiotics, while not necessary in a rabbit's diet, are often added to feeds by the manufacturer or rabbit owner, and their use undoubtedly needs to be addressed in a book on rabbit nutrition.

In most of this volume the emphasis is on the chemical nutrition of rabbits. However, as several friends pointed out to me during the writing of this book, there are other considerations that affect rabbit diet, including cleanliness of the eating area and the manner in which food is presented. Those factors will be addressed at the end of this chapter.

PREBIOTICS AND PROBIOTICS

It is difficult to read books or articles on pet care without finding references to prebiotics and probiotics, but what exactly are they? "Prebiotics" is a relatively new term that usually refers to oligosaccharides not digested by mammalian enzymes, although some other definitions are broader and include other non-living additives. The usefulness of many prebiotics comes from their ability to prevent pathogens from adhering to the gut and by stimulating the immune system. "Probiotics" are organisms—usually live organisms—that may not normally be found in the digestive system of a particular animal, but which may be able to benefit the animal through positive physiological effects when consumed.

There has been a fair amount of research done on both prebiotics and probiotics, but unfortunately not a lot of this research has been done on their effects on rabbits. Some scientists caution—and I strongly echo this caution

—that because of the rabbit's unique and sensitive digestive system, *it cannot be assumed that a probiotic or prebiotic that has been tested in other species will necessarily be safe or effective for rabbits.* For this reason, it may be best to limit use of prebiotics and probiotics to those that have been shown to at least be safe for rabbits.

Prebiotics

Theoretically, prebiotics have two potential advantages over probiotics for use in rabbits. One is that they are not affected by the strong acid of the rabbit stomach, as some probiotics can be. The other is that—oligosaccharides being a type of carbohydrate—their use does not directly introduce a potentially pathogenic organism into the rabbit.

As discussed in Chapter 3, oligosaccharides are sugars composed of several monosaccharide units. The two types of oligosacchrides that are most often used as prebiotics are fructo-oligosaccharides (FOS) and mannanoligosaccharides (MOS). MOS are often added to livestock feeds to promote intestinal health, but while studies have been done on the effects of MOS in rabbits the results are not conclusive. Some researchers have found no significant effects on cecal function when MOS was added to the diet of young rabbits, and other researchers have obtained results that could be interpreted to show MOS may have a positive effect on the rabbits' digestive system. Still other researchers have found the inclusion of MOS may increase the absorption of magnesium, help remove toxic compounds, and lower mortality rates in young rabbits.

Studies on the effects of FOS added to the diet of rabbits have also yielded varying results. FOS and *inulin*, which is a chemically similar polysaccharide, are often lumped together under the term *fructans*. They are non-starch plant storage carbohydrates found in a various plants, including grass, artichokes, chicory root, green beans, and members of the onion family. In one study on young rabbits, those fed chicory had improved cecum function, but another researcher found that the rabbits with inulin added to their diet did not have improved cecum function and had higher rates of diarrhea. Still another researcher found no statistical difference in diarrhea incidence in young rabbits given FOS.

Given the varying results of the studies and also the fact that most of the studies were done on young rabbits and may not necessarily reflect the effect of the prebiotics on older rabbits, deciding whether or not to use feeds with prebiotics or add them to your rabbits feed yourself can be difficult. Possible benefits need to be weighed carefully against possible risks, especially for very young rabbits. For a more detailed discussion on oligosacharrides see Chapter Three.

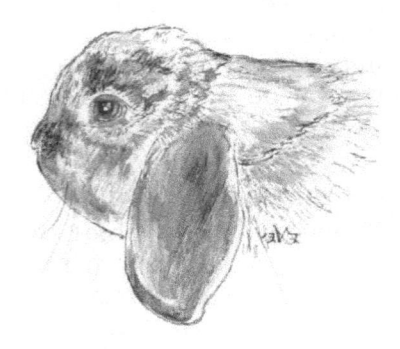

Probiotics

As of this date, there have been more studies done on the effects of probiotics on rabbits than studies on the effects of prebiotics, but again results are varied. Some researchers have found no positive or negative effects on rabbits from probiotic use; others have found positive effects, especially on young rabbits.

Probiotics are thought to cause positive effects by several mechanisms, including reducing production and/or absorption of toxins, stimulating the production of enzymes in the host animal, producing vitamins and anti-microbial substances such as bacteriosins, competing with pathogenic organisms for adhesion to epithelial cells, and by stimulating the immune system of the host. Most of the microorganisms used in probiotics are strains of gram-positive bacteria in the genera *Bacillus, Enterococcus, Lactobacillus, Pedicoccus,* and *Streptococcus.* Yeasts and a few fungi may also be used as probiotics, especially yeasts from the genus *Saccharomyces.*

Some scientists and veterinarians have questioned whether probiotic organisms are able to survive the rabbit's extremely acid stomach, are able to colonize the digestive tract if they do survive, and whether they can survive the anaerobic conditions of the cecum. These are valid concerns, especially given that the pH of a rabbit's stomach is about 1 (compared to 2 in humans). In one study on lactobacilli, some of the bacteria were found to survive both the low pH of the rabbit's stomach and the bile salts, but were still found in low numbers in the rabbits' GI tracts. The researchers concluded that the lack of adhesive capacity of these lactobacilli might keep them from colonizing the rabbits' digestive tract. However, the researchers also presented a possible solution to the problem, suggesting that giving those probiotics repeatedly might ensure enough organisms would be present for the host rabbit to benefit from the probiotic. Some organisms survive the acid stomach environment better than others; *L. acidophilus* appears to be particularly resistant to low pH. In yet another study, spores of a probiotic organism were found to be present in the intestine and cecum after feeding rabbits food containing the spores (and none were found in rabbits not fed the probiotic). No conclusions were made in this particular study regarding the organisms' ability to colonize the digestive tract after the introduction of the spores.

Most studies on the effects of probiotics on rabbits have been done on very young rabbits. In one study the researchers concluded that using a probiotic with *Bacillus subtilis* and *B. licheniformis* lowered mortality in young rabbit kits between 35 and 49 days during summer conditions; in another it was concluded that *Lactococcus lactis* reduced pathogenic bacterial colonization in young rabbits and increased protein digestibility. In a study on *B. licheniformis and B. subtilis,* the researchers found that numbers of the pathogens *Escherichia coli and Clostridium perfringens* were lowered in rabbits given the probiotic, but that the probiotics did not have any effect of lowering the numbers of *Pasteurella multocida.* In still another study, young rabbits given probiotics containing *Streptococcus faecalis, C. butyricum,* and *B. mesenterioides* had a 15% incidence of diarrhea compared to 80% in rabbits not receiving the probiotic, and the probiotic was found to be effective in preventing the growth of a particular strain of *E. coli.* Some anaerobic bacteria in the genus *Enterococcus* have been found to produce bacteriosins that are active against pathogenic clostridia in the rabbit digestive tract. Overall, the use of probiotics in young rabbits appears to be very effective in stimulating immune response in the digestive tract.

Another very positive benefit from probiotic use is the

reduction of ammonia, which can cause severe respiratory problems, especially in multiple rabbit situations. Ammonia is produced by amino acid degradation in the body and is converted to urea in the liver where it can enter the bloodstream if there are excessive amounts. Breathing excreted ammonia can cause rabbits to suffer more respiratory ills. *Lactobacillus acidophilus* has been found by researchers to reduce the amount of blood urea and cecal urea in rabbits as well as excreted ammonia. This use of probiotics could be of particular value where multiple rabbits are housed in close proximity. As noted in Chapter 7, lactobacilli may have another positive benefit for rabbits because the bacteria "eat" oxalates, phytochemicals that can affect the absorption of calcium and magnesium.

The yeast *Saccharomyces cervisiase* is sometimes used as a probiotic for rabbits, and may possibly have considerable value in protecting a rabbit from the effects of mycotoxins present in food, since the yeast has been demonstrated to have a high capacity for binding aflatoxins, ochratoxins, and tetratoxins. Some lactic acid bacteria are also able to bind aflatoxins and ochratoxins in the digestive tract.

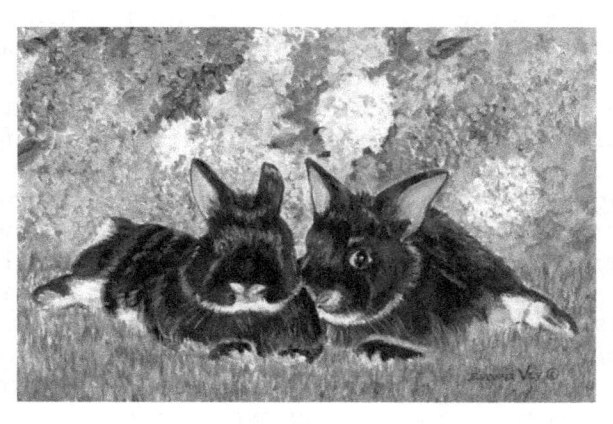

POTENTIAL NEGATIVE EFFECTS OF PROBIOTICS

Although data is starting to accumulate that probiotics may indeed confer many positive effects on rabbits, there are also possible negative effects, and these should be considered before making the decision whether or not to give a rabbit probiotics. One consideration is that the metabolic activity of probiotic organisms can sometimes have a negative effect—for example metabolic compounds produced by some probiotics can potentially degrade the mucous that protects the digestive tract (lactocbacilli do not have this effect). If the intestinal barrier is diminished, bacteria can poteantially cross the mucous membrane and epithelium and be transported to lymph nodes and other organs, possibly leading to septicemia (blood poisoning). This would be most likely to occur if there were intestinal injury or abnormal intestinal flora in the rabbit.

Another consideration is that—under the right conditions—a microorganism that is considered not pathogenic can become pathogenic. This has been demonstrated in other animals where lactic acid bacteria have been isolated from infections in the host. Bacteria that are not normally pathogenic can become opportunistic pathogens if the host has a skin injury, chronic disease, cancer, or altered metabolism from a therapeutic drug. Should this occur with lactobacilli it can be very serious as lactobacilli resist many antibiotics. In other words, although it is very unlikely to occur, it *can* occur, and if it does it could be a life-threatening situation.

DECIDING WHETHER TO USE PREBIOTICS AND PROBIOTICS

Although vidence on the effectiveness of using prebiotics on rabbits is inconclusive and touted positive effects may be questionable, for the most part prebiotcs do not appear to have many negative effects on rabbits. Scientific evidence for the effectiveness of probiotics in rabbits is still limited, there is accumulating scientific data and a great deal of anecdotal evidence as to their effectiveness. For this reason, many—although not all—veterinarians will now suggest the use of probiotics for rabbits under some circumstances. In addition to being useful for reducing mortality in very young rabbits, probiotics may be suggested for adult rabbits with certain conditions:

- gastrointestinal hypomotility (stasis) and other digestive disorders
- mycotoxicosis and other poisoning
- neoplasia (cancer)
- post-operative care

- antibiotic therapy

Each person should weigh the pros and cons of using either prebiotics or probiotics, as well as considering the health, age, and condition of their particular rabbit(s) before deciding whether the use of a probiotic or prebiotic could be beneficial. Evonne Vey, the illustrator of this book, is a strong proponent of the use of probiotics based on her personal experiences and those of others. I would agree probiotics and prebiotics can be very helpful under some circumstances (and am particularly intrigued by the use of *Saccharomyces* to bind mycotoxins), but suggest caution if considering their use for a severely immuno-compromised rabbit.

There are many probiotics on the market. Depending upon the organisms contained tin the probiotic, one might be more effective than another for a particular use. However, most of us have neither the time nor the resources to determine the best probiotic for a particular medical condition. What one can do is try a specific probiotic, and if after a couple of weeks no improvement is noticed, that probiotic could be discontinued and another tried.

YUCCA

Although yucca could be included under the heading "prebiotics," I am putting it under its own heading because it is added to so many rabbit foods. Yucca schidigera, common names Spanish dagger and Mohave yucca, contains a variety of phytochemicals including saponins, resveratrol and yuccaols. In several studies with young rabbits, yucca extract was found to reduce ammonia levels in both the blood and cecum. Additionally, yucca contains potent antioxidants and may have many other beneficial effects such as lowering cholesterol, boosting the immune system, and acting as an anti-inflammatory and anti-parasitical. In one study that compared the effects of the probiotic *Lactobacillus acidophilus* and yucca extract, the yucca was found to be more effective at reducing urea and ammonia levels, although levels were reduced by *L. acidophilius* as well. Overall, the addition of yucca extract to rabbit feed appears to have multiple positive effects.

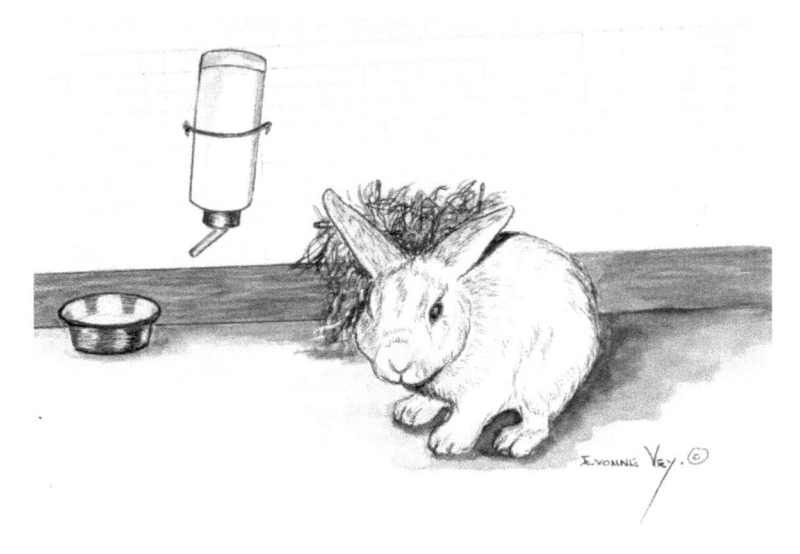

CLEANLINESS

Cleanliness is an essential but often neglected aspect of feeding rabbits. Failing to keep rabbits' food and water containers clean can lead to the growth of algae and mold and may result in food becoming contaminated with dangerous mycotoxins (see Chapter 6). Any leftover pellets should be emptied out before fresh is put in. If possible, it is best to clean food and water containers daily. I use white vinegar, which leaves a bit of a sticky residue on the containers but has an antibacterial action and has been found to disrupt many biofilm aggregations (although it is not always effective on salmonella). Scrubbing with a mild soap in water (rinse well to remove any soap residue) is also effective. A dilute solution of an iodophor such as Betadine or Vanodine or a very dilute chlorine solution can safely be used on feeding surfaces as well. Pine or similar cleaners should not be used for rabbit dishes or the areas where rabbits live since the phenols contained in these cleaners may cause harm to rabbits.

It is not only the food and water containers of rabbits that need to be kept clean; the entire surrounding area should also be cleaned since rabbits tend to spill and scatter food. This scattered food can become wet and turn into a breeding ground for mycotoxin-producing molds. The above-mentioned cleaners can be used in a rabbit's living space, and there are also special cleaners made just for cleaning where rabbits live, such as A Bunnies Friend™ Bunny odor and habitat cleaner.

The food itself—whether hay or a commercial feed—must also be kept clean and dry and away from potential contaminants such as insects, rodents, and raccoons. Wash all fresh produce intended for your rabbit, carefully removing any that has brown edges, spots or other signs of spoilage. Do not feed your rabbit any fruit or vegetable you would not eat yourself—rabbit digestive systems are actually less able to cope with spoiled greens than those of most humans.

Going to the trouble of keeping everything clean is more than worth the trouble and can save a great deal of time and money in the end by preventing many illnesses and their spread.

EFFECTS OF WEATHER

Most of us do not think of the weather and how it can affect our rabbits when we feed them. Yet the effects are very real and are something we should take into consideration when we notice changes in our rabbits' feeding habits. Kathy Smith has contributed an excellent article on this rarely-thought-of aspect of feeding rabbits:

Weather Rabbits
by Kathy Smith

It is well known that animals are more "in tune with" weather changes than most humans. Horses often "spook," letting humans know when a bad storm is coming. An amazing number of wild animals survived the December 26, 2004 tsunami in Southeast Asia by fleeing to higher ground in advance of the tidal wave.

Some rabbits seem particularly sensitive to weather changes. I call Mithril my "weather bunny" and I trust him more than any meteorologist. From the time he arrived Mithril has accurately predicted when severe weather warnings should be heeded. The night before his first Mother's Day with us (2008), I noticed Mithril acting "slightly off"—anxious and not interested in food. George was watching TV and I asked if there were any weather alerts. None. Nothing. The next morning as I drove the back road to visit my mom, there were several trees down along the road. Several times since that day I have sat in the living room watching Mithril calmly munch pellets or groom himself while listening to tornado sirens and the dire warnings of local weather forecasters. But you can bet the next time Mithril acts "weather off" like he did on May 10, 2008, he and I will go spend some quality time in the basement even if the weather people are blissfully unaware!

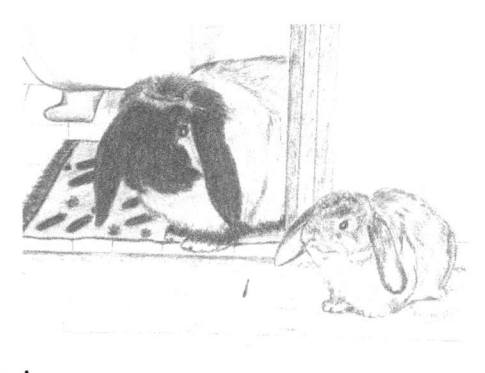

Biometeorology is the study of how both daily and seasonal weather changes influence living beings. Awareness of weather impacts on human physiology can help those of us with weather-sensitive bunnies understand what **may** be happening with them, allowing us to support our rabbit rather than annoy him during these periods.

Temperature & Humidity

If your bunnies are outdoors, you know that changes in temperature and humidity have a huge impact on their appetite and activity level. But you may also observe small but noticeable changes in your pampered indoor companions. Barring heating/air-conditioning problems or power outages, my bunnies and I keep our home in the 65-70 degree range year round. Yet I know my appetite and activity levels change depending on what it is like outside, even if the thermostat registers a constant temperature. Why should my bunnies be any different?

In hot weather, our bodies need more fluids. In cold weather they need more fuel (or calories). You may notice your rabbit showing more interest in his salad on warmer days while chowing down on pellets on cold ones, much like we humans often lean toward salads in the summer while choosing heartier meals in the winter.

In cold weather the fluid in our joints becomes slightly thicker. For most people and animals, this change goes unnoticed. But in older rabbits and those who may have suffered injuries when they were young, these changes can be painful and may lead to decreased activity and appetite.

High humidity can give you a feeling of heaviness which may decrease both appetite and desire to be active. Missouri summers are hot and humid and when humidity is high I notice Mithril does most of his eating between midnight and 8:00 a.m. As long as food is being eaten overnight and fecal output continues, I try to accept these weather-related appetite variations as normal for him.

Hot, humid weather can also make breathing more difficult, especially if there are underlying heart or lung problems. Heart disease, often undiagnosed in our rabbits, can also make it harder to regulate the body's core temperature. Remember, too, that your rabbit is spending those hot, humid days in a fur coat. Because I personally feel the heat and humidity even in the air conditioning, I will actually turn the thermostat **lower** on those miserable days and my bunnies seem to appreciate it!

Sometimes it is the suddenness of weather changes that triggers symptoms. Sharp increases in humidity or sudden drops in temperature may trigger migraines in humans who are susceptible to them. Some of our weather bunnies may be feeling migraine-like symptoms. Rapid temperature changes are thought to weaken the immune system, explaining why people often claim to "catch cold" when the weather suddenly changes. When the thermometer seems to be riding a roller coaster, try offering immune-boosting herbs like Echinacea, golden seal, olive leaf, and astragalus root.

Though I haven't followed this advice myself, I recommend keeping a weather diary for any bunny you feel is particularly weather sensitive. On a calendar, record the day's temperature (high and low) and humidity as well as notes about your rabbit's eating habits. Always remember to note when appetite returns to normal, because as you start to recognize both seasonal and weather-change patterns, this information will reassure you that things will improve.Looking back at your diary will help you relax with the normal fluctuations in your weather bunny's eating habits.

Barometric Pressure Changes and Frontal Systems
Most of us have had an older friend or relative who claims to be able to predict major weather changes and storms based on the aches and pains in their bodies. And as our bodies age, we ourselves may begin to "feel" changes in the weather.

Pain in arthritic joints or the site of an old injury can occur up to two days before weather changes arrive. It is not unusual for me to notice Mithril acting "off"—quieter than normal and less interested in food—about 48 hours before a major weather change. I have learned to look at weather.com before going into full panic mode. With Mithril, it is not unusual for his problem to resolve just **before** the front actually comes through.

Joint pain and inflammation is the most common weather-related symptom in humans. If you watch weather forecasts you know that low pressure is usually associated with storm fronts. One explanation of the link between weather changes and joint pain is that the decrease in air pressure causes the tissues around the joints to swell, irritating surrounding nerves and causing pain. Another thought is that a fall in barometric pressure causes the body to retain water, which can lead to swelling and pain. Because the pressure changes associated with storms are relatively minor, most of us (human and animal) will not experience significant pain. But for those who are more sensitive, the pain is real and the correlation too obvious to ignore.

There are other documented ways that the passage of weather fronts affects human bodily fluids:

- Blood clots faster just before a front passes and clots dissolve more easily after a cold front passes.
- Passage of a front can change levels of blood sugar, calcium, phosphates, sodium, and mag-

nesium in the bloodstream. If your rabbit gravitates to certain foods after a front passes, he may be naturally trying to rebalance nutrients.

- After a cold front passes, the volume of blood in the body decreases and the sedimentation rate, a measure linked to inflammation, is lower. Over the years, I've noticed Mithril is often perkier once a cold front passes, perhaps because he has less inflammation.
- White blood cells (WBC), which help the body fight infection, increase when the barometer falls sharply.
- Urine output increases with cold fronts and decreases with warm fronts.

In humans, warm fronts may cause irritability, fatigue, headache, increased respiration and/or heart rate, and changes in bleeding/clotting. Humans who are sensitive to warm fronts may be helped by taking vitamins A, B12, and C as well as sodium bicarbonate, potassium, and phosphorus. If you have a weather rabbit, you may want to make foods rich in these nutrients available when warm fronts are forecast.

In humans, cold fronts are more likely to cause nausea, dizziness, joint pain, asthma-like breathing difficulties, and heart problems. Humans who are sensitive to cold fronts may be helped by taking vitamins B1, D, and E as well as calcium and magnesium. If you have a weather rabbit, you may want to make foods rich in these nutrients available when cold fronts are forecast.

Other common symptoms in humans that accompany weather changes include migraines, inner ear problems, sinus pressure, and uneasiness.Your weather rabbitmay seem "off" as he copes with one or more of the symptoms discussed in this section.

We do not yet know why weather fronts cause these changes in the body. One school of thought is that passage of fronts can cause blood vessels to constrict, decreasing circulation and causing pain and other migraine symptoms (nausea, dizziness, sensitivity to light and sound, irritability, etc.). Another explanation for some weather-related symptoms is that weather changes might affect either the pressure in the brain itself or in the way the brain blocks pain. Any of these explanations could hold true for our weather rabbits as well.

Lops and rabbits with known ear problems may experience ear discomfort from weather fronts if outside air pressure changes rapidly and their ears are unable to compensate quickly enough. Most of us have felt this sense of our ears "popping" (or needing to) taking off in an airplane, ascending a steep mountain, or simply being in a fast elevator with a mild cold. If you notice your rabbit making strange mouth movements when a front is coming through, he may be working to equalize pressure in his ears.

As with humans, rabbits who are less healthy overall are more likely to suffer pain and other symptoms when barometric pressure changes. It is also likely that any medical condition that is aggravated by stress (e.g. heart disease and e.cuniculi exacerbations) can worsen when major weather fronts come through. Taken together, these two statements present us, as rabbit caregivers, with an important challenge: controlling our own anxiety about what we observe in our beloved companions. If you have a weather bunny and major weather changes are occurring or are expected in the next 48 hours, the most important thing you can do to help him is try to relax. Pamper him with favorite treats, let him know you love him, and look back at that weather diary to assure yourself that what he probably needs is just a "tincture of time."

http://www.rawfoodexplained.com/weather-and-human-well-being/the-weather-in-your-health.html

https://weather.com/health/news/13-ways-weather-affects-your-health-without-you-knowing-20140613#/1

https://weather.com/health/news/why-your-joints-hurt-when-weather-changes-20141105

http://www.webmd.com/allergies/features/the-weather-wreaking-havoc-on-health?page=2

http://www.medicinenet.com/script/main/art.asp?articlekey=52133

http://www.examiner.com/article/how-your-body-forecasts-changes-the-weather

http://www.expertparenthood.com/weather-and-the-changes-in-your-body/

THOUGHT, ENERGY AND INTUITION

Kathy Smith, author of *Rabbit Health in the 21st Century* and co-author with me of *When Your Rabbit Needs Special Care,* reminded me that rabbits, being the sensitive animals they are, can be very affected by the mental state of the person who is caring for them and providing their food. At my request she wrote the following piece to address this subject:

Energy
by Kathy Smith

Think about a time you ate a simple meal, lovingly prepared for you by a friend, spouse, parent, or child. Did you find it delicious beyond what can be explained by the ingredients? Are there certain foods you think of as "comfort food?" If you answer "yes" to either of these questions, you are already familiar with how energy can transform food. Since rabbits are highly sensitive animals, it is likely that a caregiver's frame of mind when preparing and/or delivering their meals may be almost as important as the food itself.

In its simplest form, adding this type of energy to food is about relaxing and having faith in the wisdom, resilience, and adaptability of the physical body. When making diet choices for our rabbits, we need to balance information and intuition while resisting the urge to second-guess our decisions. There is growing evidence that thoughts *can* have consequences in the material world, despite the fact that science cannot yet explain *why* this is the case. With rabbits in particular, we need to be diligent but not obsessive—the last thing any of us want to do is worry a problem into existence!

There are many ways we can consciously infuse our rabbit's food with nurturing energy. Three practices I have found especially powerful are:

- **Mindful preparation and serving.** For most Westerners, mindfulness is a vague term associated with Eastern spiritual traditions. Simply put, mindfulness can be described as intense focus on whatever one is doing at any given moment. It is the exact opposite of multitasking and, as such, may be a foreign concept to those who have only lived in the age of technology.

  Not everyone can afford organic produce, premium hay, or expensive pellets, but everyone can make the best of what they feed; and even the best ingredients can be enhanced by mindfulness. The key to this practice is to (however briefly) cease all other activity and give your full attention to the task at hand. Turn off *all* electronic distractions. Take a couple of deep breaths. Smile and focus on your current activity, whether it is assembling salads or delivering fresh hay and water. Take your time and enjoy being fully present. Try to remain in this focused state until the task is done.

- **Expressing gratitude.** Following the tradition of Native Americans, take time to give thanks both to Mother Earth and to the individual plants and minerals that you are feeding your rabbit either in raw or processed form. While washing produce or serving pellets/hay, consider offering words of gratitude to those who planted, harvested, processed, packaged, shipped, delivered, stocked and/or sold the items. By acknowledging their role in bringing these items to your home and by expressing appreciation, it is possible to help dispel any negative energy the food may have absorbed from contact with unhappy humans.

- **Blessing the food.** Asking for a blessing

is a practice that has roots in many spiritual traditions and neither requires nor rejects the concept of God. If you have childhood memories of being forced to mechanically "say grace" before you could begin to eat, keep in mind that there are other forms of blessing. As you prepare and serve your rabbit's food, make a sincere request that it be used to nourish the body in the best way possible. Depending on your beliefs, this plea can be directed to God, The Universe, Spirit, the food itself, or even the rabbit it is being served to. Blessings can range from a complex ritual (such a doing Reiki over the food) to a brief (perhaps silent) request as you mindfully serve your rabbit's meal. The key is your intention combined with a sincere belief that nourishment goes beyond what is provided by physical nutrients.

Once you tap into the power of this type of energy, you will probably develop your own unique rituals and practices. Be flexible, trusting that you are being guided to do exactly what is needed at each moment.

Kathy Smith strongly believes in using one's own instints/intuition in caring for one's rabbits, and has written the following excellent piece on the subject:

Nutrition and Intuition
by Kathy Smith

In the beginning, I knew nothing. My first bunnies—Midnight, Choca Paws, and Smokey—lived much of their lives as outdoor bunnies. Their diet was primarily alfalfa-based pellets. I didn't know they needed hay. Midnight occasionally got parsley or Brussels sprouts (his favorite!). Choca Paws regularly got parsley and (way too many) carrots. Sometimes he was allowed to graze on the ornamental kale plant on the patio. And Smokey? I cringe at the thought of admitting that his diet consisted of pellets, canned pumpkin, and appalling amounts of 7-

grain bread, banana, and yogurt (which he begged for and sucked from a syringe).

Midnight died at age six from an abdominal tumor. Smokey was eight years old when he lost his six-month battle with oral cancer. Choca Paws was almost nine when he was euthanized because of a mass in his sinus cavity. None of these rabbits ever had a single episode of GI upset. All three were lops and none of them had molar problems. When I first became an **informed** rabbit caretaker, I couldn't believe how incredibly lucky I had been. Since becoming informed, I have tried to do "everything right" and watched, green with envy, as people who did "everything wrong" had rabbits who were healthier and lived longer than mine. Today I truly believe that when we are in a state of being "blissfully unaware" of what we **should** be doing, we naturally tap into our intuition.

INFORMED INTUITION

Those of us who grew up in western cultures were raised to value information and our analytical side while ignoring (or actually resisting) intuition. At best, we spend hours, days, or even years of our lives trying to logically justify what we simply "know" to be true (what a waste of precious time and energy!). At worst we ignore that quiet, inner voice that tries to tell us when expert advice—or what has worked for us before—simply **is not working** in our current situation.

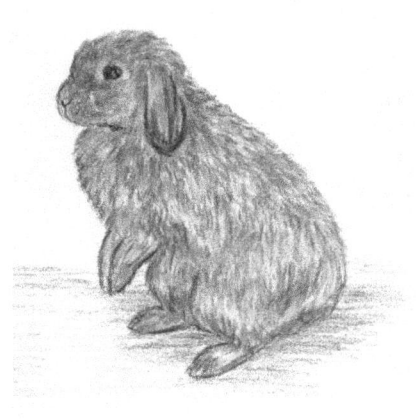

That worst case scenario is Murray's legacy. I had just learned about proper rabbit diet when The Trio came to live with me: unlimited hay, limited pellets, and lots of fresh greens. As Murray's dental and GI problems worsened, I followed conventional wisdom in the rabbit world, offering more and more variety of gourmet produce. At no point did it actually occur to me that I could (or should) try something completely different! When we become so dependent on information that we lose touch with our intuition, we put ourselves and/or our loved ones at risk.

There is an incredible amount of factual information in this book. As my eyes glazed over at the sheer volume of detail, my first thought (as a retired computer programmer) was: Wouldn't it be great if this was all programmed somewhere? A nice screen where you could enter data on each rabbit's history, medical conditions, and diets; click the "answer" button and, presto, the perfect diet would be displayed for you in a concise, printable format. Sound good? The answer to that question is a resounding "**NO**!" Why? Because it is almost certain that **not all** pertinent questions would be asked, some of your answers might be incomplete or partially incorrect, and the program (no matter how well written and tested) would still have a few bugs.

So what is the answer? If you have read this book straight through and are thinking "OK. Got everything," you can probably skip the rest of this section. If you are wondering how you will ever remember or access information when you need it, keep reading. And if you skimmed or stopped reading and skipped to this section, I urge you to go back and read, mindfully, from the beginning. Trust your inherent ability to process and retain what is (or will be) needed at a subconscious level. You don't have to **make** this happen – you simply need to **allow** it to happen naturally. Let go of your need to understand the process!

I believe there is a middle path that embraces both the intuition I had with my first rabbits and the information and lessons I have learned since then, beginning with Murray. I call this "Informed Intuition." The beautiful thing about Informed Intuition is that it is naturally inclusive of all information (even things you don't know that you know), it automatically adjusts to change, and it acknowledges that there is no single right or wrong answer. Everything that is alive is constantly changing, so what seemed to work before did work then. You did not dream it. However, you need to adapt to how things are in the present moment. The concept of informed intuition embraces both of my cardinal rules for my rabbits' diets:

- If it's not broken, don't fix it.
- If it's not working, don't keep doing the same thing

over and over expecting different results (Albert Einstein's definition of insanity). Change something.

ACCESSING YOUR INTUITION

Everyone is gifted with intuition. How easily a person is able to access it depends on many things including (but not limited to):

- **How we were raised.** For many of us, intuition was socialized out of us. A child's intuitive insights are often responded to with phrases like "don't be silly" or "that's ridiculous." The more you heard those phrases as a child, the deeper your intuition may be buried. Talents we don't value or recognize often go dormant. But with a little conscious attention we can revive them.

- **Whether we believe that intuition has value**. If you are female, stop referring to your "women's intuition" apologetically; instead, view it as a source of personal power and watch it grow and strengthen.

- **How often we use our intuition.** Like muscles, intuition is strengthened by use. The first step is actually hearing your own inner voice. For most of us, this requires temporarily quieting the outer noise that surrounds us. An easy way to start is by stopping to take a couple of deep breaths each time you get into your car alone. Once you are able to hear your own voice, the next step is having the courage to follow that voice, even when it leads you down the road less travelled. The more you follow your intuition and thank it for guiding you, the easier it will become to access it.

Most of us have some activity that automatically puts us in "the zone" where we receive answers to problems we are not consciously pondering. In this state we have quieted the analytical mind, allowing our intuitive side to step forward. Triggering activities may be meditation, yoga, vigorous exercise, our favorite artistic endeavor, gardening, cooking, sewing or almost anything we enjoy. Many people have answers come to them while taking a shower, soaking in the tub, or just before falling asleep. The possibilities are endless. Try to identify the activities that trigger this state of mind for you. Make a point to schedule time for at least one of these on a regular basis – if possible, daily.

Reconnecting with our intuition is a process requiring patience, practice, and more patience. It often consists of two steps forward and one step back. Even if you are one of those lucky people who are able to naturally access your intuitive side whenever needed, the ideas discussed below may be helpful when your intuition feels blocked (as is often the case when you are under stress or dealing with especially important, difficult, or emotionally-charged subjects).

Everything is connected energetically—you, your loved ones (human and animal), and objects.

We are all linked to each other and to a Universal Energy that transcends both time and space. We may have a term for it—the Wisdom of the Ages, the Collective Consciousness, the Akashic Record—or it may remain nameless. We are all able to connect to this vast knowledge-base, *whether we believe in it or not*. We do not need to understand how it works. How many of us truly understand how our cars, the electric outlets in our homes, or our computers work? But we use them, don't we? Here are some tools that can help us utilize that great resource that is our intuition.

The Written Word

When faced with challenging situations, many people will focus on a question, randomly open a book, place their finger somewhere on the page, and find deep meaning in whatever is written there. Richard Bach's wonderful book *Illusions* describes this process in detail, making use of another of his books *The Messiah's Handbook*. Many people use the Bible (or other sacred text) or their favorite spiritual anthology. Others turn to the dictionary or even the daily newspaper.

If your rabbit is having a problem or you are wondering about making dietary changes, you can try the above technique using this book. Focus on the issue for a moment or two; then open this book to a random page. It may immediately be very clear to you why a particular page was chosen. Even if what your read doesn't **seem** relevant, I urge you to" sit with it" for a while: open your mind, soften your focus, and see what comes to you. Once you get a message, trust it is real, thank the source for giving direction, and take action.

Card Decks

The use of cards decks for accessing intuition taps into the same energies described above. Whether you enjoy the occasional tarot card reading by a psychic, consider the concept silly, or have "ick" feelings about such readings, you can truly benefit from creating and using your own Bunny Nutrition card deck. You can make your cards quickly and inexpensively; or you can turn it into an artistic endeavor. Either way, making your own cards allows you to blend your personal energy with the information from this book.

I suggest making a card for each food item you might want to feed your rabbit. Index cards work great and are inexpensive. As you go through the tables in this book **consider** each item and make a conscious choice whether to make a card for it. It is perfectly OK to reject any item. In fact, this is your natural intuition kicking in. However, before excluding an item, take a moment to ask yourself why you are making that decision and whether that reason comes from you or an outside authority. If in doubt, make the card. You can choose to set it aside, temporarily or permanently, at any time in the future. The following are examples of my personal thought processes for items I had the initial impulse to exclude:

- **Collard greens.** Murray developed sludge immediately after the first time I fed collard greens. This is an experience I personally don't want to risk repeating. Intellectually, I know that there was probably no direct cause-and-effect relationship; at a visceral, emotional level, however, the two events are tightly linked. I acknowledge (to myself and others) that this feeling has very little to do with collard greens and everything to do with **me**. However, as long as collard greens continue to have this emotional "charge", I would not include this item in **my** card deck.
- **Kiwi.** I have no idea how to pick a good kiwi. However, maybe I could learn. I could make a card for it and decide before a reading whether to include it.

- **Radicchio**. Now that I am retired, this is no longer in my price range. Also, none of my current rabbits have any interest in it. However that could change. I could make a card for it for possible future use, but exclude it with my current family.

- **Shepherd's purse.** I have never seen this for sale anywhere. When I spoke to Evonne Vey while writing this section, she told me it was useful for urinary blockages and the homeopathic tincture should be in everyone's first aid kit. I will purchase that for emergencies. However, my first holistic vet, Dr. Randy Kidd, told me that most animals will naturally gravitate to what their bodies need and, as a result, it has been my policy not to force herbal remedies on my bunnies; instead I **offer** appropriate herbs in their most natural form. I have added shepherd's purse it to my list of things to look for next time I'm in an herbal store. I would create a card for this item once I find that type of source for it.

- **Spinach.** I've tried this several times over the years. None of my bunnies ever liked it. I would not make a card for it at this time.

- **Watermelon**. I don't like watermelon and I no longer have enough bunnies to make it practical to buy one just for them. Evonne Vey reminded me that watermelon is helpful for several urinary issues (including stones) and that it is sometime available by the slice. After our conversation, I checked to see if (like strawberries) it is available year-round, It is not. Unfortunately, my furkids don't want to hear that a treat they enjoy is "not available at this time." For now, I would not make a card for watermelon. However, if someone brings me a piece of watermelon this summer, I will accept it graciously and find out how the rest of my family feels about it.

When making your cards, I recommend writing on only one side of the card, consistently choosing either the lined or unlined side. You can simply write the name of the food or you may choose to make some notes on its nutrients. Many items are listed in multiple chapters of this book; by making a single card for each item, creating your deck may be a way for you to restructure the information for yourself. This might be an important step if you are one of us who still sometimes (or always) needs logical validation of an intuitive insight. If, during this process, you get a gut feeling (good or bad) about the food and a particular health issue, be sure to make a note of that feeling and indicate that this was **your** intuition. When you have finished going through all the tables, it is a good idea to alphabetize your cards, check for duplicates, and ensure you have only one card for each food item.

Simply by making the cards—with however much information you choose to include—you will be tapping into universal energy and **creating exactly what you need** for future use. If you are creative, artistic, or know you process information better visually than verbally, you may want to include a picture of the food on the information side of the card. If you feel like drawing, go for it—whether you think of yourself as artistic or not! If you don't want to draw, seed catalogs are a great source of small pictures. You can leave the "back" of the cards plain or choose some **uniform** design (rubber stamps work well) for the back of the cards. Remember that when drawing from your deck, you don't want the back of the card giving you clues to what is on the other side.

Once your card deck is complete, there are many ways to use it. I always suggest sitting with the cards, taking a couple of relaxing breaths, and focusing on a specific issue before each use. You can decide ahead of time the number cards you need to draw **or** draw cards until you feel "done." Or you may choose to spread the cards on the floor in front of your rabbit and let her/him tell you what s/he needs! Feeling blocked about what to put on your grocery list for your bunnies? Draw a few cards from your deck. Not sure what to put in tonight's salad? Pull the cards for what is in your refrigerator or pantry, lay them in front of your rabbit, and let her/him tell you what s/he is hungry for. Use your imagination and have fun, knowing the possibilities are endless and you cannot do it "wrong."

Whether you choose to work with the written word, cards, or "nothing," remember that the intuitive mind will tap into whatever it has access to when it needs to communicate with you. Whenever there is a noticeable repetition of words or images, your intuition is trying to get your attention. Treat it as an ally: heed what is saying and thank it for appearing to you.

Nurturing and Nutrition

Oliver was one month shy of this 10th birthday when he arrived at my house on August 11, 2003. At the time, he was the oldest bunny I had ever shared my home with. Sarah, his original mom, arrived at my door with Oliver's carrier in one hand and a bag of one of the "gourmet" foods in the other. I was still in the stage of believing that because I was now bunny-educated, I had all the answers. Oliver's pellets were in the trash before Sarah's car was out of my driveway. It would be some time before the full irony of that arrogant move sank in. No, I don't think I should have given Oliver those pellets. But it was Sarah's bunny, not mine, who was almost 10 years old.

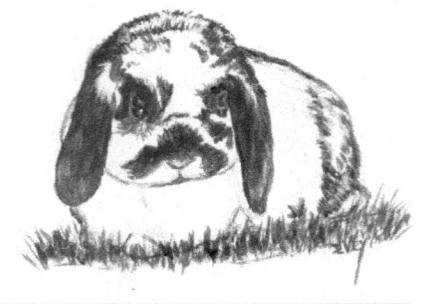

Almost ten years later, I am only beginning to comprehend the lesson from Oliver and Sarah. We may not be able to provide perfect nutrition for our rabbits (or other loved ones) because of incorrect or incomplete information, limited access to fresh foods, or a shortage of money. What we are unable to do nutritionally can, in part, be compensated for with true nurturing—fully feeding the soul. Looking back, I know that Sarah truly nurtured Oliver, from the moment she brought him home through her realization that she could no longer give him the life he needed. Every moment of every day we choose whether to be nurturing to ourselves and our loved ones. The words nurture and nutrition have a common root—*nutrire*, to nourish. Do the best you can with nutrition, but always choose to nurture those you love.

References

Abaza, I. and H. El-Said. 2005. Effect of using Yucca schidigera as feed additive on performance and growth of growing rabbits. *Proceedings*: 4th International Conference on Rabbit Production in Hot Climates, Sharm El-Sheikh.

Abdelhamid, A. M. 1990. Effect of feeding rabbits on naturally moulded and mycotoxin-contaminated diet. *Arch. Anim. Nutr.* 40: 55–63.

Amber, K. H., H. M. Yakout, and S. Rawya Hamed. Effect of feeding diets containing yucca extract or probiotic on growth, digestibility, nitrogen release and caecal microbial activity of growing New Zealand White rabbits. *Proceedings*: 8th World Rabbit Congress, Puebla.

Brewer, N. R. 2006. Biology of the Rabbit. *J. Am. Asso. Lab. An. Sci.* 45(1): 8–24.

BSAVA Manual of Rabbit Medicine and Surgery. Second Edition. 2006. Edited by Anna Meredith and Paul Flecknell. Glouster: British Small Animal Veterinary Association.

Cheeke, P. R., S. Piacente, and W. Olaszek. 2006. Anit-inflammatory and anit-arthritic effects of yucca schidigera: A review. Accessed link.springer.com/article/10.1186%2F1

Chrenkova, M., L. Chrastinova, M. Polacikova, Z. Formelova, A. Balazi, L. Ondruska, A. Sirotkin, and P. Chrenk. 2012. The effect of Yucca schidigera extract in diet of rabbits on nutrient availability and qualitative parameters in cecum. *Slovak. J. Anim. Sci.* 45(3): 83-88.

Copeland, D., M. McVay, M. Dassinger, R. Jackson, and S. Smith. 2009. Probiotic fortified diet reduces bacterial colonization and translocation in a long-term neonatal rabbit model. *J. Pediatr. Surg.* 44(6): 1061–1064.

Eiben, Cs., T. Gippert, K. Godor-Surmann, and K. Kustos. 2008. Feed additives as they affect the fattening performanace of rabbits. *Proceedings*: 9th World Rabbit Congress, Verona.

Falcao-e-Cunha, L., L. Castro-Solla, L. Maertens, M. Marounek, V. Pinheiro, J. Freire, and J.L. Mourao. 2003. Alternatives to antibiotic growth promoters in rabbit feeding: A review. *World Rabbit Sci* 15: 127–140.

Fortun-Lamothe, L. and S. Boullier. 2007. A review on the interactions between gut microbes and digestive mucosal immunity. possible ways to improve the health of rabbits. *Livest. Sci.* 107(1): 1–18.

Harkness, John E., Patricia V. Turner, Susan Vande Woude, and Colette L. Wheeler. Fifth Edition. 2010. *Biology and Medicine of Rabbits and Rodents.* New York: Wiley-Blackwell.

Ishibashi, N. and S. Yamazaki. 2001. Probiotics and safety. *Am. J. Clin. Nutr.* 73(suppl): 4655–4705.

Kamra, D. N., L. C. Chaudhary, R. Singh, and N. N. Pathak. 1996. Influence of feeding probiotics on growth performance and nutrient digestibility in rabbits. *World Rab. Sci.* 4(2): 85–88.

Kritas, S. K., E. Petridou, P. Fortomaris, E. Tzika, G. Arsenos, and G. Koptopoulos. 2008. Effect of inclusion of probiotics on micro-organisms content, health and performance of fattening rabbits: 1. Study in a commercial farm with intermediate health status. *Proceedings:* 9th World Rabbit Congress, Verona.

Linaje, R., M. D. Coloma, G. Perez-Martinez, and M. Zuniga. 2004. Characterization of faecal enterococci from rabbits fro the selection of probiotic strains. *J. Appl. Microbiol.* 96(4): 761–771.

Matusevicius, P, R. Sliaudaryte, Z. Antoszkiewicz, and A. Bednarska. 2004. A natural way to improve productivity of rabbits using probiotic Yeasture. *Veterin. Zootec.* 26(48): 1–3.

Matusevicius, P., L. Asmenskaite, A. Zilinskiene, A. Gugolek, M. O. Lorek, A. Hartman. 2006. Effect of probiotic Bioplus 2B® on performance of growing rabbits. *Veterin. Zootec.* 36(58): 54–59.

Pearce, M, I. Shahin, and D. Palcu. 2010. Available solutions for mycotoxin binding. Meriden Animal Health Limited. Accessed July 15, 2010 at: http://en.engormix.com/MA-mycotoxins/articles/available-solutions-mycotoxin-binding_l500.htm

Saunders, Richard A. and Ron Rees Davies. 2005. *Notes on Rabbit Internal Medicine.* Oxford: Blackwell Publishing.

Shrivastava, AK, K. K. Tiwari, R. Kumar, and R. R. Jha. 2012. Effects of feed additives on body weights of different ages in rabbit. Scho. J. Agri. Sci. 2(11): 277-282.

Tachikawa, T., G. Seo, M. Nakazawa, M. Sueyoshi, T. Chishi, and K. Joh. 1998. Estimation of probiotics by infection model of infant rabbits with enterohemorrhagic *Escherichia coli* O157:H7. *Kansenshogaka Zasshi* 72(12): 1300–5.

Yu, B. and H. Y. Tsen. 1993. Lactobacillus cells in the rabbit digestive tract and the factors affecting their distribution. *J. App. Microb.* 75(3): 269–275.

Chapter 10

FACTORS AFFECTING RABBIT DIET & DISEASE

Today's rabbit owners are not the first to wish to feed their rabbits good diets. In the 1880 volume *The Practical Rabbit Keeper* by Cuniculus, there is a detailed discussion on various foods to feed rabbits. I found particularly fascinating a week's suggested menu for novice rabbit keepers. The diets listed contain a fairly wide variety of foodstuffs, and include some foods that must be prepared by the owner. For example, for Tuesday it is suggested the following be given: morning—roots, crushed oats, and tea leaves; afternoon—green food and hay; evening—mash of potatoes and meal.

Apparently some of those who kept rabbits in the 1800's succeeded quite as well in feeding and taking good care of their rabbits as we do today. A few years ago a photographer in England was walking in the woods and stumbled over what appeared to be a small tombstone. Intrigued, the photographer cleaned the gravestone and discovered—much to his surprise—that it was for a rabbit that had lived to be thirteen years old! Clearly the little rabbit had received good food and care to live so long.

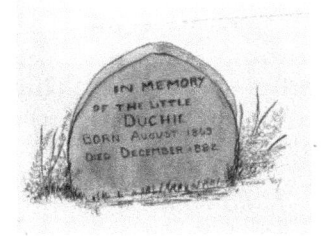

We are fortunate that feeding rabbits is now much easier in that we can purchase pellets and hay and other foods. But we still wonder, as did rabbit owners in the 1800's, "What is best to feed my rabbits?" If you have read the rest of this volume before turning to this chapter, you will know that this is not a simple question and that the answer depends upon the age, breed, health, gender, and housing of the rabbit, among other factors.

After the first edition of this book a few readers complained that information was scattered throughout the book rather than being gathered in one place. The reason the information is found in multiple places is that information on diet and any particular nutrient is best read in context—in other words, understanding the role of a nutrient in diet is important for understanding why certain amounts and/or proportions are needed in rabbit diets. While I have bowed to reader demand and am presenting simpler, less technical information on diet in this chapter, I urge readers to refer to other chapters for additional information on the interactions between nutrients and physical health.

I also must begin this chapter with a strong caution: *any diets mentioned in this chapter are only suggested starting points*. Remember that rabbits are individuals and that what works for one may not work for another. Despite the desire we may have for simple answers, there are none when it comes to rabbit nutrition. Each rabbit's age, breed, health, genetics, environment, activity, etc. must be taken into consideration when determining the best diet for that particular rabbit.

LIFE STAGES AND DIET

Rabbits require different diets for optimal health at different times of their lives. Young rabbits especially, with their developing digestive systems, require that close attention be paid to their diets because they are prone to life-threatening illnesses if they receive certain foods in excess. Older rabbits also need different amounts of various nutrients than a healthy rabbit in its prime, as do pregnant and lactating does.

Pregnant Does

Pregnant does require more food. Attempts to keep a pregnant doe on the same diet as a non-breeding doe will lead to serious problems for both the doe and the developing kits. A pregnant doe will need her usual rations increased by two-thirds to three-fourths. Very small breed does, wool breeds, and rabbits living in colder temperatures may need their rations doubled (or more). Pregnant does also need slightly higher amounts of fat (3-6%) and calcium (0.75-1.1%) in their diets. Supplements of vitamins E and C may also be beneficial. For more detailed information see pages 27, 51 and 72.

MILK FEVER. Right before giving birth (kindling) and afterwards, the mother rabbit can have a sudden drop in plasma phosphorus, calcium, and magnesium and develop what is commonly called called milk fever (hypocalcemia). The first symptom is often anorexia, followed by muscle tremors and ear flapping (the neuromuscular system is affected). If immediate action is not taken this will progress to convulsions and the doe will die. An injection of calcium gluconate almost always relieves symptoms within two hours, but oral administration does not have the same effect as injected calcium gluconate, so it is important to get the doe to a veterinarian immediately upon development of symptoms.

Lactating Does

At about five days after giving birth a lactating doe will need her rations increased another two-thirds to three-quarters from what they were during her pregnancy. Again, does of very small breeds, wool breeds, and rabbits living in colder temperatures will need their rations increased even more or an energy deficit may develop. If adjustments are not made to the diet to correct an energy deficit, the condition will progress to hepatic lipidosis and death.

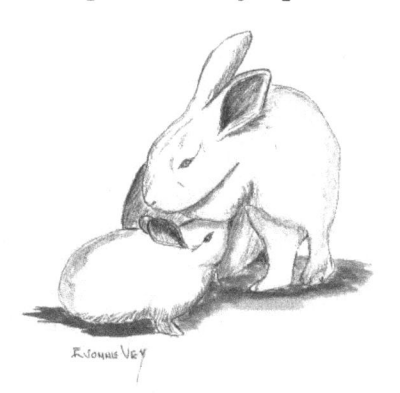

Lactating does need more fat and calcium in their diet than non-breeding does, and additional vitamin E may be beneficial. Lignin, which can be beneficial to kits, has a negative effect on milk production in does. For more detailed information see pages 27, 51 and 72.

Young Rabbits

Young rabbits will start to nibble on solid food shortly after their eyes open, which is usually about ten days after birth (longer for hand-raised rabbits). The digestive systems of young rabbits are extremely sensitive, and any sudden changes to their diet from this time to 8-12 weeks can result in pathogenic bacteria gaining dominance in the gut, which in turn can lead to sickness and death. The developing digestive system of rabbit kits is so sensitive that it is not unusual for litters to have mortality rates of 14-20% after weaning.

Ideally, the diet for young rabbits should be a

consistent low-protein (12-14%), low-starch, high-fiber (16-20% crude fiber) diet consisting primarily of a little grass hay and a good-quality commercial pelleted feed. Any overload of fructose or starch is particularly dangerous. Young rabbits still on their mother's milk have a high ability to digest the milk sugars (lactose and galactose), but little ability to digest fructose. After they are weaned, the ability of rabbit kittens to digest the milk sugars decreases and their ability to digest fructose increases. The instability of the cecal microflora at this critical time makes young rabbits very susceptible to digestive problems. High glucose or fructose in the diet can allow pathogens to proliferate and colonize the digestive tract. Toxins from these organisms are often lethal to kits.

Fiber is critical for young rabbits, and it is particulary important they receive a balance of digestible and indigestible fiber. Indigestible fiber helps reduce disgestive problems and digestible fiber (pectins and xylans) both helps prevent digestive illnesses and has a very important role in the development of the gut immune system. Recommended levels are 16-20% crude fiber (28-30% NDF, 10-12% NDSF). Soluble fiber, or NDSF, is usually added to the diet in the form of feeds containing beet pulp. See Chapter 3 for the definitions of NDF and NDSF, as well as additional information on fiber.

High dietary lignin, which is essentially indigestible, has been found to have a positive effect on growing kits at about 6g per day. While lignin and indigestible fiber are highly important in the baby rabbit's diet, too much insoluble fiber can cause digestive problems if the protein level is higher than the digestible energy. This can lead to the growth of excessive amounts of harmful microflora in the gut and excessive ammonia (see p. 51). A bit of straw provides extra lignin to the diet.

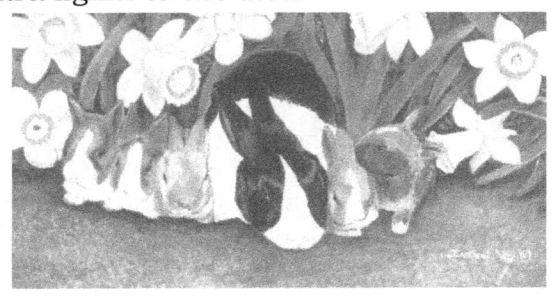

Some researchers have found that adding fructo-oligosaccharides (FOS) and mannanoligosaccharides (MOS) can have a positive effect (see pp) Adding vitamin E to the diet (about 8-9mg per 100g of feed) may help enhance their immune system.

Since the ideal diet for young rabbits is not the same as for the does, it is recommended that feed in reach of the kits be tailored to their needs, and higher-energy foods for the doe be placed where she will be able to reach them but the kits won't.

Experts disagree on when small pieces of succulent foods such as grass and greens should be added to a young rabbit's diet. Some argue for adding these items to the diet late in the kit's development—even after 12 weeks—while others argue that kits need some of these foods early so that the gut develops the proper microflora to handle green foods. I believe the answer is in the quantity given and would suggest providing very tiny amounts (a few grass blades or very small amounts of other greens) beginning a few days after the eyes open. See pp. 25, 26, 52, 72 and 142 for more information.

FEEDING ORPHANED RABBIT KITS

Hand-raising orphaned rabbit kits or kits not being fed by the mother is notoriously difficult. The survival rate is very low; as little as 6-10 percent of hand-raised kits survive. For this reason, *if there is a wildlife rehabilitator, rabbit rescue, or other rabbit organization near you, I highly recommend contacting them to see if they can refer you to a person who is experienced in giving such care.* However, not everyone lives where this is possible, and the following information is provided for emergency situations where experienced help cannot be found. The greatest dangers in hand-raising kits come from over-feeding and from the kit aspirating some of the formula, so great care should be taken to avoid both.

Rabbit milk is much richer than cow's milk. Rabbit milk contains about 10-20% fat, 10-15% protein, and 1.8% lactose; cow's milk contains about 4% fat, 3% protein, and 4.7% lactose. For this reason cow's milk is not a good substitute for a mother rabbit's milk. Several companies make a milk substitute specifically for rabbits, which is best to use if one needs to hand-raise a rabbit kitten. If one rescues a rabbit that turns out to be pregnant I suggest purchasing such a substitute to have on hand before the doe has her kits. For situations where one has not had time to prepare there are several options. Cheeke (1996) gives a recipe of one part water, one part evaporated milk; add to each cup of that mixture one egg yolk and one tablespoon corn syrup. However, in an absolute emergency, kitten milk replacer, human infant formula, goat's milk, or even cow's milk can be used, preferably with one tablespoon whipping cream added to each cup of formula or milk. The mixture should be kept in the refrigerator but should not be fed cold to the kit. Heat formula to a temperature that feels warm on the underside of your wrist.

Before trying to feed the orphan, be sure your hands are thoroughly cleaned. Do not kiss or hold the kit to your body, as this could introduce dangerous bacteria. If the kit is under four days old it can be placed on its side on a soft cloth placed over a heating pad set on low (do not put the kit directly on the heating pad as this can cause serious burns); if older than four days it is best to feed the rabbit in an upright position (this helps prevent aspiration of fluid). Be aware that even very young kits are likely to wriggle and hop. Do not overheat the kit, but feed in a warm area of the room (kits up to 7 days do best with temperatures around 80° F, kits from 1-8 weeks at temperatures from 68-72 degrees).

Authorites differ as to recommendations on the frequency of hand-feeding kits. A doe will feed her kits frequently the first day she begins to nurse, but after that only once or twice a day. For this reason, it is often recommended that a person only hand-feed twice a day, at morning and evening. But because of the difference in the composition of doe's milk versus formula, some vets and experienced rabbit kit foster mothers recommend more frequent feedings in order to provide adequate nutrition and prevent bloat in the kits.

Although it is unlikely to be available in an emergency, adding one teaspoon of freeze-dried or powdered colostrum from capsules to each two tablespoons of formula mixture is recommended for the first ten days. A purchased probiotic biotic gel or powder can be added to the formula at the rate of 1cc probiotic per 10cc formula after the kit's eyes open. Giving these probiotics earlier is not always advised, as they can affect the pH of the stomach to the detriment of a very young kit.

Eyedroppers are not recommended for feeding as it is too easy to get too much in the kit's mouth too quickly. For very young rabbits under four days old it is sometimes recommended that they first be fed by placing drops of the formula on a clean finger and allowing the kit to lick it off. A bottle specifically for feeding kits is best, but a doll's baby bottle can work, as can a 1-cc syringe. Do not squirt milk into the mouth with either; formula should be be fed very slowly in small amounts, making sure to point the syringe or bottle tip to the side of the mouth, not to the back of the throat.

If the kitten raises its head and sneezes, or milk bubbles develop on the nose or at the mouth, clear the milk away immediately with a cloth or bulb. After each feeding it is necessary to wipe the perineal area carefully with a warm wet cotton swab or gauze pad in order to stimulate urination and defecation.

Suggested amounts to feed kits per 24 hours, by age (use bottom of range for smaller breeds, top of range for larger breeds):

- Up to 4 days, 4-6cc total, divided among 8 feedings.
- 5 to 10 days, 6-10cc, divided among 6 feedings.
- 10 to 15 days, 12-16cc, divided among 3 feedings.
- 16 days to 3 weeks, 18-30cc, divided between 2 feedings
- 3 weeks to 6 weeks, about 30 cc, divided between 2 feedings.

Normally rabbits depend totally on their mother's milk for about ten days, at which time their eyes open and they they may begin to nibble on solid food. Hand raised kits in general do not develop as fast as those raised by natural rabbit mothers, so these dates may lag behind by as much as a week.

Older Rabbits

Feeding older rabbits can be tricky. Their metabolism changes, as does their behavior, and they become prone to various diseases and conditions such as arthritis, pododermatitis (sore hocks), urine burn, and kidney disease. They bodies don't utilize nutrients as well as they did when younger, and may produce less of needed compounds. For this reason, foods with relatively high amounts of copper, manganese, magnesium, zinc, vitamin E, and flavonoids may be helpful to older rabbits. See the appropriate disease headings at the end of this chapter for information on other nutrients that may help diseases and conditions that affect older rabbits.

I asked Kathy Smith if she would be willing to write a piece on caring for your older rabbit for this book and was thrilled when she sent me the following outstanding piece:

ELDER BUNS
by Kathy Smith

As caregivers, we need to be in touch with the stage of life our rabbit acts like he is in rather than what the calendar says. Age is just a number. My French lop Thumper began looking old when he was only five. Chip, his Holland lop companion, was still bouncing off the walls at age ten. We live in a culture that loves babies, reveres youth, and looks at the aging process with fear and distaste. The first (and hardest) step in helping your rabbit enjoy the latter part of his life is to manage your own emotional reactions to signs he is aging.

As you notice age-related changes in your rabbit's physical abilities, observe how readily **he** adapts. As long as the change occurs gradually, your rabbit will probably not be upset about changes in his appetite or things he can no longer do – and he will not want you to be upset either. Our rabbits can teach us so much about aging with grace and dignity! Becoming a senior citizen should be viewed as an accomplishment for you and your rabbit, not a condition that can be (or needs to be) "fixed."

Your rabbit will let you know when he is ready for you to use the information in this section. Along with changes in appetite and/or food preferences, other visible signs that your rabbit is reaching the winter of his life may include reduced activity, longer and/or deeper periods of sleep, sagging skin, an overall frail appearance, and diminished senses (vision, hearing, taste, and smell). By accepting these changes as part of a normal process, you can learn to work with your rabbit's shifting dietary needs and preferences to improve quality of life which, in turn, often extends quantity of life.

If your rabbit has let you know it is time to pay attention to this section, you have probably noticed a decrease in his activity level. While this is a normal part of the aging process, you may want to have your veterinarian check for chronic inflammatory conditions like arthritis, which can cause pain and reduce mobility, or chronic low-grade infections which can cause anemia and reduce energy levels. Whether you and your veterinarian choose pharmaceutical therapy will depend on both the severity of the condition diagnosed and how your rabbit has responded to medications in the past. As the body ages it metabolizes drugs differently, creating a Catch-22: NSAIDs prescribed for arthritis may accelerate weakening of the kidneys or cause GI issues; antibiotics may cause GI upset or further decrease appetite by causing food to "taste funny." For my super-drug-sensitive bunny Mithril, the homeopathic anti-inflammatory T-Relief (formerly Traumeel), immune boosting herbs like Echinacea, golden seal, and olive leaf, and regular chiropractic care have kept his chronic inflammation at a manageable level with minimal use of drugs.

As your rabbit's activity level decreases with age, he will probably eat less. This is actually good as it helps keep weight at a healthy level. Resist the urge to encourage your rabbit to continue eating at his old rate. An elderly rabbit who eats with a "young bunny" appetite is likely to become obese. As long as your rabbit is eating regularly, producing fecal pellets, and maintaining a fairly steady weight, try to relax with the changes in his appetite and eating habits.

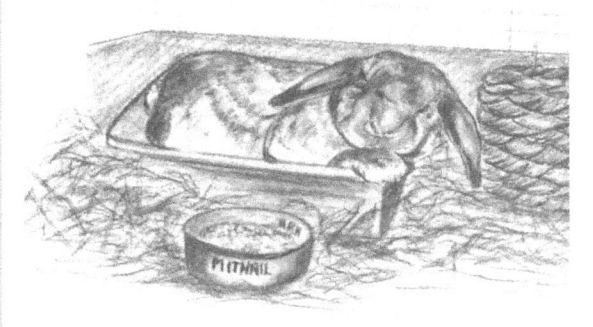

As he ages it is not unusual for a rabbit to stop eating one or more of his favorite foods, either temporarily or permanently. When this happens, try not to panic. It helps to understand that metabolism changes with age, and liver and kidneys may begin to function less efficiently. This can impact both digestion and how food tastes long before abnormalities show up in blood work (though you may still want to have baseline lab work done). Changes in kidney function may cause some foods to no longer "taste right" to your rabbit. Or foods may no longer agree with your bunny, either causing GI upset or simply no longer providing enough energy/nutrition to make eating them worth the effort. On the flip side, foods that your bunny previously turned his nose up at may become his new favorite as he ages. In the last months of his life, Apollo continued to love his dandelions, but added baby kale, carrots, and strawberries (all previously rejected) to his Top Five list. You may also want to offer small amounts of herbs like dandelion root, burdock root, and milk thistle seeds to help support both liver and kidney function.

As our bunnies age, we often notice a decline in their eyesight and hearing. What we may not realize is that the senses of smell and taste are also becoming weaker, influencing which foods really appeal to our bunnies. When Lauren reached age 10, she stopped eating lettuce, but continued to enjoy the fragrant herbs like parsley and cilantro. You may want to cautiously explore new herbs like fresh dill, basil, and mint and other fresh produce items with a more pungent smell.

Be creative in **slowly** offering new bunny-safe foods to see what appeals to your senior bunny. A good starting place is the produce you already have, either for yourself or other bunnies in your household. Periodically re-try those tried and true favorites your bunny has recently rejected. Choose a few never-tried items from this book, or let your nose (and your intuition) guide you through the produce aisle of an organic food store. If you've had your bunny since he was young, think about bunny-safe foods he enjoyed in his youth that you stopped feeding because he was putting on weight. Offering such foods as an occasional (or regular) treat can sometimes reignite an interest in food.

While much concern is expressed about overweight rabbits, I have personally seen more of the opposite problem in my own geriatric rabbits. Several of my older bunnies have looked boney with sagging skin and an overall frail appearance. All had good appetites and many were on the plump side of normal in their youth. The good news is that all the bunnies I remember as looking old, thin, and frail at the end of their lives had that same look for at least two or three years. Oats can help keep weight on and are a good source of energy. Try offering small amounts of canned pumpkin which is high in fiber. Not all bunnies like the taste, but mine who did eagerly lapped it off a saucer and none of those bunnies ever looked bony! You can also try limited amounts of favorite fruits as well as almonds and sunflower or pumpkin seeds. As always, introduce new items one at a time in moderate quantities and watch carefully for signs of GI upset.

As your rabbit ages, pellets become increasingly important as a source of energy and balanced nutrition. If you have been feeding the same pellet for years and your rabbit eats eagerly with little or no GI upset, now is **not** the time to change! Remember, "If it's not broken, don't fix it." However, if you've always insisted on timothy pellets and your rabbit eats them grudgingly, consider adding (or gradually changing to) alfalfa pellets. If you have always limited pellets and your rabbit is losing weight (or even looking thin and frail), increase the amount of pellets you feed or consider free-feeding pellets. If your rabbit is having GI issues, consider trying an extruded "pellet" as they are said to be easier to digest. For Lauren who stopped eating most greens and was never able to eat hay, pellets were her primary food source for the final 2½ years of her life. She was not overweight and, interestingly, around this same time she stopped needing to have her molars filed. Sometimes it is good to trust that our rabbits will eat what their body needs most, especially in the later stages of their lives.

Aging rabbits may begin to eat less hay or stop eating it entirely. If this happens, see your veterinarian to rule out dental problems. Also, check the hay you are feeding to see if it still smells fresh and fragrant. If it smells "wrong", pitch it immediately. What you will probably find, however, is that it smells fine, just not as strongly fragrant as when you first got it. As your bunny's sense of smell becomes less acute, you may need to order hay more often but in smaller amounts. I also recommend offering more than one type of hay. Even if you are feeding the most expensive gourmet timothy hay, your bunny may want some variety. For years Mithril has demanded a "hay buffet" (four or five popcorn tins in the living room, each with a different type of hay). In addition to timothy, try orchard grass, meadow grass, bluegrass, and/or brome. If you've always fed first cutting, try second or even third cut. Mithril's all-time favorite hay is a 2nd cut timothy with clover. It is very fragrant and used to trigger my allergies much worse than it does today. It is even OK to mix in a small amount of alfalfa hay occasionally. Some online vendors will send small samples of several of their hays either free or for a nominal fee—it never hurts to approach them with your dilemma and ask! If possible, have at least three different hays available for your senior rabbit to choose from at all times, even if (or **especially** if) you are fairly certain he isn't eating much hay.

At some point, you may find yourself waking your rabbit up to remind him to eat or to feed him. He may go for long periods without moving much if at all. The message I have gotten from my bunnies at this point is "Everything takes so much energy." For each food item you offer these rabbits, they seem to carefully weigh whether the amount of energy (or pleasure) they receive from the food is greater than the amount of energy they have to expend to eat it. For some rabbits this means the end is near. For others, it is signals the start of a roller coaster ride that can last months or even years.

If you are lucky enough to be on the roller coaster with your rabbit, it will help to embrace the concept of "the new normal." This means letting go of everything you think you know about "correct" rabbit care and listening to what your rabbit needs and wants right now, today. This will be different each day for each rabbit. Accepting the "new normal" means knowing that on any given day your rabbit may sit in one spot and refuse to eat hay or pellets or greens or all of the above. Fecal pellets may be scary-small and/or ill-formed. There may be precious few of them, none in the litter-box, and you'll be thrilled to find them wherever they are! While you sleep your bunny may or may not eat the salad you left for him or a few of his favorite pellets. Tomorrow may be better or worse, and either way it will probably be OK.

At this point some rabbits will sometimes, but not always, appreciate being syringe fed Critical Care, pumpkin, baby food, or a home-made recipe. Often with Mithril I can simply sit on the floor and offer the syringe of Critical Care. Sometimes he sucks it eagerly. Other times I find I do have to restrain him a bit, but I don't force. This is the point in his life where "no means no."

You can also coax some rabbits to start eating by hand-feeding them their favorite greens or other treats. I can sometimes get Mithril to start eating his salad by hand-feeding a few pumpkin seeds. During Murray's last months he allowed me to hand-feed special imported (Canadian) extruded pellets one pellet at a time. Princess Pandora loved banana so much that I was once able to tempt her to eat some hay by pulling individual strands through a piece of banana. That hay jump-started her appetite, and she was fine for several months. Be creative about ways to tempt your bunny to eat. Know that this will always be a moving target, so don't discourage easily and don't get too comfortable with any one solution!

Some rabbits don't want to be "fussed over" and all rabbits at this stage of life will have times that they seem to refuse everything you try to tempt them with. When this happens, put everything they might be tempted by (water, pellets, hay, and produce) within easy reach of all their favorite hangouts and leave them in peace. Although Mithril accepts the syringe feeding, most of what he eats on his own is eaten while I sleep or when I'm away from home for several hours. Occasionally he will munch pellets while I'm in the room – there is no more beautiful sound in the world right now! Make a point of savoring such moments with your aging rabbit.

At some point, your elder rabbit's body **will** start shutting down. When this happens, it is important not to interfere with the process. What we call supportive care for bunnies who are recovering from an injury or illness – sub-q fluids, force feeding, even some medications – can actually prolong the dying process, perhaps making it unnecessarily painful. Trust that there is amazing wisdom and protection from pain in the body's natural shutdown process. And always keep food and water within easy reach, just in case you are wrong about being at the end of that roller coaster ride.

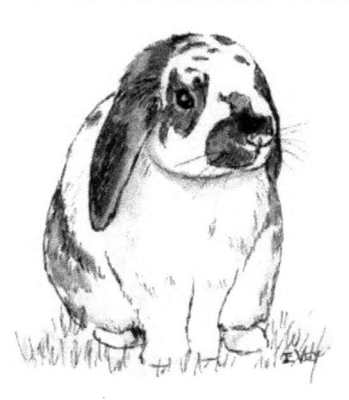

RABBIT BREEDS AND DIET

The breed of rabbit can affect the optimal amounts of nutrients in a rabbit's diet. This is especially true of large, very small, and long-haired rabbits, which have much different energy needs than do rabbits of average size and smooth coats.

Small rabbits

Small breeds such as Netherland Dwarf and Polish may be especially prone to energy deficits if given only hay or if they are given too few pellets. Because of their small size and high metabolism, very small rabbits need slightly higher-energy diets. A diet that does not provide enough energy leads to needed energy being taken from body tissues (ketones will be found in urine when this happens), and if the process is not interrupted, hepatic lipidosis and death may result.

In *Rabbit Medicine and Surgery for Veterinary Nurses*, Fraser and Gileg give the following equation for determining the maintenance energy requirement (MER) for rabbits: MER = constant (k) X body weight. (k= 100 for adults, 200 for growing rabbits, and 300 for lactating rabbits).

Wool breeds

Long-haired, wool-producing rabbits such as American Fuzzy Lops, Jersey Woolies, and the angoras generally require higher levels of fat (4-8%) and protein (17-20%) in their diets than shorter-haired rabbits. Giving seeds (e.g. sunflower) and nuts (e.g. walnuts) is often helpful to provide these rabbits the extra protein and fats they require because of their wool. Providing a nutritionally-complete concentrate (pelleted) feed is also important (as is daily grooming!).

Some people with wool breed rabbits worry that feeding concentrate foods will predispose the rabbits to wool block. However, because of the higher nutritional needs wool rabbits have, it is not usually a good idea to give limited pellet diets or hay-only diets. Some rabbit experts suggest that leaving the concentrate out of long-haired rabbits' diets one day a week and giving only hay for that one day will have the same effect as feeding mostly hay every day, but will keep the nutrition of the diet at adequate levels. Wool rabbits can also be given a higher-fiber pellet, one containing 18-20% crude fiber.

Large breeds

Not long before I wrote this section I attended a lecture on raptors. The wildlife biologist giving the speech told about an orphaned Harris Hawk that had been found by some people who took it home and raised it, feeding it chicken they bought in a grocery store. When the young hawk reached adulthood its legs fractured under the weight of its body because the minerals and other nutrients that are contained in the bones and fur of their natural prey (and were necessary for proper development) were not present in the grocery chicken.

A similar result can happen to large rabbits, especially Flemish Giants, if they are not given enough protein and other nutrients for proper bone development when young. Their bones can fracture (often hairline fractures) from their body weight when they reach adulthood. One person who has raised Flemish Giants for many years shares her experience in providing the nutrition necessary for the proper development of Flemish Giants:

> I feed our Flemish Giants an alfalfa-based pellet from weaning on. I prefer a well-balanced pellet with 17% protein, 20+% fiber, and no more than 3.5% fat. I give free access to clean hay (alfalfa/timothy mix) from the time they leave the nestbox. I "free-feed" all lactating mothers, and also all babies until they are 8–9 months of age. Babies right out of the nestbox get rolled oats mixed with their pellets for 3–5 weeks, gradually lessening the oats and increasing the pellets. I do not feed greens, fruits, or treats until the baby is 4+ months.
>
> Adult Flemish—non-breeding does and all bucks from 9 months of age—get 1 ½ cups of pellets a day plus hay. Greens and fruits are given 1–2 times a week (usually 1/3 cup as a treat), and can include fresh comfrey, parsley, clover, dandelion leaves, apples, oranges, fresh papaya, mango, kale, spinach, and carrot tops (once in a while carrots). I have almost no issues with stasis.

The Flemish Giant has a very rapid rate of growth from birth through 8 months of age. Most Flemish are born weighing about 3–4 oz., and by 8–9 weeks weigh 5 lbs. From 8 weeks to 8 months, the rabbit can gain ½ to ¾ lb. per week, and is not considered full grown until 14 months of age. Flemish Giants are expected to achieve an adult weight of 14–20 lbs, and need a bone structure that will support this weight.

I strongly feel the Flemish Giants need a higher protein level than the smaller rabbits that mature quicker. I have found that Flemish fed greens too early and in too great a quantity, especially if the greens comprise the bulk of the diet, tend not to reach full size and seem to have a propensity to bone fractures. As adults, these rabbits experience frequent leg and spine fractures that are difficult to set and to heal. Their weight seems to be too much for their skeleton to carry, especially if active.

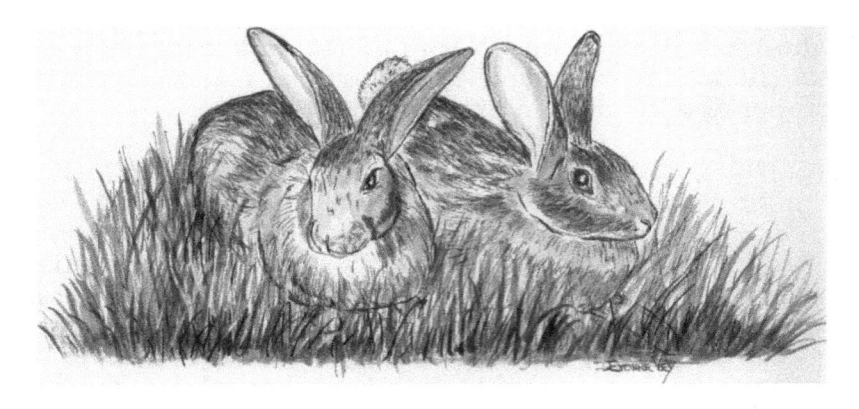

COMMUNITY RABBITS

Rabbits are now the third most popular companion animal in many countries around the world. Unfortunately, as their popularity has grown, so has the number of pet rabbits that are dumped. Many people have the mistaken idea that a rabbit released into a woodland or vacant lot will have a "free" and "happy" life, but this perception is far from the truth. Although rabbits have instincts, survival skills have to be learned, and domestic rabbits have not had that opportunity. Furthermore, their color patterns make them easy prey for predators of all kinds, and they are vulnerable to parasites and disease.

If a dumped rabbit is fortunate enough to be released into an area that can provide some of its needs, other dumped rabbits will probably find their way there as well. If any of the rabbits have not been neutered or spayed they will soon breed and a community develop. The rabbits will burrow and nibble on vegetation, sometimes creating a "nuisance." In such situations local governments may opt to kill the rabbits rather than seek more humane (and more costly) options. Trap-neuter-return programs, along with supplemented feeding, can sometimes help prevent the colony from becoming a problem. Long-time rabbit advocate Debby Widolf is devoting her time and energies to increasing awareness of this problem and providing information regarding possible solutions.

Feeding Colonies of Community Domestic Rabbits
by Debby Widolf

Feeding colonies of community rabbits can present the volunteers and caregivers with challenges depending on how many rabbits there are, the current environment and weather, the availability of natural food sources, and whether there are very young rabbits, lactating or pregnant mothers. Consideration must also be given to where the food sources are located, the vulnerability to predators (humans included), whether volunteers will have the cooperation of the property holders, and the practical questions of what the financial resources are, whether the colony will need to be moved, the numbers of volunteers you will be able to count on, and their commitment to the care. How the feeding and watering is managed is dependent upon all these variables.

In a temperate climate where dense food sources are plentiful and a large foraging area is present, most of the rabbits' basic food needs may be met for a limited time. As the colony grows however, natural food resources become scarce even in the best of conditions. Where there are seasonal changes, finding nutritious food as harsh weather arrives leads to stress, disease and death of many unmanaged colonies of domestic rabbits. Most often these rabbits are in need of nutritional food and a clean water source.

As a beginning, large groups of rabbits can be fed bales of alfalfa hay or alfalfa blend hay and survive on this food. The hay must be protected from getting wet, moldy, and being used as a nesting place by other animals. Two "X" bases made out of wood and two-inch wire can be constructed with a hinged metal lid on top to keep the hay dry and a few inches off the ground. A quick container can be made out of a large Rubbermaid tub with lid. Anchor the inside of the tub to the ground. Make a 4-5 inch hole in both ends a couple inches off the ground and keep the tub stuffed with fresh hay.

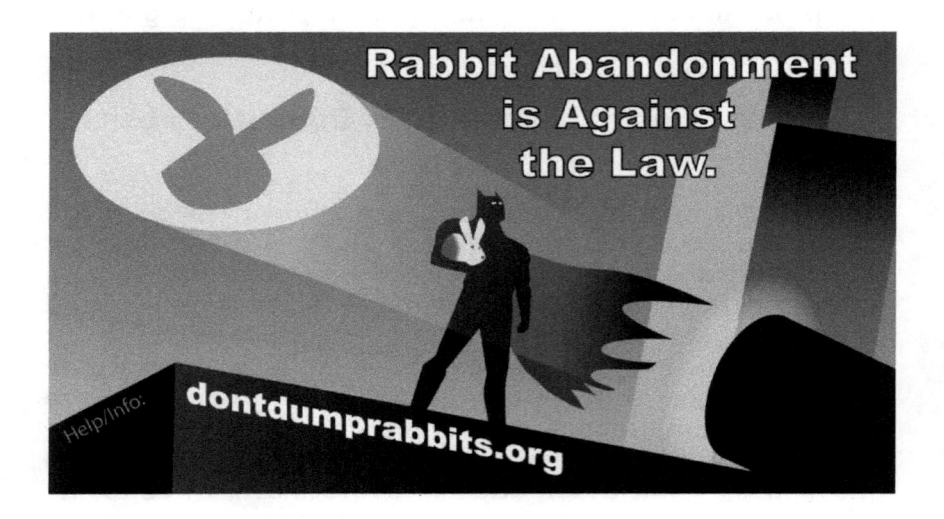

Nutrition for TNR Colonies and Community Rabbits

When feeding colonies of domestic rabbits that live outdoors in a wild state it is first necessary to forget all one has learned about feeding companion rabbits, for the nutritional needs are quite different. To begin with, colonies of rabbits usually consist of rabbits of varying ages, breeds/mixes, and health, and—especially when the colony is is first discovered—some females may be pregnant or lactating. Since it is not possible to feed each community rabbit individually, the food provided to the colony needs to meet the minimal nutritional requirements of all these rabbits. Secondly, the rabbits in outdoor colonies expend a great deal more energy than companion rabbits. Dominance encounters, fleeing from predators, and surviving harsh weather all utilize a great deal of energy. If food is inadequate, rabbits become weak and more likely to die from disease and predators.

Generally, providing colony rabbits that are living outdoors with adequate nutrition means providing high-protein high-energy foods (although this may vary a little by the location of the colony and what plants are growing in the environment). In most cases, a good alfalfa hay with lots of leaves (the more leaves the more protein, fat, and carbohydrates) is the best choice. If it is possible to provide pellets to a community of rabbits, alfalfa-based pellets will provide better nutrition. If the colony is located somewhere with lots of greenery for the rabbits to forage on, the alfalfa hay can be mixed with grass hay (again the more leaves the higher nutrition), but in arid areas where the native vegetation is sparse the hay provided should be primarily alfalfa.

Keeping both hay and pellets protected (see Debby Widolf's article above) is extremely important since toxins from molded hay and pellets can be deadly to the rabbits. Because of the rapidity with which it can spoil outdoors, fresh produce is not recommended for community rabbits unless there are enough volunteers to check on it daily and remove any that is beginning to rot. In areas with raccoons, hay and other food should be checked for contamination by raccoon feces, and any so contaminated removed, as the droppings may carry a parasite (raccoon roundworm) that can be deadly to rabbits.

In addition to a high-energy staple such as alfalfa hay or pellets, it is essential to provide adequate clean water. Rabbits that depend upon hay and/or pellets as a primary source of food need more water than rabbits whose diets consist primarily of succulent green plants. Adequate water also helps keep the urinary tract healthy, especially when a rabbit is consuming a lot of high-calcium alfalfa hay and pellets. It is important to arrange with volunteers to clean water receptacles on a weekly basis to prevent the buildup of biofilm (the slimy coating that develops on the surface of water containers with time) to help prevent problems with toxins and disease.

DIET AND DISEASE

Dental Health and Diet

One issue that comes up when discussing rabbit diet is that of dental disease. Many domestic rabbits suffer from dental disease, particularly acquired dental disease (ADD) at one time or another in their lives. Different veterinarians and researchers have presented various theories as to the primary cause of dental disease, including genetics, tooth wear, and nutritional deficiencies, and have often done research the results of which support their theory. Compelling evidence for metabolic bone disease (MBD) brought on by nutritional deficiencies as a primary cause of ADD has been published, as have results of studies showing that the motion of the rabbit's jaw when chewing has great impact on tooth wear and health. Trauma, neoplasia (tumors), and genetic factors may also contribute toward ADD.

In one interesting study published by Harcourt-Brown, pet rabbits kept free-range had no dental problems while hutch-kept rabbits did. Higher PTH (parathyroid hormone) levels were found in the hutch-kept rabbits, along with lower blood calcium concentrations. Harcourt-Brown's conclusion from this particular study was that ADD was related to husbandry and to alterations in calcium metabolism. Crossley has published various articles on the effects of tooth wear and dental health, showing that the type of food consumed affects the lateral motion of the rabbit's jaw. Hay and natural vegetable foods cause wider lateral movements and less vertical motion; grains and pelleted feeds have the opposite effect, reducing lateral movements and increasing vertical motion. Additionally, more time is spent chewing fibrous foods than is spent chewing concentrate feeds. He suggests that diets primarily composed of pelleted concentrates result in abnormal tooth wear, potentially leading to ADD. Another author points out that a hungry rabbit does not chew food adequately, leading to less wear.

In all truth, I have seen domestic rabbits from 10–14 years old that had been fed almost exclusively on pellets and had no dental disease. I have also seen rabbits kept free-range that did have dental disease. I do not think there is one primary cause of ADD. In my personal opinion, dental disease in rabbits may be caused by a multiplicity of factors, and interplay among those factors. There is strong evidence for a genetic cause of much dental disease, especially in dwarf and lop rabbit breeds. Nutrition, especially the lack of calcium and vitamin D, as well as other minerals, clearly plays a frequent role in the development of acquired dental disease in pet rabbits. Pet rabbits are often kept indoors most of the time and fail to have adequate exposure to direct sunlight to prevent deficiencies of vitamin D. Lack of proper chewing motion (whether from hunger or type of feed) may at times be a cause of ADD in itself, or may exacerbate problems developing from nutritional deficiencies.

Feeding a rabbit a nutritionally complete diet and making sure the rabbit has exposure to direct sunlight may help prevent or delay acquired dental disease, as may providing the rabbit hay and fresh vegetable foods. I do not believe tooth wear is a reason to limit the amount of concentrated pellets fed to a rabbit; rather I believe the rabbit should be fed hay and fresh foods in addition to the pellets. A rabbit that is not fed adequate nutritionally-dense foods may become hungry; with the result that food, including hay, will be chewed less, potentially affecting wear. Wild rabbits of the same genus and species often eat a variety of foods, including occasional grains which cause the same chewing motions as do pellets. Providing a variety of foods that require both chewing motions would logically come closest to mimicking the diet of wild rabbits. I believe that common sense and moderation provide a more healthful answer than excluding potentially beneficial (and needed) rabbit foods such as pelleted concentrates. (Not to mention that pelleted feeds, if fresh, provide a good source for vitamin D for rabbits that are not exposed to direct sunlight.)

Special foods for rabbits having difficulty chewing

If a rabbit has to have his or her teeth worked on, has a facial abscess, or has any other problem that gives the rabbit a sore mouth, it can be very difficult to persuade the rabbit to eat enough. Lisa Hodgson, editor/publisher of the British rabbit magazine *Bunny Mad!*, shares some recipes that may help rabbit caretakers persuade a reluctant rabbit to eat:

Mom's Medicinal Mashes
by Lisa Hodgson[6]

Nursing a rabbit that struggles to eat due to dental problems, painful abscesses and other health issues can be difficult. Getting them eating is key and these recipes may just help as they require little chewing and contain healthy and appetizing ingredients.

The mash has been our saviour through many illnesses and was inspired by my first dental bunny, Fern. By sharing them with you we hope to help other bunnies through their difficult times.

Carrot Crush
Ingredients:
- 1 X large peeled tomato
- 1 X 10 cm piece of carrot
- 1 X 4 cm piece of broccoli
- 1 X 4 cm piece of cauliflower
- 2 X sprigs of parsley
- 15 ml of water

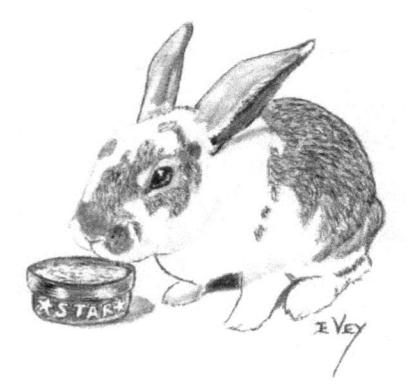

Green Dream
Ingredients:
- 1 X small leaf kale
- 2 X small leaves of pak choi (bok choy)
- 2 X sprigs of coriander
- 2 X sprigs of mint
- 1 X 4 cm piece of broccoli
- 1 X 3 cm piece of cucumber
- 15 ml of water

Banana Brunch
Ingredients:
- 1 X 8 cm piece of banana
- 10 tablespoons of oat bran
- 15 ml of water

---

[6] Hodgson, Lisa. 2012. Mom's Medicinal Mashes. *Bunny Mad!* Issue 15. Reprinted with permission.

Bran Bliss
Ingredients:
- 1 X 8 cm piece of carrot
- 3 X sprigs coriander
- 10 tablespoons oat bran

- Simply measure out your ingredients and chop vegetables into small pieces.
- Add all ingredients to a blender. I use a Kenwood mini chopper which is perfect for small portions.
- Blend for 10 to 20 seconds or until consistencey is smooth. If texture looks dry add a little more water.

Top Tips:
- Use your imagination and try out your own special recipes using your rabbit's favourite foods.
- A very sick rabbit will not always feed from a bowl, so put a little on a spoon or your finger and offer it to them...they often can't resist!
- If your rabbit is very sick you can help aid digestion by adding a small amount of Fibreplex or probiotics, but never add medications.
- Green Dream and Carrot Crush can also be used to syringe feed which helps provide some variety. Syringe feeding should only be attempted on the advice of your vet.
- The oat bran recipes are wonderful for helping gain weight.

Please note: If your rabbit won't eat, please treat this as an emergency and seek veterinary attention. New foods should always be introduced gradually. These recipes are a supplement and should only be given as part of a healthy diet. Oat bran is not suitable for overweight rabbits as it may cause weight gain.

Kathy Smith has also had 'dental bunnies,' and shares her experience (and a recipe for a fruit smoothie) with one of them:

As I write this at the end of March 2013, Ms Holly is celebrating 8 ½ years as part of my family. Not bad for a West Virginia "meat farm" bunny. She and her littermate Theodore (who died while I was writing this) were rescued in September 2004 and arrived at my home in late October of that year.

In May 2011, Holly was acting slightly "off." As we headed to the vet, I expected her to need molars filed. What I didn't expect was to hear Dr. Allan say, "Her mouth is a mess." During the next 4 months we began routine dental work every 6-8 weeks. She did fine at first. In July she had an abscessed tooth, was slow to bounce back from anesthesia, and had appetite loss from the antibiotics. When Dr. Allan went on vacation in August, the "backup" vet plans we discussed were only for euthanasia. The one saving grace was that Ms Holly thought canned pumpkin was bunny ice cream. She couldn't get enough of it and it became a staple in her diet (and Theodore's).

In September 2011, Holly went back for dental work. The abscess was gone, points were manageable, and she did fine under anesthesia. But about four hours after coming home from the vet she was leaning against her x-pen clearly telling me she wanted to die. I made her a promise that if she chose to live, we would deal with her teeth on her terms. My intuition told me to offer her (via syringe) some of the smoothie I was making for myself every day. I now add 2-3 teaspoons of this to about ½ cup softened Kaytee Rainbow Exact and give to her every day:

 1 cup apple juice (no sugar added)
 2-3 handfulls fresh blueberries
 12 large or 15 medium strawberries
 2 small-to-medium bananas
 12-15 ice cubes

Blend on "smoothie" setting until...smooth. I have a large blender. If yours is smaller, you can make ½ recipe (or even smaller amounts, though making only 2-3 teaspoons is probably not an easy option).

It is hard to believe that the Holly who lives with me today is the same bunny I had practically given up for dead a year and a half ago. She not only chose to live, she chose to thrive. She seems to have "aged backward" from that moment when she chose life. When we moved to our new home in April 2012, she really came out of her shell. Until the death of her brother, when I took food downstairs to them, she would greet me at the gate to her and Theodore's area. She then faced a terrible dilemma...do I come out and explore or do I pounce on the food?

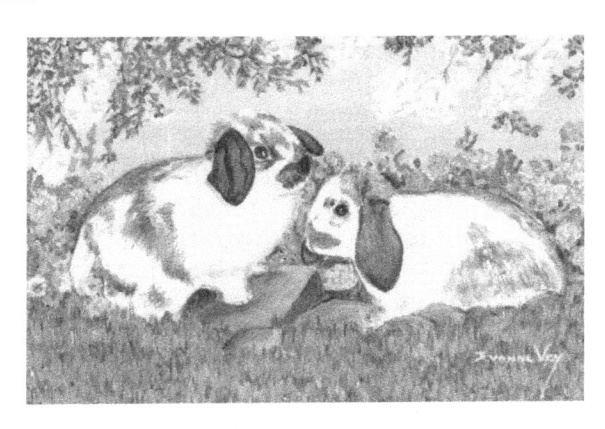

Overweight and Underweight Rabbits

Rabbits are not naturally slim animals, but animals of a medium build. Australian rabbit expert Christine Carter, author of *The Wonderful World of Pet Rabbits,* gives some hints for determining whether a rabbit is a healthy weight:

DO YOU HAVE A FAT OR SKINNY RABBIT?
by Christine Carter

It sounds strange but is true: skinny and obese rabbits (purebred and crossbred) do exist. Unfortunately, owners are often unaware that their poor bunny could be undernourished or burdened with excessive weight, possibly with serious consequences. Apart from lethargy, fat rabbits are susceptible to serious medical conditions, including heart, liver, and kidney disease, chronic diarrhea, splayed legs, heat stress in hot weather, arthritis in their later years, and breeding and birthing difficulties. It is important not to be complacent or blasé about whichever way the weight scales tip, for in reality the rabbits are likely to be silently suffering. It is their birthright to enjoy a natural state of health and vitality.

Check your rabbit's condition by popping him on a piece of carpet (or similar item to prevent slipping) and run the palm of your hand over the length of his backbone. It the spine feels prominent, he needs an immediate increase in protein, usually via pellets. If his pellet intake seems adequate, yet he has a hearty appetite and is still relatively skinny you should investigate further for an explanation. For instance, he may be malnourished because of teeth problems. If on the other hand your rabbit has a heavy, fat stomach, and extra-large dewlap (storage of fat under the chin or chest), loose, hanging flab on hips and shoulders, immediately decrease his daily ration of pellets or whatever fattening foods may be the cause of the excess weight. Do not starve a bunny to effect a quick weight reduction. Both losing weight and gaining weight should be gradual processes.

Older rabbits may need more food to maintain their weight, as may some with chronic illnesses. Lactating does and young rabbit kits also need more food.

Behavior can be the key to knowing if your rabbit is receiving enough food. A rabbit that wolfs food down without thoroughly chewing each bite may not be getting enough food, and swallowing food that is not chewed enough leads to less nutrients being extracted and a higher chance of bowel obstruction. A rabbit that chews excessively on non-food items such as toys or furniture may simply be hungry, and not receiving enough nutrient-dense food. One day one of my rabbits started chewing on the wooden edge of his condo. He had plenty of hay, a bonded mate, and toys. I added more hay and more toys, but his chewing continued. Then I noticed that his bowl of pellets was empty. I gave him a few more pellets and he stopped chewing the wood. I added another two tablespoons per day to his diet and the wood-chewing never resumed.

DIGESTIVE ILLNESSES AND DIET

Digestive ills are often the first sign of a serious problem with a rabbit's health. If your rabbit ceases to produce any feces, has true diarrhea, becomes bloated, and/or refuses to eat and sits hunched and grinding teeth, take the rabbit to a veterinarian immediately. Do not attempt to deal with potentially life-threatening conditions by yourself. Murray states that assuring adequate pain relief to rabbits with GI disease is critical. He points out that rabbits appear to be exceptionally sensitive to the physiologic effects of pain, which may lead to suppression of the immune system, anorexia, and hypomotility, which may have the effect of exacerbating gastro-intestinal disease.

In general, digestive trouble decreases when both indigestible and digestible fiber and fiber from multiple botanical origins are included in the diet. Rabbit diets with crude fiber content of less 6-10% *and* diets with a crude fiber content of more than 20-22% lead to more digestive upsets. Anything that creates *dysbiosis,* or an imbalance in the microflora, can lead to digestive illness. Too little fiber can alter GI tract con-ditions so that pathogenic organisms proliferate; excessive dietary fiber can alter the digestible energy of the diet, creating an energy deficit and a protein surplus. A protein surplus leads to excessive proteolytic enzymes and the production of too much ammonia, which is another road to digestive ills. Fiber also affects the mucosa of the gut, which is important in immune response. It has been found that including 20% soluble fiber (pectins, xylans) in diets that had been based on insoluble fiber improved the health of the mucosa and thereby improved the immune response.

It is important that rabbits' diets be *balanced.* For optimal digestive health they need to receive indigestible fiber, digestible fiber, protein, and other nutrients in both the proper amounts and proper proportions. Giving balanced diets to rabbits may help prevent most digestive illnesses, for diet and nutrition have greater roles in preventing than in curing digestive illnesses. One way to tell if your rabbit is receiving a good diet is by fecal pellets Australian rabbit expert Christine Carter points out that the appearance of a rabbit's droppings can give a good indication of the quality of the diet it is receiving:

Rabbit droppings—proof of the pudding
by Christine Carter

Rabbit droppings are the tell-tale signs that indicate whether our pet is on a good or poor diet. We should observe their droppings—otherwise called scats or rabbit raisins—because the food ingested will influence the resulting output. The diet for all rabbits should consist of high fibre, moderate protein and low carbohydrate.

Rabbit droppings have a characteristic odour, colour, shape and size, and when not normal, signal possible digestive problems and hence the need to improve bunny's diet. An ideal specimen looks a little flattened, smooth, slightly glossy, and if broken apart is dry and fibrous. A protein rich, low fibre diet will produce small (sometimes misshapen) dark brown to black coloured droppings, whereas a healthy high fibre diet produces much larger, dry, tan-coloured droppings.

Both samples pictured in this illustration were produced from one rabbit that came to stay with me for several weeks as a boarder. At first, bunny consistently produced the droppings depicted in the illustration on the left because the owner only supplied her pet with rabbit pellets and small amounts of vegetables. The samples produced on the right are much larger because I supplied handfuls of tall wheat grass, lots of oaten hay, vegetation and only a quarter a cup of pellets per day on his menu. The droppings just grew in size as the amount of vegetation was gradually increased. Be concerned if you see tiny faeces samples; if the cause is not a fur ball it could be the result of a low fibre diet.

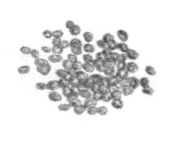

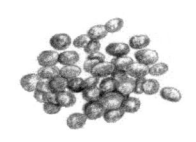

As well as the solid, regular droppings, you may occasionally find unusual smelly droppings excreted by your rabbit. While the bulk of food fibre produces hard droppings, small particles pass into the caecum, which can be thought of as a fermentation vat. During the digestive process, the partly digested food is formed into edible caecal pellets. Caecal pellets are dark brown, soft, moist and often described as looking like a tiny bunch of grapes, or similar in appearance to a loganberry.

Rabbits normally consume their caecal pellets as they are produced and owners rarely notice the practice, as at the time it would appear as if bunny were just washing herself. To some owners the habit could be regarded as distasteful but caecal pellets are highly nutritious and are an essential part of a rabbit's good health. The little pellets are clustered together (covered in mucous to protect them from stomach acids) and contain good gut bacteria, B-complex vitamins, vitamin K, fatty acids and essential amino acids.

Eating these special pellets is called 'coprophagy' or 'caecotrophy' and lack of consumption in the long term may result in malnutrition and vitamin B deficiencies as well as a predisposition to digestive upsets. Individuals most at risk are obese rabbits, rabbits with a fur ball (wool block), excessively large dewlaps, or malocclusion.

Sometimes caecal pellets are mistaken for a touch of diarrhoea, especially after finding them squashed on the hutch floor or perhaps stuck on the rabbit's bottom. If bunny also produces a fresh supply of firm droppings then you can be reassured that it's not diarrhoea. Rabbits can over-produce caecal pellets; overeating commercial rabbit pellets, seeds, lucerne, vegetables and any other foods high in protein and carbohydrates, or low in fibre, may cause this. To effect a natural balance to your rabbit's digestive system it is best to assess and adjust bunny's diet. Cut back on rich foods and increase fibre intake with grass and hay (oaten hay is particularly relished by bunnies) and keep in mind it will take a few days to have an effect on the droppings.

Uneaten cecotrophs

Rabbits may fail to eat all the cecotrophs they produce because they are on a high-protein diet or simply a diet that is nutritionally complete (researchers found rabbits receiving commercial feeds eat fewer cecotrophs). The main problem uneaten cecotrophs creates for an otherwise healthy rabbit is a sanitary one, for uneaten cecotrophs may soil both the rabbit's fur and environment and attract flies. Reducing the protein in the rabbit's diet may help to reduce the number of uneaten cecotrophs.

Other rabbits may be unable to consume their cecotrophs because of paralysis, arthritis, or another disease or medical problem that reduces their appetite or makes cecotrophs difficult to access. In these cases uneaten cecotrophs can be collected and offered to the rabbit (try not to damage the protective mucus covering in the process).

Dysbiosis ("poopy butt")

Dysbiosis, whether intestinal or cecal, is caused by an imbalance of microflora. Cecal dysbiosis is more common and, in general, is a less serious condition. The rabbit produces malformed, unusually soft, and sometimes less odorous cecotrophs that may become smeared onto the perineal area. In the 2nd edition of the *Textbook of Rabbit Medicine*, Varga lists change of diet, lack of dietary fiber, succulent foods, and stress as common causes. Rabbits are sensitive, and stress or changes in diet or routine may cause changes in the cecal microflora. Any new foods, especially produce, should introduced into a rabbit's diet with care. Start with small amounts and slowly increase them over time, as too-rapid changes in digestive microflora may occur as the microbial population tries to adjust to the new foods. Rabbits may also have individual sensitivities to chemical compounds found in a particular produce item. In these cases it is best to remove the item from the rabbit's diet.

Some people have claimed to have success treating cecal dysbiosis with edible clay and products such as Bio-Sponge, but caution should be observed if giving a clay-based product because of the potential for cecal impaction (p.292). When a rabbit is producing soft cecotrophs, keep the perineal area cleaned, for if the cecotrophs mat and dry on the fur they can block the anus and/or attract flies, which may lay eggs on the rabbit.

Less often, an obstruction in the GI tract, internal abscesses, kidney/liver disease, or another medical disease or condition may cause cecal dysbiosis. Very little undigested sugar and starch reach the cecum (chapter 3) and are unlikely to cause cecal dysbiosis.

Intestinal dysbiosis is less common in rabbits than cecal dysbiosis, but can occur as a result of inappropriate antibiotic therapy and may also develop in advanced stages of GI slowdown (p. 293). Signs may include true diarrhea (watery or mucoid), pain, listlessness, and low body temperature. This can be a very serious condition and a veterinarian should be consulted.

Rarely, a rabbit may produce fecal pellets that are of a pasty consistency; however, these tend to still hold their shape and are almost never a cause of what many rabbit caretakers call "poopy butt."

Diarrhea

True diarrhea is a medical emergency. There will be NO normal stools produced, neither hard feces nor cecotrophs. The diarrhea may be watery or contain blood or mucous. *Get any rabbit with true diarrhea to a veterinarian immediately.* The primary role of diet is in prevention. By providing diets that are adequate in both indigestible and soluble fiber, and making any changes to diet very slowly, the incidence of diarrhea can be reduced.

Young rabbits are at especially high risk of developing diarrhea due to changes in their digestive tracts and diet after weaning. Following are several diarrheal diseases of rabbits that are affected by diet:

COCCIDIOSIS, INTESTINAL

Although rabbits are affected by about twelve species of coccia, intestinal coccidiosis is most often caused by the intestinal protozoal parasites *Eimeria magna* and *E. irresidua*. The parasites are most often found in the intestine but may be found in the cecum in heavy infestations. Infections may be of more than one species since different species will colonize different areas in the intestines. Coccidiosis can be fatal to very young rabbits, although older ones often survive. Signs vary and are often subclinical. Clinical signs are most often seen in young rabbits and may include anorexia, dehydration, and mild intermittent to severe diarrhea that may be tinged with blood and/or mucus. The severity of the disease depends upon the species involved, the age of the rabbit, and the health of the rabbit's immune system.

Younger rabbits are most often exposed to the parasite in their immediate environment; but it is possible for an older pet rabbit to contract this parasite by being fed grass with oocysts that is collected outdoors where wild rabbits graze.

Giving rabbits pomegranate peel extract and feed additives based on natural oregano and garlic oils have been found to reduce the intensity of coccidial infections and to protect against the secondary viral and bacterial infections that are often responsible for mortality from this disease.

COLIBACILLOSIS

Colibacillosis is an enteritis caused by overgrowth of

pathogenic strains of *Escherichia coli*. Diets that require high hydrochloric acid content for digestion promote the growth of this pathogen. If a rabbit has an infestation of coccidia it may predispose them to colibacillosis. The disease mostly affects the colon and cecum.

There are two types of colibacillosis that affect rabbits: one type mainly affects rabbits from one to two weeks old, and a sign is a severe, watery, yellowish diarrhea. Mortality is high. The second type mostly affects rabbits from 4 to 6 weeks old and is a diarrheal disease similar to enterotoxemia (see entry below). Signs vary from mild diarrhea and weight loss to severe watery diarrhea and death. A high-fiber diet helps protect weaned rabbits from this disease.

ENTEROTOXEMIA

Enterotoxemia is a deadly diarrheal disease primarily affecting rabbits between four and eight weeks old, although older pet rabbits can be affected, especially if they are on a course of antibiotics. The disease causes an enteritis of the intestine and cecum that is triggered by proliferation of *Clostridium* species in the intestine. The clostridia then produce exotoxins which penetrate the mucosal barrier, enter the bloodstream, and cause toxicosis, or poisoning. The iota-like toxin produced by the bacterium *C. spiroforme* is a potent and fast-acting toxin. Signs include lethargy, rough coat and greenish-brown diarrhea. Affected rabbits usually die within 12 hours. A rabbit kit may look healthy in the evening and be dead at morning.

Newly-weaned rabbits are most likely to contract this disease and mortality is very high. Adult rabbits are more resistant, but may also contract this disease, especially if they are on a course of antibiotics. Signs include anorexia, lethargy, and a watery brown diarrhea that may have some blood and/or mucus in it. Antibiotics are rarely helpful in treating enterotoxemia. Treatment may include giving fluids and edible clay or cholestyramine to bind toxins. If giving edible clay, give only a sprinkle in the rabbit's food or water and do not give for more than three days as it can contribute toward impaction of the cecum.

Factors that may contribute toward the development of this disease include an unbalanced diet, a low-fiber diet, a high-carbohydrate diet (*C. spiroforme* needs glucose to produce its toxin), GI hypomotility, and antibiotics. Diets that are high in indigestible fiber reduce the incidence of this disease, especially in young rabbits. Giving young rabbits hay and/or straw may help prevent the disease. Providing extra fiber may also help prevent the disease from developing in older rabbits on antibiotics, as may adding probiotics to the drinking water. Pomegranate extract may inhibit enterotoxin production.

MUCOID ENTEROPATHY
Mucoid enteropathy is not the same thing as **mucoid enteritis**, which is a diarrheal disease in which there is mucus in the diarrhea. Mucoid enteropathy differs in that there are few of the inflammatory changes that characterize mucoid enteritis. In mucoid enteropathy large amounts of mucus are produced in the colon and impaction of the cecum and/or terminal part of the small intestine occurs in 75% of the cases. There is no evidence of an infectious cause, but both too little fiber (less than 6%) and a diet with over 22% fiber predispose rabbits to mucoid enteropathy. Other predisposing factors are not entirely understood but may include pathogens, enterotoxins, and GI hypomotility. Young rabbits are most commonly affected by this condition, especially if they are receiving low-fiber high-carbohydrate diets. However, older rabbits under stress can also be affected by mucoid enteropathy.

Signs of mucoid enteropathy include abdominal distension, subnormal temperature, depression, anorexia, a solid impacted cecum, bloated abdomen, and a distinctive "splash" in the gut. Rabbits may sit hunched, grinding teeth, head hanging over a water bowl. They may drink more or less than normal. Normal feces cease to be produced; hard feces cease entirely or may be gelatinous or mucus-covered, there may be diarrhea in the early stages, in later stages copious amounts of mucus may be excreted (alone or with fecal material) and eventually all production of feces may cease. Affected rabbits are usually dehydrated, but there will be excess water in the stomach, which produces the typical "splash."

Treatment may include rehydrating with electrolytes and adding salt to food (not to the water or by salt wheel). Stress and antibiotic treatment may predispose rabbits to mucoid enteropathy, as may too little or too much fiber in the diet. The chances of a rabbit becoming affected by mucoid enteropathy can be reduced by providing a diet with crude fiber over 15% but less than 22% of the diet. Water should always be available, any changes to the diet made slowly, and stress minimized.

Impaction of Cecum

Impaction of the cecum is not the same condition as mucoid enteropathy, although about 75% of rabbits suffering from mucoid enteropathy have impacted cecums. Cecal contents are solid and dry. There are several factors that may contribute to this condition, including stress, dehydration, not enough fiber in diet, too much crude fiber in diet (over 20-22%), fiber and lignin particles less than 0.3mm in length, too many foods high in pectins and gums, consumption of bulk laxatives (methylcellulose. psyllium) or clay (cat litter or edible clay).

Like GI hypomotility, this condition may not be noticed in its early stages, or according to Harcourt-Brown, may be mistaken for dental disease since affected rabbit may pick at food and drop it without eating. Other signs may include weight loss, lethargy, sitting in a hunched stance, an enlarged cecum, reduced fecal pellets or none at all, and voiding mucus.

Impaction of the cecum is very difficult to treat. Veterinarians may attempt to soften the cecal contents and prescribe motility drugs (e.g., Cisapride, Reglan). Liquid paraffin and prostaglandin are other treatments a veterinarian may suggest. It is important to coax affected rabbits to eat with healthy treats such as fresh greens that provide water and nutrition.

The main role of diet is in preventing this condition. Be sure your rabbit is given a balanced diet with both indigestible and digestible fiber as well as other nutrients and water. If a rabbit is taking some edible clay for removal of toxins for another disease, do not give the clay for too long a period, as it can contribute to cecal impaction.

Megacolon Syndrome

Megacolon is a condition in which feces chronically accumulate in the colon, where they become abnormally liquefied. The rabbits may produce large amounts of messy and odorous soft fecal material (sometimes called "cowpiles" or "cowpies") that becomes a sanitary problem. There is a genetic predisposition to this disease in rabbits homozygous for the English Spot gene and in albino rabbits. Researchers found that rabbits affected by megacolon have fewer nerves to parts of the gastrointestinal tract, which affects the rate and strength of the contractions. The rabbits also have significantly reduced sodium absorption rates across the wall of the cecum, which reduces the dry matter content of the digesta and increases the mineral content. In the proximal parts of the large intestine, digesta is abnormally liquefied. The rabbits are susceptible to motility difficulties and gas.

Rabbits with a genetic predisposition to the disease may develop it at different ages, depending upon environmental factors such as diet, stress, and age. The age of four years appears to be a common age for signs to appear, although some rabbits with a genetic disposition to the disease may never develop it at all. Rabbits that do not have a genetic predisposition can also develop the syndrome if the spine is damaged or if nerves to the digestive tract are severed during an operation.

At the time of this writing there appears to be no accepted course of treatment for the megacolon syndrome. Some veterinarians suggest feeding higher amounts of hay, while others suggest providing a varied diet including pellets, soft green hay, fresh greens, nuts and seeds. Motility drugs may be prescribed. Giving small amounts of fresh herbs (basil, thyme, oregano) may help inhibit growth of intestinal pathogens and simthicone can help reduce gas.

Gastrointestinal hypomotility ("stasis")

Some veterinarians dislike the use of the term "stasis" for this disorder as gastrointestinal hypomotility is not truly a stasis (cessation of movement) but a slowing down. It may occur as a primary condition and lead to bacterial imbalances in the gut, or the slowdown may be secondary to a bacterial imbalance. When it occurs as a primary condition, the normal intestinal movement slows, types of fiber are no longer separated well, and bacteria begin to multiply. The contents of the gastrointestinal tract become compacted as the rabbit drinks less, painful gas accumulates in pockets, and toxins from multiplying bacteria accumulate. An imbalance of electrolytes (minerals that carry an electric charge) occurs. Symptoms of GI hypomotility include anorexia, enlarged abdomen, gradual reduction in amount and size of fecal pellets, pain, dehydration, weight loss, and lethargy. Stress (even simple stresses such as a change in routine) and disease may help precipitate GI hypomotility, as may a lack of exercise.

This digestive disorder is again best *prevented* by diet, a diet that has a balance of both indigestible and digestible fiber provided by plants of different botanical origin. It is also important that rabbit's diets have enough water, and enough fat in them to stimulate the production of motilin in the digestive tract. Although the overall effect of a high fiber diet is to speed transit time through the digestive system, indigestible and digestible fiber have opposite effects—indigestible fiber slows the rate of transit of digesta in the stomach and intestine and speeds its time in the cecum while digestible fiber increases the rate of transit through the stomach and slows it through the cecum. Rabbits need both fibers for good digestive health.

Grass hay contains both indigestible and soluble fibre, but is lacking in many necessary micronutrient vitamins and minerals, as well as other compounds. Diets comprised only of grass hay may predispose rabbits to GI hypomotility, as well as other digestive ills such as cecal impaction and mucoid enteropathy.

Gas may occur along with GI hypomotility, and giving simethicone as soon as the signs of GI hypomotility are noticed may help. Pressure from gas can press on the pylorus, preventing emptying of the chyme into the intestine. A veterinarian may prescribe intestinal motility drugs and/or fluids for GI hypomotility. Water is important because if water is lacking in the rabbit's diet, it is pulled from the digestive tract, making the digesta even dryer, impacting the intestine and increasing hypomotility, or the slowing down of the movement of digesta through the rabbit gastro-intestinal tract. As the rabbit eats less, cecal pH increases, causing cecal dysbiosis. Changes in water and electrolyte balances may even lead to hepatic lipidosis and death if the process is not interrupted. Therefore, it is important that rabbits in the early stages of GI hypomotility be coaxed to eat.

In the early stages of GI hypomotility a rabbit will still

produce hard feces, although the feces may be smaller and harder than normal. At this early stage it may help to give a teaspoon of aloe juice (has a protective effect on the lining of GI tract—fresh aloe may be used if the leaf is peeled and the reddish vein removed) along with a teaspoon of olive oil (provides good fatty acids), and two teaspoons of pureed pumpkin (provides fiber, nutrients, and phytonutrients) every two hours or so. Some veterinarians may also recommend fresh or frozen (unpasteurized) pineapple juice for its bromelain content in the event a mat of hair is contributing to the hypomotility. If the condition progresses to where the rabbit's hard feces are very tiny and few in number, it is important to take the rabbit to a veterinarian before functional obstruction develops (see below).

Obstruction: acute bloat and blockage

Blockages of the gastrointestinal tract are very serious in rabbits, and as with most digestive ills in rabbits, prevention is key. Too little or too much of either type of fiber and lignin can be a cause of functional blockages, as can fiber and lignin that is less than 0.2 mm in length. Total obstructions can be caused by a rabbit eating too fast and failing to chew food thoroughly, especially items such as seeds, dried peas, corn, or beans. Wood toys and indigestible items such as plastic and carpet fibers may also cause functional or complete blockages.

Bloat occurs as gas accumulates in large amounts in the GI tract. Acute bloat, however, occurs as a result of a physical obstruction or severe GI hypomotility. True obstructions are usually high in the gut, near the pyloric opening (at the bottom of the stomach) or within the first six inches of the small bowel. Because of the obstruction, gas and liquids cannot pass normally and begin to accumulate in the stomach, distending it. As the stomach expands, it presses on other internal organs and causes extreme pain to the rabbit. It is critical that treatment of this condition include pain relief.

What one veterinarian terms "functional obstructions" may cause similar effects. In the end stages of GI hypomotility the digesta becomes compacted and almost ceases to move, which also causes accumulation of gas and fluid although there is not a complete blockage.

Functional obstruction may also occur at the pylorus from normal ingested food that is not chewed thoroughly, as well as in the intestine from the impacted contents that collect when intestinal contractions slow. These latter may occasionally move out on their own, causing periodic episodes of pain and anorexia until they have passed into the colon. (Once in the colon many of these blockages will no longer be as obstructive, since the colon is larger.) Bloat and acute bloat are extremely painful, may cause the rabbit to go into shock, and in some cases may cause rupture of the stomach or other organs.

A rabbit with acute bloat from a complete GI obstruction can go from perfectly well to critically ill within an extremely short period of time, and die within 12-24 hours of onset of symptoms if there is no successful intervention. *If you see several of the following signs in your rabbit, it is an extreme medical emergency and the rabbit must receive immediate veterinary attention to have any hope of survival:*

- Sudden refusal to eat or drink
- Extreme pain (rabbit will often sit hunched, grinding its teeth)
- Loud gurgles and/or sloshing water
- Distension of abdomen with tight feel
- Abrupt cessation of fecal pellets
- Shock
- Sudden onset—rabbit was fine one minute, near collapse the next

I wish to give a caution regarding chew sticks and wood toys for rabbits: I have never lost a rabbit to GI hypomotility or complications from it, and in fact I have almost never had a rabbit go through an episode of GI hypomotility. But I have lost two rabbits to lignin-related obstructions: one to a functional obstruction caused by the rabbit eating too many fresh apple twigs and one to a total blockage and acute bloat after the rabbit consumed pieces of a wood toy. Excessive chewing of willow twigs may pose risks in addition to that of obstruction due to the aspirin-like compound salicylic acid that is present.

Please watch your rabbits carefully if you give them wood toys, and if a rabbit begins to eat too much of the sticks or toy take them away.

Kidney/bladder disease

Rabbits are able to filter 45–60% calcium out of their blood (compared to 2% for most other mammals). They resist hypo- and hyper-calciuria by rapid changes in PTH secretion and calcitronin, but when the reabsorption capacity of the kidneys is reached, calcium precipitates out as crystals of calcium carbonate. This is what causes the cloudy and gritty qualities of rabbit urine, which are normal. Jenkins suggests there is a difference between this normal calciuria (calcium crytals in urine) and "sludge," which Jenkins calls microurinary calculi, or MUC. These tiny calculi form in response to cystitis or other conditions (e.g. lack of exercise, dehydration), and can accumulate as bladder "sludge" or aggregate to form uroliths. Other predisposing factors to MUC or stone formation include infections, arthritis, dehydration, nutritional imbalances, lack of exercise, and genetics.

Although in the past rabbits with sludge and/or uroliths were often told to reduce the calcium in the rabbit's diet, many veterinary health professionals now recognize that fluid intake and exercise may be more important than the intake of calcium, and Jenkins states that rabbits on low-calcium diets may actually have greater amounts of MUC. Increased fluid intake reduces the concentration of the urine and keeps the urinary tract flushed out, and exercise helps keep particles from remaining in the bladder. Giving potassium-magnesium citrate to dissolve sludge or stones is recommended by some veterinarians.

Prolonged high dietary calcium intake of more than 40 g/kg, or 4%, can also lead to calcinosis, or the calcification of soft tissues (esp. aorta and kidneys) in rabbits, and this calcification is increased if vitamin D is supplemented in the diet. Rabbits with severe calcinosis may become anorexic and become emaciated. Prolonged excesses of dietary calcium also impair the absorption of zinc and phosphorus in the rabbit. If dietary phosphorus levels are already low, a phosphorus deficiency may be created.

Foods that are high in calcium include parsley, spinach, carrot tops, mustard greens, borage, kale, dandelion greens, chicory, and lamb's quarters. However, it should be recognized that many of these greens, including alfalfa and spinach, have high levels of oxalate. This reduces the amount of calcium that is actually usable, or *bioavailable,* to the rabbit because much of it is bound as insoluble and indigestible calcium oxalate (see Chapter 5). For example, 60–70% of the calcium in alfalfa hay is bound in calcium oxalate. (Fiber content may also affect bioavailability of nutrients, including calcium.) This means that foods such as alfalfa and spinach that have high oxalate content will not provide as much calcium to a rabbit as would appear from the food's content of that mineral. Phytates and acetates (see Chapter 8) may also form complexes with calcium and also reduce the bioavailability of calcium.

Recommended dietary calcium levels for rabbits are: 0.22 % for normal growth, 0.35–0.4% for maximum bone density in growing rabbits.

Kidney failure is not uncommon in rabbits, especially as they get older. Various foods may help chronic kidney failure, including dandelion root, cleavers, and marshmallow root. Fluids are very important in rabbits suffering from kidney disease. If the rabbit is not drinking enough, trying adding a few drops of fruit juice to the water or present it in a different way. Some rabbits may prefer to drink from a bowl rather than a bottle, or vice versa.

Other Disease and Diet

The following suggestions made for diet additions that might possibly help rabbits suffering from various medical conditions do not guarantee the prevention or cure of any disease. However, adding a few vegetables or fruits containing the suggested nutrients are unlikely to be harmful and may have the potential to help prevent or ameliorate the effects of some diseases. The use of nutrients to promote health and aid in the cure of disease is common to many cultures, and the scientific bases for many traditional plant cures have been discovered.

Always consult a veterinary professional regarding any suspected medical problems in your rabbits. When used as a *complementary* form of health care, nutritional healing can be a valuable component of holistic care.

ARTHRITIS AND JOINT PROBLEMS
Older rabbits may develop joint problems, including arthritis, which can greatly impact their quality of life. Adding a few foods that are good sources of copper, manganese, silicon and/or zinc may help improve general joint health and help your older rabbit keep his mobility longer. Rosmarinic acid, a phytonutrient found in many fresh herbs, has anti-inflammatory effects that may help reduce the pain of arthritis and similar conditions.

Many of the flavonoids, a large class of phytonutrients particularly abundant in fruits (see Chapter 8) may also have anti-inflammatory effects, including chalcones, luteolin, naringenin, and proantho- cyanidins. Feeding arthritic rabbits some fresh herbs and vegetables containing these substances may help reduce arthritis pain.

Supplements of glucosamine and chondroitin, natural components of cartilage, have been found to be effective in reducing the pain of osteoarthritis in humans, and some vets have reported them effective in rabbits as well. Supplements produced specifically for improving joint quality in companion animals are available from companies such as Oxbow.

CANCER
There is evidence that selenium and molybdenum may help prevent the development of many cancers. These are minerals naturally found in many foods, but excessive amounts of foods containing theses minerals should not be given, because they can have negative effects consumed in high amounts. Vitamin A precursors (alpha-carotene, beta-carotene, and beta cryptoxanthin; see Chapter 8) may help to prevent some cancers from developing in rabbits. Many of the flavonoids, a large class of phytonutrients (see Chapter 8) may help prevent development and even combat already-formed tumors. Garcinol, a phytonutrient in magosteen, has also been found to have anti-cancer effects.

CARDIOVASCULAR DISEASE
As more companion rabbits live longer lives, heart disease has become more common. Atherosclerosis, or a

deposition of fat in arteries, is relatively rare in rabbits but may occur in some older companion rabbits. Several minerals may help slow the development of athersclerosis: copper, iodine, magnesium, selenium, silicon, and zinc. Adding a few foods that contain moderate to high amounts of these minerals may help keep your rabbit free from life-threatening atherogenic plaque buildup in the arteries (however, remember selenium can be toxic in high amounts). Excessive amounts of iron in the diet may contribute to atherosclerosis in rabbits (although some iron is essential and moderate amounts beneficial) so care should be taken not to give too many foods high in this mineral.

Vitmain E and Vitamin C have also been found to be helpful in preventing the atherosclerosis in rabbits. Several phytonutrients, including pthalides, resveratrol, and many of the flavonoids (see Chapter 8) fight cardiovascular disease, the first by reducing blood pressure and stress, and the others by slowing the buildup of arterial plaques and/or preventing blood clot formation.

FREQUENT INFECTIONS

If your rabbit has frequent respiratory or other infections, he may need a boost to the immune system. Adding a few foods with moderate to high amounts of vitamin A, magnesium, selenium, silicon, and zinc will help stimulate the immune system. Moderate amounts of iron-rich foods may help also, although high-iron foods should be given sparingly since excessive dietary iron may promote atherosclerosis.

MUSCULAR WEAKNESS/"FLOPPY RABBIT"

Although there are several potential causes of what is sometimes called "floppy rabbit syndrome" in rabbits, it is often a lack of adequate micronutrients that causes a rabbit's muscles to become weak. The rabbit may be unable to stand at all, or may stagger and fall. In cases where the rabbit is unable to stand, they will usually continue to eat and drink if the food and water is placed directly under their mouth. Severe deficiencies (or excesses) of both vitamin A and vitamin E can result in such muscular dystrophy in rabbits, and a lack of potassium may also lead to muscular weakness and even cause the heart mucle to lose some contractile force. Too much calcium and/or chronic choline deficiency may also lead to muscle weakness. Should your rabbit develop a sudden muscular weakness, it may help to give a few foods high in vitamins A and E, choline, and potassium, along with seeking a professional veterinary opinion.

SKIN AND FUR
Changes in the skin and/or fur are often one of the first signs of nutrient deficiencies in rabbits. Be on the watch for such signs and correct any deficiencies before more serious problems develop. (Most fur problems brought on by nutrient deficiencies ordinarily disappear after the deficient nutrient is restored in adequate amounts.) Signs include:

- Fur falling out or turning grey before old age: copper, magnesium, or zinc deficiency may be partly responsible.
- Dry scaly skin: copper or zinc-rich foods may help improve skin tone and health.
- Fur dull, lacking in luster: vitamin A, vitamin E, or the fat necessary for their absorption may be deficient in diet.
- Chewing fur or rough coat: adding protein and/or magnesium to the diet may help.

STRESS
Rabbits—like people—can suffer from physical and emotional stress which may be brought on by heat, illness, changes in their environment or other stresses, including picking up on stresses their owner may be experiencing. The phthalide group of phytonutrients is helpful in reducing stress, as is vitamin C. Although rabbits manufacture their own vitamin C and do not have to consume it, many studies have shown that dietary vitamin C can help reduce stress in rabbits, including heat stress and the stress of pregnancy or illness. Noni juice, which is very high in vitamin C, has been found to have calming effects on rabbits.

Foods with specific vitamins, minerals, and phytonutrients
Following is a list of some essential nutrients and phyto-

nutrients and a listing of foods that contain relatively high amounts of them. Other foods may also contain these nutrients, as well as additional nutrients, but the listed sources are foods that may safely be given to healthy adult rabbits in moderate amounts and which are easy to find.

Remember that when adding any new food to a rabbit's diet it is best to give only very small amounts at first in order to allow the rabbit's digestive flora to adjust. If a rabbit appears to have a sensitivity to, or does not want ot eat a particular food, discontinue it and try a different food that contains the desired nutrient.

VITAMINS:

Vitamin A: dark leafy greens (e.g. spinach, red leaf lettuce, parsley, arugula), yellow-orange fruits and vegetables (e.g. carrots, gac, pumpkin, mango)

B-Vitamins: cecotrophs, leafy greens

Vitamin C: leafy greens, apricot, mango, noni, papaya.

Vitamin E: alfalfa, dark green vegetables, fresh young grass.

MINERALS:

Copper: beets, green leafy vegetables, broccoli, oranges.

Iodine: green leafy vegetables.

Iron: berries, dandelion, green leafy vegetables, mint, watercress.

Magnesium: apples, banana, green leafy vegetables.

Molybdenum: dark green leafy vegetables.

Potassium: apricots, banana, oranges, ribwort plantain, pumpkin, spinach.

Selenium: bananas, bramble leaves, broccoli, mint, parsley.

Silicon: apples, cherries, fresh grass, grass hay, pumpkin.

Zinc: green leafy vegetables, mint, dandelion greens, pumpkin.

PHYTONUTRIENTS:

Coumarin: apricolts, cherries, strawberries.

Flavonoids: apples, berries, red grapes.

Garcinol: mangosteen.

Geraniol: blueberries, carrots, cilantro, oregano.

Limonene: ashitaba, celery, mints.

Lutein: broccoli, carrots, lettuce, spinach.

Lycopene: watermelon, pink guava, gac.

Phthalides: celery (chop stems in small pieces for rabbits) and loveage. Some greens and herbs, such as parsley.

Resveratrol: blue and purple berries, red grapes.

Rosmarinic acid: mints, oregano, rosemary, sage.

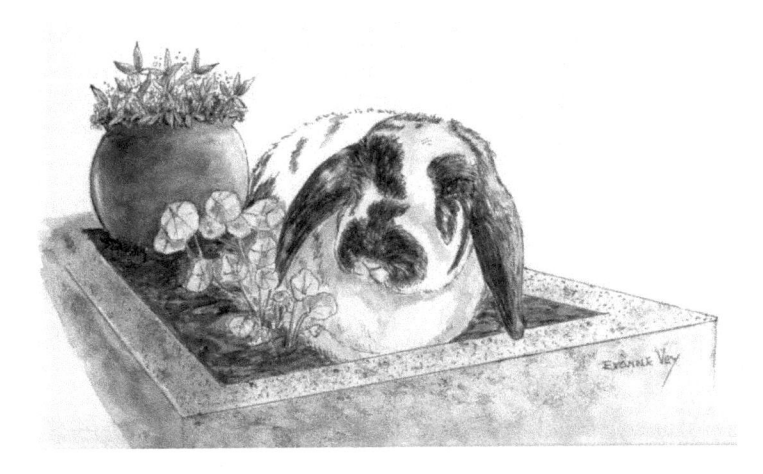

References

Note on Chapter 10 references: Rather than repeat references for information taken from other chapters in this book, I have chosen to include only a few selected references plus references for information not found in previous chapters. For complete references, see the reference lists for chapters 2, 3, 4, 5, 6, 8, and 9 in addition to those below.

Agnoletti, F. 2012. Update on rabbit enteric diseases: Despite improved diagnostic capacity, where does disease control and prevention stand?

Proceedings: 10th World Rabbit Congress. Sharm El-Sheikh, Egypt.

Beltz, K. M., M. M. Rosales, and E. Morales. 2005. Histological and Ultrstructural Findings in Commercial Bred Rabbits Exhibiting Severe Diarrhea. *Scan. J. Lab. Anim. Sci.* 32(4): 243-250.

Bodeker, D., O. Turck, E. Loven, D. Wieberneit, and W. Wegner. 1995. Pathophysiological and functional aspects of the megacolon-syndrome of homozygous spotted rabbits. *Zentralbl. Veterinarmed. A.* 42: 549-559.

BSAVA Manual of Rabbit Medicine and Surgery. Second. edition. 2006. Edited by Anna Meredith and Paul Flecknell. Glouster: British Small Animal Veterinary Association.

Brown, S. 2009. Intermittent Soft cecotropes in Rabbits. Accessed 2/22/13 at http://www.veterinarypartner.com/Content.plx?A=3012&S=1&SourceID=43

Capello, Vittorio and Margherita Gracis. 2005. *Rabbit and Rodent Dentistry Handbook.* Lake Worth: Zoological Education Network.

Carabano, R., I. Badiola, S. Chamoro, J. Garcia, A. I. Garcia-Ruiz, P. Garcia-Rebollar, M. S. Gomez-Conde, I. Gutierrez, N. Nicodemus, M. J. Villamide, and J. C. de Blas. 2008. Review: New trends in rabbit feeding: influence of nutrition on intestinal health. *Span. J. Agri. Res.* 6(special issue): 15-25.

Carpenter, J. W. 2010. Diagnosing and Treating gastric ileus/stasis in rabbits. *Proceedings:* CVC, Baltimore, USA.

Chiou, P. W., B. Yu, and C. Lin. 1998. The effect of different fibre components on growth rate, nutrient digestibility, rate of digesta passage and hindgut fermentation in domestic rabbits. *Lab. Anim.* 32: 276-283.

Chute, D. J., J. Cox, M. Archer, R. J. Bready, and K. Reiber. 2009. Spontaneous Rupture of Urinary Bladder Associated with Massive Fecal Impaction (Fecalona). *Am. J. Foren. Med. Path.* 30(3): 280-283.

Crossley, D. 2010. Dental Anatomy of Rabbits and Rodents. Accessed 11/14/2010 http://www.lafebervet.com/small-mammals/?p=2624.

Crossley, D. A. 2005. Pathophysiology of Continuously Growing Teeth. *Proceedings;* Exotics Conference, Ljubljana. Accessed 11/15/10 at http://vetdent.eu/cpd/cpddownloads/notes-elodontpahtophysiology.pdf

Drs. Foster and Smith Educational Staff. 2015. Enterotoxemia (Antibiotic-associated Enteritis) in Hamsters, Rabbits, and guinea pigs.

Acessed 4/7/16 at http://www.peteducation.com/articvle.cfm?c=

Fraser, M. and S. J. Gerling. 2009. *Rabbit Medicine and Surgery for Veterinary Nurses.* Chichester: Wiley-Blackwell.

Gidenne, T. and F. Lebas. 2002. Role of dietary fibre in rabbit nutrition and in digestive troubles prevention. *Proceedings:* 2nd Rabbit Congress of the Americas. Habana City, Cuba.

Gomez-Conde, M. S., S. Chamorro, P. Eiras, P. G. Rebollar, A. Perez de Rozas, C. de Blas, and R. Carabano. 2007. Neutral detergent-soluble fiber improves gut barrier function in twenty-five-day-old weaned rabbits. *J. Anim. Sci>* 85(12): 3313-3321.

Grunkemeyer, V. 2013. Clinical Approach to Ileus in Rabbits and Guinea Pigs. North Carolina University CVM.

Fontanesi, L., M. Vargiolu, E. Scotti, R. Latorre, M. S. Pellegrini, and M. Mazzoni. 2014. The KIT Gene is Associated with the *English Spotting* Coat color Locus and Congenital Megacolon in Checkered Giant Rabbits (*Oryctolagus cuniculus*). Accessed 3/9/16 at www.ncbi.nlm.nih.gov/pmc/articles/P

Haligur, M., O. Ozmen, and N. Demir. 2009. Pathological and Ultrastructural Studies on Mucoid Enteropathy in New Zealand Rabbits. *J. Exo. Pet Med.* 18(3): 224-228

Harcourt-Brown, F. M. 2002. *Textbook of Rabbit Medicine.* Oxford: Butterworth-Heinemann.

Harcourt-Brown, F. M. and S. J. Baker. 2001. Parathyroid hormone, haematological and biochemical parameters in relation to dental disease and husbandry in rabbits. *J. Small Anim. Pract.* 42(3): 130–136.

Harcourt-Brown, T. R. 2007. Management of Acute Gastric Dilaiton in Rabbits. *J. Exo. Pet Med.* 16(3): 168-174.

Harkness, J. E., P. V. Turner, S. VandeWoude, and C. L. Wheler. 2010. *Biology and Medicine of Rabbits and Rodents,* 5th edition. Danvers: Wiley-Blackwell.

Jenkins, J. R. 2010. Evaluation of the Rabbit Urinary Tract. *J. Exo. Pet Med.* 19(4): 271-279.

Jenkins, J. R. 2004. Gastrointestinal Diseases. *In: Ferrets, Rabbits and Rodents: Clinical Medicine and Surgery.* 2nd edition. K. E. Qusenberry and J. W. Carpenter, eds. St. Louis: Saunders.

Kowalska, D., P. Bielanski, P. Nosal, and J. Kowal. 2012. Natural alternatives to Cocciostats in rabbit nutrition. *Ann. Anim. Sci.* 12(4):

561-574.

Lowe, J. A. Pet Rabbit Feeding and Nutrition. In: *Nutrition of the Rabbit*. Carlos de Blas and Julian Wiseman, eds. Wallingford: CABI Publishing.

McNitt, J. and P. Cheeke. 1996. *Rabbit Production*, 7th edition. Danville: Interstate Printers and Publishers.

McWilliams, D. A. 2001. Nutritional Pathology in Rabbits: Current and Future Perspectives. Paper: Ontario Commercial Rabbit Growers Asso. Congress.

Martorelli, J., D. Bailon, N. Majo, and A. Andaluz. 2012. Lateral approach to nephrotomy in the management of unilateral renal calculi in a rabbit (*Oryctolagus cuniculus*). *AVMA* 240(7): 863-868.

The Merck Veterinary Manual. Ninth edition. 2005. Edited by Cynthia M. Kahn. Whitehouse Station: Merck and Co., Inc.

Moore, L. and K. Smith. 2008. *When Your Rabbit Needs Special Care: Traditional and Alternative Healing Methods*. Santa Monica: Santa Monica Press.

Murray, M. J. 2005. Rabbit Gastro-Intestinal Disease. *Proceedings:* North American Veterinary Conference, Orlando, Florida

Pakandl, Michael. 2009. Coccidea of rabbit: a review. *Folia Parasit.* 56(3): 153-166.

Patton, N. M., K. W. Hagen, J. R. Gorham, and R. E. Platt. 2008. *Domestic Rabbits Diseases and Parasites*. PNW 310-E. Corvallis: Oregon State University.

Pelton, Vicki. 2009. *How to Care for Newborn Rabbits (up to 2 months old)*. Accessed 3/20/16 at www.curiousbunny.com/newborn_rabbits_detail.pdf

Rodriguez-Romero, N., L. Abecia, M. Fondevilla, and J. Balcells. 2011. Effects of levels of insoluble and soluble fibres in diets for growing rabbits on faecal digestibility, nitrogen recycling, and *in vitro* fermentation. *World Rabbit Sci.* 19: 85-94.

Rosell, J. M., R. Garriga, J. Martinez, M. Domingo, and L. F. de la Fuente. 2012. Calcinois in Female Rabbits. *Proceedings:* 10th World Rabbit Congress, Sharm El-Sheikh, Egypt.

Selim, N. A., A. M. Abdel-Khalek, S. A. Nada, Sh. A. El-Medany. 2008. Response of growing Rabbits to Dietary Antioxidant Vitamins E and C. 1. Effect on Performance. *Proceedings:* 9th World Rabbit Congress, Verona, Italy.

Stenglein, M. D. E. Velazquez, C. Greenacre, R. P. Wilkes, J. G. Ruby, J. S. Lankton, D. Ganem, M. A. Kennedy, and J. I. DeRisi. 2012. Complete genome sequence of an astrovirus identified in a domestic rabbit (*Oryctolagus cuniculus)* with gastroenteritis. *Virol. J.* 9: 216-225.

Subramanian, S., D. S. Kumar, and P. Arulselvan. 2006. Wound Healing Potential of *Aloe vera* Leaf Gel studied in Experimental Rabbits. *Asian J. Biochem.* 1(2): 178-185.

Varga, Molly. 2015. Emergency management of gut stasis in rabbits. *Companion An.* 20(1): 20-25.

Varga, Molly. 2014. *Textbook of Rabbit Medicine,* 2nd edition. Oxford: Elsevier.

Verstraete, F. J. M. and A. Osofsky. 2005. Dentistry in Pet Rabbits. Continuing Education Article #2, CompendiumVet.com. Accessed 11/14/10 at http://cp.vetlearn.com/Media/PublicationsArticlePV_27_09_671.pdf

Vidal, J. E., B. L. McClane, J. Saputo, J. Parker, and F. A. Uzal. 2008. Effects of *Clostridium perfringens* Beata-Toxin on the Rabbit Small Intestine and Colon. *Infect. Immun.* 76(10): 4396-4404.

Wang, X., M. Ma, L. Sun, C. Wang, Y Zhu, and F. Li. 2012. Effects of different protein, fibre and energy levels on growth performance and the development of digestive organs in growing meat rabbit. *Proceedings:* 10th World Rabbit Congress. Sharm El-Sheikh, Egypt.

Warfield, Kristen. 2019. Man Finds Tombstone in Middle of Woods with Sweetest Message on It. *the dodo.* Accessed 3/2/19 at http://www.thedodo.com/close-to-home/man-discovers-pet-rabbit-headstone

Wieberneit, D., N. Mahdi, K. Zacharias, and W. Wegner. 1991. The problem of spotted breeds of rabbits. 1. Fattening and body condition at slaughter, organ parameters. *Dtsch. Tieraztl. Wochenschr.* 98: 352-54.

Wieberneit, D. and W. Wegner. 1995. Albino rabbits can suffer from megacolon-syndrome when they are homozygous for the "English Spot" gene (EnEn). *World Rab. Sci.* 3(1): 19-26.

White, R. N. 2001. Management of calcium ureterolithiasis in a French lop rabbit. *J. Sm. Anim. Pract.* 42(12): 595-598.

Wilbur, J. L. 1999. *Pathology of the Rabbit.* Washington DC: Dept. of Veterinary Pathology, Armed Forces Institute.

APPENDIX I

Possible signs of nutritional deficiencies and excesses

Sign	Possible nutritional deficiencies	Possible nutritional excesses
anorexia	vit. A, B-complex, Ca, Zn, soluble and/or insoluble fiber	vit A, Vit D, soluble and/or insoluble fiber
weight loss	vit B_3, B_6, Mg, Zn, sugar, starch, soluble fiber, protein	vit. D, insoluble fiber
poor growth of kits	choline, Cu, Mg, Zn, fat, protein, soluble fiber	vit. A, Mo, NaCl
GI hypomotility	fat, soluble and/or insoluble fiber	protein
impacted cecum		insoluble fiber
intestinal dysbiosis	vit. A, soluble and/or insoluble fiber	vit. A, protein
diarrhea	vit. B_3, Mo	vit. D, Mo, insoluble fiber
increased urination		protein
edema	choline, Mg	
respiratory difficulty	vit. K	
eye ulcers	vit. A	vit. A
sores around mouth	Zn	
dermatitis	vit. B_2, B_6, biotin, Cu, Zn, fat	
poor wound healing	vit. E, Mn, Zn, fat, protein	
depressed immune sys.	Fe, Se, Zn	
fur chewing	Mg, fiber	
fur loss (alopecia)	biotin, Cu, Mg, Zn, fat, protein	
graying of fur	folate, Cu, Zn	
reddening of fur	protein	
fur texture change	vit. E, Mg, fat	
muscle tremors	Ca	

incoordination	vit. E	
muscle weakness	vit. A, vit. B1, choine, vit. E, vit. K, protein, K (potassium)	vit. A, vit. D, vit. K
floppy rabbit syndrome	vit. A, choline, vit. E	vit. A, vit. D
paralysis	choline, vit. E, vit. K, protein	vit. D
convulsions	vit. B_6, Mg	
head tilt, neurological	vit. B-complex	
kit morbidity	vit. E, Cu, Mg, soluble and insoluble fiber	I, Mn, sugar, starch, protein
excitability	Mg	Cu
lethargy	vit B_5, folate, vit. B_{12}, Co	
brittle bones	vit. D, Ca, Mn, Si	
bone loss and/or softening	vit. B12, vit. D, Ca, Co, P, Si	
arthritis, joint pain	essential fatty acids	Cu, Mo
hypertension	K (potassium)	fat
heart damage	choline, vit. E, K (potassium), vit. E, Mg	Fe, fat
kidney damage	choline	vit. D, vit. K, Ca, K (potassium), Si, protein
liver damage	choline, vit. E	fat, protein

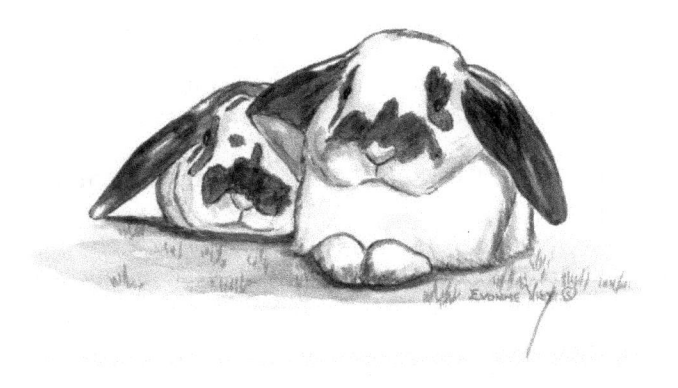

APPENDIX II: BUNNY-SAFE TREATS

Given that this is a volume on rabbit nutrition, I felt I should include an appendix listing at least a few businesses where good bunny-safe treats can be purchased. I know there are many other businesses in addition to those I have listed where a person can buy excellent bunny treats. However, I feel I can only list those I have purchased from myself and have been very satisfied with both the service and products.

BUNNY BUNCH BOUTIQUE (www.BunnyBunchBoutique.com)

When I started Bunny Bunch Rabbit Rescue over thirty-five years ago I learnt about the proper diet for rabbits and realized nothing healthy was being sold for rabbits in the stores. Not even hay. So I set out to change that by starting Bunny Bunch Boutique online.

I started making safe healthy chews and toys for rabbits. Being an avid gardener I started planting flowers, bushes and trees to make organic treats for rabbits. Every weekend I took rabbits to different adoption events and started setting up all my products for sale. Before long they were in great demand. I also opened two brick and mortar stores in Southern California, and will be opening a third in the Los Angeles area in 2019.

Having 200-300 rabbits in the Bunny Bunch Rescue I have a lot of rabbits to keep happy and healthy. So I shop for the best hay I can find. We offer timothy, Bunny Bunch Blend, Orchard, Alfalfa, and a variety of Herb and Flower hays. I even do custom mixes for picky eaters. Exotic vets send clients to us to make up special hay mixes for clients who have senior rabbits or picky eaters. All hay is packaged at our facility when ordered, so it never sits packaged getting old. It is always fresh and delicious.

I also have a line of natural organic treats made of organic, edible flowers and leaves. These are a great way to give treats that are good for your rabbit. Willow wreaths, twigs and leaves are something rabbits love too. We harvest willow several times a year and always have it available. If your rabbit is older, I have a special pellet for weight gain and offer supplements for seniors and other conditions.

I love rabbits and I have spent my life rescuing and learning all about them. A healthy diet really makes a difference to a long healthy life. I have had several rabbits live to fifteen years old.

ELLIOT'S AWESOME TREATS – EAT (Facebook, email bunnybinks@gmail.com)

Elliot's Awesome Treats are edible wild greens and twigs which are grown organically in Kettering, Ohio, then hand-picked and dried. These tasty treats offer great nutrition and health benefits, provide variety in the diet and are typically higher in phytonutrients than traditional cultivated crops. Pytonutrients are chemical compounds associated with positive health effects; cultivated plant foods typically have had at least some of the nutrients bred out of them in favor of higher yields, increased cold tolerance, etc.

For example:
- Spinach (a cultivated crop) contains 1800 IU of provitamin A per 100 g.
- Violets (a wild edible plant) contain 20,000 IU of provitamin A per 100 g.

Wild foods can be valuable adjunct therapies for a poorly bunny, guinea pig, or other pet; they are not a substitute for veterinary care, but when used correctly they can provide additional support for other therapies that have been prescribed.

Edible sild foods add variety ot your bunny's diet, and most bunnies seem to prefer wild greens in their dried state (possibly the natural flavors are concentrated by drying). Sometimes a few dried leaves of plantain (an excellent source of fiber) or thistle is just the thing to tempt a poorly bunny into eating again.

EAT twigs are softer woods (Rose of Sharon) and twigs such as mint, chicory, and primrose, which are easier on the teeth of older pets with dental/chewing issues.

EAT owner Phyllis O'Beollain has been gardening organically for over 35 years and has lived with house rabbits for over sixteen years. A fan of herbal therapy, she uses her gardening experience to grow her own wild edibles, thus ensuring their quality and potency.

THE WELL KEPT RABBIT (www.thewellkeptrabbit.com and on instagram @thewellkeptrabbit)

The Well Kept Rabbit really started back in 2009 with shop owner Anna's first bunny, Jujube, who sparked her love affair with bunnies. Anna quickly became a rabbit advocate, eventually training to become an Educator with the House Rabbit Society. It shocked her that the majority of the treats and toys found in pet stores were filled with disturbing ingredients dangerous for bunnies and other small pets to be consuming. She felt inspired and began crafting healthy, organic treats and toys for her bunnies and other small pets to enjoy! These days she spends her time at home with her four bunnies (aka taste testers and quality control team) crafting up new healthy treats for bunnies and other small pets.

"At the Well Kept Rabbit we focus on extensive research to create unique appealing products while never abandoning our promise to to use only safe, healthy ingredients. We maintain the highest standards for all our goods, never using preservatives, additives, coloring, etc. All of our beautiful colors are crafted using different blends of natural foods that are safe for your small pet to consume. Ultimately, we aim to encourage and even revolutionize a more holistic approach to small pet care."

ACRONYMS AND ABBREVIATIONS

ADD: acquired dental disease
ADF: acid detergent fiber
ALA: alpha-linoleic acid
ATP: adenosine triphosophate
DE: digestible energy
DF: dietary fiber, digestible fiber
DHEA: dehydroepiandrosterone
DON: deoynivalenol
EFA: essential fatty acid
FOS: fructo-oligosaccahride
GI: gastrointestinal
GOS: galacto-oligosaccharide
HC: hemicellulose
HDL: high-density lipoprotein
IU: international unit
LDF: low dietary fiber, low-digestible fiber
LDL: low-density lipoprotein
MBD: metabolic bone disease
mcg: microgram
ml: milliliter
MOS: mannanoligosaccharide
NDF: neutral detergent fiber
NDN: non-dietary nitrogen
NSAID: non-steroidal anti-inflammatory drug
OPC: oligocentric proanthocyanidin
OTA: ochratoxin A
ppm: parts per million

PTH: parathyroid hormone
SCFA: short chain fatty acid
VFA: volatile fatty acid
VFI: voluntary feed intake

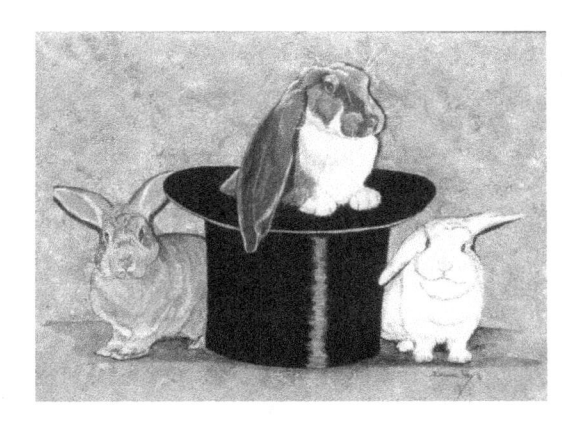

INDEX OF TABLES

Percent sugar and starch content of selected foods   38

Percent soluble and insoluble fiber content of selected foods   46

Fat content of selected foods   63

Protein content of selected foods   67

Fat-soluble vitamin content of selected foods   80

Water-soluble vitamin content of selected foods   86

Oxalate, calcium, and phosphorus content of selected foods   95

Mineral content of selected foods   102

Comparison of three rabbit pellet ingredients tags   128

Typical nutrient content of selected hays   134

Nutrient and phytochemical composition of selected vegetables and herbs   186

Nutrient and phytochemical composition of selected fruits   192

Nutrient and phytochemical composition of selected grains, nuts, and seeds   195

Nutrient and phytochemical composition of selected legumes   196

Selected plants potentially toxic to rabbits   227

Possible signs of nutritional deficiencies and excesses   308

GENERAL INDEX (page references to tables are italicized)

acai, 190, *192*

acetic acid, 22

alfalfa,
    hay, 39, *134, 196*
    pellets,
    sprouts, *69, 80,196*

aflatoxin B$_1$, 156

alkaloids, 226
    pyrrolizidine 181, 214

alopecia, *See* fur loss

almond, *46, 69, 80*

amino acid, 66
    essential, 66
    limiting, 69

ammonia, 69, 236, 238, 262

amylose, 40

angel's trumpet, *228*

angelic acid, 217

angelica 179, 188, 189

anorexia, *308*

anthocyanidins, 174

anthocyanin, 174

antioxidants, 78, 79, 183

apple, *46*, 173, *192*, 296
    seeds, 172

apricot, *46, 69*, 191, *192*

apigenin, 175

arginine, 69

arthritis, 203, 267, 299, *399*

arugula, *186*, 188, 200

ashitaba, 174, 179

Aspergillus, 156, 157

aster, 194

atherosclerosis, 66, 299

atropine, 226

avocado, *227*

azalea, *229*

Bacillus, 234

Bacteriodes, 26, 44

banana, *46, 69, 192*

bark,
    apple, 179
    cherry, 179
    pear, 179
    willow, 296

barley, *69*, 179, *195*

basil, *69, 186*, 189, 268

beans, 39, 176, 179
    castor, 176, *227*

beet, 170
    greens, 178, *186*

bentonite, 154, 161

Bermuda grass, 133, *134*

betacarotene, 79

betacyanin, 170

betaxanthin, 170

betalains, 170

bilirubin, 19

biliverdin, 19

biotin, 83

blackberry, 214

bladder sludge, 92, 297

bleeding heart, *227*

bloat, 295

blueberry, 173, 181, 190, *192*

bluegrass, Kentucky, *134*
bok choi, 188
borage, common, 213
bran, wheat, *46, 69*
bread, 42, *46, 69*
brewer's yeast, 83, 97, 99
broccoli, *46, 69, 186,* 188
brome grass, 133, *134*
bromelain, 190
buckeye, 228
burdock, 224
butyric acid, 22
cabbage, *46,* 175, *186,* 188
    family, 29, 39, 175, 200
    Napa, 188
    rosette, 188
caffeic acid, 170
caladium, 227
calcium, 91-94, *95*
canavanine, 170
cancer, 203, 299
cantaloupe, *46*
capeweed, 227
Carafate, 160
carambola, 191
carbohydrates, 30-54
    complex, 31
    simple, 30
cardiac sphincter, 18
cardiovascular disease, 203, 297, 300
carnation, 194
carotenes, 171
carotenoids *See* carotene
carrot,
    root, *46, 69, 186*
    tops, *69, 186*
cat's ear, 223
catechins, 174
cauliflower, *46*
cecal dysbiosis, 288
cecotrophs, 23
    and B-vitamins, 81
    excessive, 68
    soft, 288
    uneaten, 287
cecotrophy, 23, 67, 68
cecum, 21, 22
    impacted, 292, *308*
celery, *69,* 179, *186,* 188
cellulose, 45-47
chaconine, 172, 182
chalcones, 174, 299
chard, Swiss, 170, *186,* 200
cherry, *46, 69,* 172, *192*
chicory, 37, 200
chickweed, 202, 214,
cholesterol, 61, 65
cholestyramine, 290
choline, 77, 83
chrysanthemum, 194
chyme, 19
cilantro, *69, 186*
citrinin, 156
clay, edible, 154, 290
Clostridium, 33, 235, 290
clover, *134,* 172, *196,* 215
cobalt, 94, *102*
coccidiosis, 289
coenzyme Q10, 90, 91
colibacillosis, 290

collards, 171, 253

colon, 20, 21

community rabbits,
  feeding,
  nutrition,

copper, 94, *102,* 302

coprophagy, 23

cornflower, blue, 198

cottonseed, 125, 176

coumarin, 172, 303

cranberries, *69,* 143, 174, 181, 184, 190, *192*

crocus, autumn, 227

cruciferous vegetables, *see* cabbage family

cucumber, *46, 69*

currants, 183

cyanocobalamine, 83

cysteine, 66

daisy, 194
  Marguerite, 194
  Michaelmas, 194

dandelion, *69, 186,* 202, 215

daphne, 227

dates, *46, 69,* 83, 174, *192*

datura, 228

death camus, 227

dehydration, 149

delphinium, 227

dental disease, acquired, 278-279

dermatitis, *308*

dextrins, 43

diarrhea, 289-292, *308*

dicoumerol, 215

dieffenbachia, 227

diet, rabbit
  balanced, 137, 285
  and breed, 272-274
  and elder rabbits, 265-271
  grass-hay-only, 136, 137
  of lactating does, 261
  of pregnant does, 260
  of orphaned kits, 263-265
  of young rabbits, 26, 27, 142, 261, 262
  variety in, 118
  of wild rabbits, 9-13

digestive system, rabbit, 16-27
  adult, 16-25
  young, 25-27

digestive illness, 203, 284, 285, 289-296

dill, *186,* 189, 267

disaccharides, 32

dock, 223

dogbane, 227

dragon,
  fruit, red, 170
  tree, 227

duodenum, 20

dysbiosis,
  cecal,
  intestinal,

drugs/nutrients
  interactions, 61, 181, 104-109

emu bush, spotted, 229

endive, 200

Enterococcus, 153, 234

enterotoxemia, 288

ergot, 156

escarole, 200

Escherichia, 23, 235

Eubacterium, 153

eucalyptus, 228

fats, 60-65

deficiency, 63
in rabbit diets, 60-64
monounsaturated, 60
polyunsaturated, 60
saturated, 60
unsaturated, 60

fatty acids,
decanoic, 25
essential, 60, 64
linoleic, 65
linolenic, 65
ocanoic, 25
omega-3, 60, 65
omega-6, 60
short chain, 45
trans, 61
volatile, 22, 31

feces
hard, 23
healthy, 285-287
mucoid, 288, 291, 292
soft, 23, 288

feeds, 118-128
extruded, 120, 121
labels of, 123-128
pelleted, 119, 123

fennel, 201, 223

fern, bracken, 227

fescue, meadow, 133, *134*

fever, 203
milk, 260

fiber, 43-52
insoluble, 43-45
in rabbit diet, 52-54
particle size, 51, 292, 295
soluble, 43, 45
terms, 49-51

flavanols, 174

flavanones, 175

flavonols, 174

flavones, 175

flavonoids, 172-75, 185, 303

flax, 228

floppy rabbit, 300, *309*

flowers, in rabbit diet, 194, 198

folate, 83

folic acid, 83

foxglove, 171, 228

free radicals, 78, 91

fructans, 233

fructo-oligosaccharides, 36, 223

fructose,

fruit, 142-44, 190, 199
dried, 191
exotic, 191
pectin,

fumosin B$_1$, 157

fundus, 18

fur/hair, 203, *308*
chewing, 301, *308*
condition of, 155, 228
graying of, 228301, *308*
loss, 301, *308*
reddening of, 70, *308*

Fusarium, 158

fusus coli, 21

gac, 171

galacto-oligosaccharides, 36

gall bladder, 19

gallotannins, 184

garcinol, 303

garcinones, 184

gastrointestinal hypomotility, 293, 294, *308*
and fat,

Georgina gidyea, 228

geraniol, 169, 201, 303

geranium, 194, 198

geum, 194

glucose, 32

glucosinolates, 175
gluten, 70, 71
glycine, 66
glycoalkaloids, 182
glycoproteins, 176
glycosides
    cardiac, 171
    cyanogenic, 172
    goitrogenic, 175
goji berries, 171, 191
goitrogens, 175
goldenrod, 198
gossypol, 176
grains, 144, 195
grapes, *46, 69*, 184, *192*
grass, fresh, 138-41
    container, 140, 141
    moveable pen for, 138
    in wild rabbit diet,
groundsel, 223
guava, 171, 190
gums, 45
hay, 131-137
    alfalfa, *46*, 132
    choosing, 133-35
    grass, *46, 69*, 132-6
    nutrition from, 131
headtilt, *309*
hemicellulose, 45-47
hemlock, 180, 212, *229*
herbs, 141, 189, 201
histidine, 66
hollyhock, 194, 198
honeydew melon, *192*
horse chestnut, 228
hydrangea, 228
ileum, 20

indole-3-carbinol, 176
infections, frequent, 203, 300
inulin, 37, 38
iodine, 96, 97, 185, 302
iron, 97, *102*, 302
isoflavone, 175
isoleucine,
isothyocyanates, 176
ivy, English, 228
jejunum, 19, 20
jimson weed, 228
Johnson grass, *229*
juglone, 181
jute, 228
kale, *69, 187,* 200
ketones, 25, 270
kidney disease, 297, 298
kits, rabbit
    diet of, 26, 142, 261
    digestive system of, 25-27
kiwi, *46,* 253
knotweed, 216
Lactobacillus, 153, 178, 234
lactones, 179
lactose, 32
lamb's quarter, 202, 216
lantana, 228
larkspur, 227
lectins, 176, 177
legumes, 171, 179, 196
lettuce, *46*
    leaf, *187,* 200
    prickly, 223
    Romaine, *69, 187*
leucine, 66

Leuconostoc, 153

lignin, 45, 46, 262

lignocellulose, 48

lily-of-the-valley, 171, 228

limonene, 169, 201, 303

lipase, 61

lipids *See* fats

locust, black, 227

loveage, 179, 202, 217

lupine, 228

lutein, 303

luteolin, 175

lycopene, 66, 171, 303

lysine, 66, 69

magnesium, 97, *102*, 302

mallow, common, 217

manganese, 98, *102*

mango, *46*, 174, *193*

mangosteen, 184, 190

mannanoligosaccharides, 36, 233

marigolds,
    cape, 194
    common, 194
    pot, 194

megacolon syndrome, 293

melilotin, 215

methionine, 66, 69

milkweed, 229

minerals, 77, 78

molasses, 33, 90

mold, 152, 153

molybdenum, 98, 99, *102*, 302

monosaccharides, 32

montmorillonite, 154

motilin, 61

mucoid enteritis, 291

mucoid enteropathy, 291

mustard greens, *69*, 171

mycotoxicosis
    signs of, 158, 159
    treatment of, 159-161

mycotoxins, 152-161

myricetin, 175

nasturtium, 194

naringenin, 175

nectarine, *193*

nettles, 224

niacin, 82

noni, 301

nuts, 144, 145

oak, 184, 229

oatgrass hay, 133, *134*

oats, *46, 69*, 179 *195*

ochratoxin A, 157

oleander, 229

oligonetric proanthocyanidins, 183

oligosaccharides, 36-39

orange, *46, 69*, 171

orchardgrass, 133, *134*

oregano, 170 *187*

oxalates, *95*, 177

oxalic acid, 177

Oxalobacter, 178

palmitrin, 61

pancreas, 20

pansies, 194

pantothenic acid, 82
papain, 142
papaya, 171, *193*
parsley, *69, 187*
Pasteurella, 235
peach, *69, 193*
peanuts, *196*
pear, *46,* 174, *193*
pectin, 43-45
Pedicoccus, 234
Penicillium, 157
pellets, commercial, 120-29
    amounts rabbit diet, 127
    extruded, 120, 121
    free-feeding vs. limited, 127
    grass-based vs. alfalfa-based 122, 123
    labels, 123-128
peppermint, 181, *187*
pepsinogen, 18
perilla, *187,* 189
Peyer's patches, 19
phenols, 169, 226
phenylalanine, 66
philodendron, 229
phloridzin, 179
phosphorus, 99
phthalides, 179, 303
phytates, 179
phytochemicals, 166-201
phytonutrients, 166-201
phytic acid, 179
phytosterols, 175, 180
pineapple, *69,* 190, *193*
pine nuts, 145

piperdine, 180. 181
plantain, ribwort, 202, 218
plants,
    cultivated, 184-204
    edible wild, 212-224
    toxic, 212, 225-229
plums, *46*
polysaccharides, 39-52
pomegranate, 184, 190, *193*
porphyrins, 24
potassium, 100, *102*, 302
prebiotics, 232-234, 238
prickly pear fruit, 170, *193*
privet, 229
proanthocyanidins, 174, 220
probiotics, 232-235
Proprionibacterium, 153
protein,
    cecotrophs, 67
    deficiency, 70
    excess in diet, 68, 70
    limiting, 69
    recommended, 71, 72
pumpkin
    canned, 171, *187*
    seeds, *69, 195*
purslane, 178, *187*, 202, 219
pylorus, 19
pyridoxine, 82
pyrrolizidine, 181
quercetin, 174
quinones, 181
raffinose, 39
raisins, *46*
rapeseed, 176
raspberry, *46, 69, 193,* 214
    leaf, 214

respiratory disease, 84, 203, *308*
resveratrol, 181, 303
retinoic acid, 79
retinol, 79
rhododendron, 229
rhubarb, 174
riboflavin, 82
ricin, 178
rocket, *See* arugula
rose, 194
    Christmas, 171
rosemary, 170 *187,* 201
rosmarinic acid, 170, *187,* 201
ryegrass, 133, *134*
rutin, 174
Saccharomyces, 161, 234, 236
sacculus rotundus, 20
sage, 170, 201
salicylic acid, 181, 182
sansiveria, 229
saponins, 182
sarsaponins, 182
seaberry, 171, 184, 190
seeds, in rabbit diet, 144, 145
selenium, 66, 100, 102, 302
shepherd's purse, *202, 219,* 253
shisho, 199
silica, in grasses, 101
silicon, 101, *102,* 302
silybin, 175
silymarin, 218
sneezeweed, 229

sodium, 101
solanine, 182
sorghum, 183, 229
sorrel, 176
soybeans, 175, *196*
spinach, *46, 69, 187,* 200
    Ceylon, 189
    water, 189
Staphylococcus, 184, 190
starch, 40-43
stachyose, 39
starweed, 214
starwort, 214
stock, 194
stomach, 18, 19
    acidity, 19
    of rabbit kit, 25
straw, wheat, *69,* 135
strawberry, *46,* 220
    leaf, *193,* 220
stress, 203, 301
    heat, 85, 301
    and vit. C, 84, 301
    and noni, 301
Streptococcus, 153, 234
sucralfate, 160
sucrose, 32
sugars, 32-36
    in adult rabbit diet, 33
    in young rabbits, 32, 33
sunflower, 194, 199, 220
    seeds, *46, 69,* 179, *195*
tangerine, *193*
tannins, 183
    condensed, 183
    ellagic acid, 184
    gallo, 184
    hydrolysable, 184
tarragon, 181

teeth, 18

terpenes, 169, 226

thiamin, 82

thistle
    milk, 218
    sow, 218

threonine, 66

thyme, *187,* 189

timothy, 132, 133, *134*

tomato, *46,* 171, 181, *193*

trefoil *See* clover

tricothecenes, 158, 161

tryptophan, 66

turnip weed, 224

tyrosine, 66

ulcers, eye, 308

urea, 69, 238

urease, 69

urine, 24, 25
    color, 24
    excessive, *308*
    sludge, 297

urinary tract disease, 203

uroliths, 178

valine, 66

vegetables, 185
    sensitivity to, 188, 288
    and young rabbits, 142

verbascose, 39

vermiform appendix, 22

violets, 194

vitamins, 77-89
    A, 79, *80,* 302
    B-complex, 81-87, 302
    C, 84, 85, 302
    D, 85, 88
    E, *80,* 88, 89, 302
    K, *80,* 90

vomitoxin, 158

wallflower, 194

walnut, *46, 69,* 181, *195*
    black, 227

water, 147-151

watercress, *69*

watermelon, *46, 69,* 171, *193*

weather, and feeding, 240-45

weight, of rabbits, 263, 284, *308*

wheatgrass
    fresh, *69,* 140
    hay, *134*
    slender, 133

willow twigs, 296

wireweed, 216

wolfberry, 171, 191

wounds, healing of, *308*

xanthones, 184

yarrow, 199

yeast
    brewer's, *Saccharomyces,*

yew, 229

yucca, 182, 238

zeaxanthin, 171

zeolite, 154

zinc, *102,* 104, 302

zucchini, 181, *187*

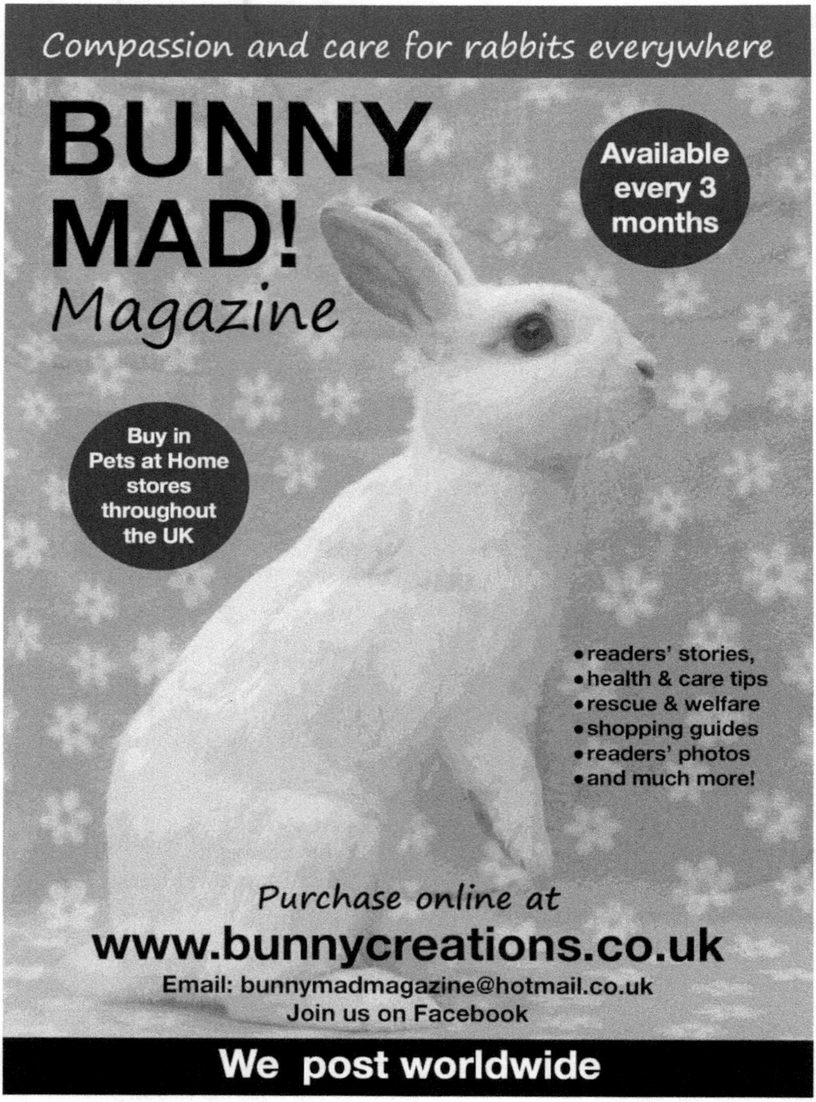
Compassion and care for rabbits everywhere
BUNNY MAD!
Magazine
Available every 3 months
Buy in Pets at Home stores throughout the UK
• readers' stories,
• health & care tips
• rescue & welfare
• shopping guides
• readers' photos
• and much more!
Purchase online at
www.bunnycreations.co.uk
Email: bunnymadmagazine@hotmail.co.uk
Join us on Facebook
We post worldwide

CPSIA information can be obtained
at www.ICGtesting.com
Printed in the USA
LVHW080959160719
624096LV00002BA/201/P

9 780368 770531